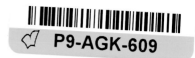

P9-AGK-609

RENEWALS 458-4574

DATE DUE

THE FAMILY MENTAL HEALTH ENCYCLOPEDIA

Other books by Frank J. Bruno

The Story of Psychology (1972)

Think Yourself Thin (1972)

Psychology: A Life-Centered Approach (1974)

Born to Be Slim (1978)

Behavior and Life (1980)

Adjustment and Personal Growth (1983)

Dictionary of Key Words in Psychology (1986)

THE FAMILY MENTAL HEALTH ENCYCLOPEDIA

Frank J. Bruno, Ph.D.

WILEY

JOHN WILEY & SONS
New York • Chichester • Brisbane • Toronto • Singapore

To my son Franklin,
whose sense of humor
has a positive effect
on my own mental health

ISBN 0-471-63573-1

Printed in the United States of America

10 9 8 7 6 5 4 3 2 1

PREFACE

The mind is its own place, and in itself
Can make a heaven of hell, a hell of heaven.

John Milton, *Paradise Lost* (1667)

How will *The Family Mental Health Encyclopedia* be useful to you?

Mental health, when it is present, is often taken for granted. However, when mental health is lost or diminished, much has been taken away from the quality of life. We all need to know as much as we realistically can know about how mental health is maintained.

A mental health problem is quite likely to touch you, a member of your family, or a friend. Here are just some of the mental disorders that plague the human race: alcoholism, Alzheimer's disease, anorexia nervosa, anxiety disorders, attention deficit disorders, bulimia nervosa, conduct disorders, depression, mental retardation, organic mental disorders, sexual disorders, and schizophrenia. This encyclopedia provides accurate information about the causes, behavioral aspects, and treatments of these disorders.

Mental health professionals such as psychiatrists, clinical psychologists, counselors, and social workers sometimes seem to speak a language all their own. In your dealings with them, you may find yourself hearing about alienation, anxiety, brain pathology, confabulation, dementia, hysteria, Korsakoff's psychosis, mutism, obsession, reality contact, and so forth. This book is a reliable guide to the meaning of such terms.

Drugs are often prescribed for mental disorders. It is important that you learn about both the benefits and the adverse side effects associated with frequently prescribed drugs.

Some mental disorders may respond well to counseling and psychotherapy. It is helpful to know something about these interventions and their underlying assumptions.

Every time you look up information about a mental health subject, you learn just a bit more about human nature.

The Family Mental Health Encyclopedia is a convenient reference book that will answer questions that may arise about mental health, mental disorders, causes of distress, and kinds of therapy.

What is the prevalence of mental disorders? As already indicated, a mental disorder is quite likely to touch you, a member of your family, or a friend. How does this general statement translate into actual statistics?

The National Institute of Mental Health recently concluded an extensive study suggesting that within a defined 6-month time span approximately 20% of the population suffers from a mental or behavioral disorder. This percentage at first seems incredibly high until we note that 5 or 6% of the population abuses alcohol and other drugs. Eight percent of the population has severe bouts of anxiety. Another 6% frequently suffers from depression. (Schizophrenia, popularly known as madness, is *not* the principal mental disorder. Its prevalence is about 1%.)

Here is another way of indicating the high incidence of mental health problems: In the United States alone, approximately 200 million prescriptions a year are written for drugs used to treat mental disorders.

Finally, one of the saddest facts of all is that many mental disorders are never treated. It is estimated, for example, that only about one-third of persons suffering from depression receive treatment. And only about 18% of persons with alcohol and drug abuse problems receive treatment. Schizophrenia has one of the best treatment rates. Approximately one-half of the persons suffering from it are treated.

For more complete information concerning the prevalence of particular mental disorders, see the appropriate entries in the encyclopedia.

In order to provide you with a *useful* reference book, the encyclopedia contains several important features.

Writing style. Every effort was made to make the writing clear and to the point. Although many specialized terms and subjects are both defined and discussed, they are dealt with in ordinary language. The unfamiliar is made intelligible through the pathway of the familiar. Where necessary, examples are used.

Technical terms. When technical terms appear in the body of a subject entry, they are always italicized and defined at the point of use. Again, the focus is on making mental health topics clear and intelligible.

Subject entries. The core of the encyclopedia consists of approximately 700 subject entries. These vary in length from a single paragraph to short articles. A wide spectrum of mental health subjects is included, all of them of practical interest.

Name entries. There are a number of name entries for persons who have made significant contributions to the study of mental health. The focus is not on biographical aspects of their lives but on their teachings—what we can learn of value from them.

Cross-references. Almost every entry ends with several cross-references directing you to relevant collateral information elsewhere in the encyclopedia. Thus subjects do not stand in isolation but are supported by a network of associated facts and ideas.

Index of authorities. At the end of the encyclopedia, you will find an index of authorities. Its purpose is to guide you to specific pages where the ideas and discoveries of psychiatrists, psychologists, and other researchers who have made important contributions to the field of mental health are cited.

What is mental health? It is easier to talk about mental illness, psychopathology, and the negative aspects of human behavior than it is to speak of mental health itself. The abnormal, the odd, and the deviant exert a strange fascination. However, it is to our advantage to remember that the study of the abnormal exists as an instrument to bring us from the darkness of behavioral pathology to the light of normal behavior.

Thus we need a working definition of mental health to guide us as we study how it is maintained, lost, and restored. This then shall be our definition of mental health in this book: *Mental health is a state of well-being characterized by rational thinking, emotional maturity, and effective action.*

The subject entry *mental health* in the encyclopedia proper adds to this definition with examples and a discussion.

In short, *The Family Mental Health Encyclopedia* is a home reference book filled with practical information. The kind of material contained in it is, of course, of general interest. However, the encyclopedia will be of particular value to you during times of mental and emotional crises, times when you need facts at your fingertips.

Above all, the encyclopedia is *useful*.

FRANK J. BRUNO

Upland, California
March 1989

ACKNOWLEDGMENTS

A number of people have helped me make *The Family Mental Health Encyclopedia* a reality. My thanks are expressed to:

Herb Reich, Senior Editor at John Wiley & Sons, for recognizing the merits of the book, and for being an encouraging and creative editor.

Judith Overton, Editorial Secretary to Herb Reich, for her practical assistance during the preparation phase of the manuscript.

Robert Chadwick for excellent copy editing.

Phyllis Brooks for carefully supervising production.

My wife Jeanne for our many meaningful discussions about adjustment, personal growth, and mental health.

My son Franklin for our frequent conversations about words, language, and meaning.

My colleague George K. Zaharopoulos for his steadfast encouragement of my writing projects.

My niece Deanna for her advice and information concerning certain word processing procedures.

F. J. B.

A

abnormal behavior: Any behavior that deviates in a significant way from a *norm*, a standard of reference used by a given group. Such behavior is often seen by a particular family, religious organization, or nationality as odd, eccentric, or peculiar. Abnormal behavior is not in and of itself undesirable or "sick." Sometimes it can be quite creative, constructive, and positive in nature.

If abnormal behavior is destructive to a group or self-destructive, we can speak of behavior that is both abnormal and maladaptive. It is this kind of behavior that people are often speaking of when they use the unadorned word *abnormal* in reference to behavior. Such usage is, however, colloquial and a bit careless.

See also *abnormal psychology*; *maladaptive behavior*.

abnormal psychology: The study of the abnormal behavior of human beings. This field of psychology takes as its goals the description, diagnosis, explanation, and treatment of various kinds of mental disorders. Although it is true that abnormal behavior is not in and of itself "sick," nonetheless the field of abnormal psychology, as it is usually construed, tends to focus its interest on pathological states.

Abnormal psychology is similar to, but not identical with, psychiatry. It is correct to say that abnormal psychology makes a contribution to psychiatry.

See also *psychiatry*.

abreaction: In psychoanalysis, the discharge of an emotion associated with a memory that is both repressed and painful. The basic assumption is that an emotion can become "strangled" if it is linked to an idea that is forbidden conscious expression. And these strangled emotions, until released, have an adverse effect on one's health. More specifically, they are believed to contribute to a neurotic process.

In practice, an abreaction is usually intense and involves the vivid recall of a seemingly forgotten experience. Frequently these are experiences from early childhood. The patient is sometimes said to relive the experience. For example, Prudence, a patient in psychoanalysis, recalls a childhood incident in which her mother slapped Prudence across the face and called her a stupid child for a minor infraction. Prudence remembers that she wanted to scream at her mother, "I hate you. I hate you." But because she was a "good" girl, she bit her tongue and said nothing. Now, in therapy, she gives expression to the forbidden emotion.

An abreaction is a part of a general process of cleaning out, or purging, of ideas and memories from the unconscious mental level. This process is known as *catharsis*, and the concept of catharsis played a significant role in early psychoanalytic therapy.

See also *catharsis*; *Freud, Sigmund*; *psychoanalysis*.

addiction: A state in which one's behavior is characterized by a habit of great strength. In everyday conversation, the word *addiction* tends to imply the habitual use of a drug such as alcohol or heroin. However, it is possible to speak of a person who is addicted to lying or cheating.

Some addictions are thought of as positive ones. There are, for example, people who must take a daily walk. The psychiatrist William Glasser, father of reality therapy, notes that it is possible to get as "hooked" on a beneficial behavior pattern as on an undesirable one.

See also *drug addiction*.

adjustment: A dynamic process making it possible for the individual to live in harmony with both the physical and the social environments. For human beings, adjustment should not be thought of as an end state but an ongoing series of transactions designed to balance the needs and demands of existence. The term *well-adjusted person* is often used to describe one who is particularly adept at finding the harmony described previously. Strictly speaking, we should refer to the *adjusting* person in contrast to the *adjusted* one.

The term *adjustment* found its greatest vogue several decades ago. In more recent times, there has been emphasis on the concept of *self-actualization*, suggesting growth as a person in contrast to the more static concept of adjustment. It must be honestly admitted that sometimes the processes of adjustment and self-actualization are in conflict. Adjustment tends to suggest balance, maintaining the status quo. Self-actualization may require a giving up of long-standing adjustments.

However, the concept of adjustment should not be abandoned. It is essential for human beings to attain at least moderate levels of adjustment, or they find it very difficult to go on. Life is distressing, and there is emotional suffering when adjustment fails.

The dilemma presented to each of us can be framed as follows: How is it possible to both adjust and grow as a person? The answer depends on the individual and the particular circumstances of his or her life.

See also *maladjustment*; *self-actualization*.

adjustment disorder: A kind of mental disorder characterized by great difficulty in social functioning. The individual with an adjustment disorder will have serious problems in either getting along with others or maintaining the ability to continue functioning in a vocation. Depression, anxiety, disturbances of conduct, physical complaints, inability to work or study effectively, and withdrawal from social contacts are frequently associated with this disorder.

The diagnostic category *adjustment disorder* is used as a clinical label only if a psychosocial stressor can be identified. For example, the individual has recently lost a job or been through a divorce. If the reaction to such a psychosocial stressor seems clearly excessive and inappropriate, then it is correct to speak of an adjustment disorder.

See also *life change units (LCUs)*; *psychosocial stressors*.

Adler, Alfred (1870–1937): Father of a school of psychology and psychotherapy known as *individual psychology*. Adler was an early associate of Sigmund Freud but broke off professional relations with Freud in a dispute over the primacy of the sexual drive. Freud saw sexual problems as the principal source of neurotic disorders. Adler, borrowing from the teachings of the philosopher Friedrich Nietzsche, contended that the frustration of the *will to power* was a primary cause of neurotic disorders.

Adler asserted that the will to power is an inborn drive in the direction of competence, mastery, and superiority over others. When the will to power cannot overcome obstacles in its path, the result will be an *inferiority complex*, a set of related ideas making the individual feel inadequate and incompetent in some important area of personality development. For example, one can have an inferiority complex concerning one's mathematical ability.

Adler pioneered innovations in psychotherapy, recommending friendly face-to-face contact between therapist and patient in contrast to reclining on a couch and free associating. He argued that the human being is a *creative self*, a conscious personality capable of expressing autonomy and overcoming life's many problems. Ideas such as this one indicate that Adler anticipated later developments in both existential and humanistic therapies.

See also *existential therapy*; *humanistic therapy*; *individual psychology*; *psychoanalysis*.

adrenal glands: A pair of endocrine glands playing important roles in the body's capacity to handle stress. Each adrenal gland is located above a respective kidney. A gland's *cortex* is its gray external layer. The cortex produces a group of hormones called *corticoids*, hormones capable of reducing inflammation.

A gland's *medulla* is its brown center. The medulla produces the hormones epinephrine (adrenalin) and norepinephrine (noradrenaline). Both of these hormones help the body prepare for action, particularly when there is a real or imagined danger. For these reasons, the adrenal glands play a significant role in stress-induced diseases. When the individual experiences excessive and/ or chronic stress, the capacities of the adrenal glands may be overtaxed. Illness and even death may be related to adrenal depletion.

See also *behavioral medicine*; *endocrine system*; *general adaptation syndrome*; *psychosomatic disorders*.

adrenocorticotrophic hormone (ACTH): A hormone secreted by the frontal portion of the pituitary gland. ACTH plays a significant role in the body's reaction to stress. Let us say that one feels threatened in some way. The pituitary gland responds with an increased secretion of ACTH. This circulates in the bloodstream and acts upon the adrenal glands, stimulating them to respond by releasing their own hormones. ACTH is, in effect, the brain's messenger to the adrenal glands. The study of ACTH and the hormones of the adrenal glands have added to our understanding of the physiological processes involved in various diseases complicated by stress.

See also *adrenal glands*; *general adaptation syndrome*; *psychosomatic disorders*.

affect: As used in the context of clinical psychology and psychiatry, affect pertains to the core of an emotional state. It is helpful to associate this usage with the familiar word *affection*. Emotional reactions ranging from euphoria to depression are aspects of one's affect.

Mental health professionals often speak of *appropriate* and *inappropriate affects*. Laughing or giggling when a social situation demands tears or a sad expression is an example of inappropriate affect. It is also possible to speak of *blunted affect*, a flatness of emotional response. For example, a schizophrenic woman was told that her mother had died that morning. Her response, without a change in expression, was, "Oh, I see." A moment later she

asked what was planned for dinner that evening. Significant disturbances of affect should be taken seriously. They are often among the signs suggesting the presence of a mental disorder.
See also *anhedonia*.

affective disorders: See *mood disorders (affective disorders)*.

agitation: A state of pathological excitement. Signs of agitation include restlessness, inability to concentrate, inability to relax, and excessive psychomotor activity (i.e., moving about in an aggressive or disorganized manner). Agitation may be associated with more than one mental disorder. Schizophrenic patients may become upset by their delusions or hallucinations. Mentally retarded persons often have a low frustration tolerance and may become agitated if their momentary wishes cannot be satisfied. Children suffering from the hyperkinetic syndrome are somewhat more prone than average to agitation.

Mental hospitals use various strategies to control agitation. Restraints, sedatives, seclusion rooms, warm baths, patient activities, and so forth sometimes have a positive effect.

See also *delirium; dementia*.

agoraphobia: An anxiety disorder characterized by a set of related fears. A common one is the fear of being alone. Another common fear is of public places, particularly ones where a person can easily feel "trapped" or overconfined (e.g., a crowded stadium). Fear of travel any significant distance from home is also common. In extreme cases, some homemakers have made themselves into house prisoners.

Persons suffering from agoraphobia recognize that their fears are irrational, and this often depresses them. Also, if they do act in contradiction to the fears, they often resort to magic rituals, obsessive-compulsive behaviors, as a kind of "protection" against imagined dangers.

Agoraphobia is explained in two general ways. A person may have a bad experience in a crowd or on a trip, even a short one, away from home. This bad experience makes the person *hypersensitive* to the stimuli associated with the bad experience. In other words, a conditioned fear becomes established. A second way to explain agoraphobia is in terms of its symbolical meaning. It is possible that the agoraphobic behavior is a disguise for an unacceptable wish. For example, Lynn unconsciously wishes to leave her husband—"walk away from the marriage." Her moral code and the guilt arising from this code make her repress her wish. The repression of the forbidden wish is aided by the conscious phobia of leaving home.

In view of the fact that explanations of agoraphobia tend to be psychological, the treatment of agoraphobia is also usually psychological. Desensitization therapy, a kind of behavior therapy, is often used to treat agoraphobia. On the other hand, if it is believed that the agoraphobia has a symbolic basis, some form of insight therapy may be called for.

See also *anxiety disorders*; *desensitization therapy*; *insight therapy*; *obsessive-compulsive disorder (obsessive-compulsive neurosis)*.

alcohol amnestic disorder: A disorder characterized by the damage to the central nervous system and memory impairment. The older, more traditional name for this disorder is Korsakoff's psychosis. Its symptoms were originally noted by Sergei Korsakoff, a Russian neurologist, in the late 1800s. The principal cause of alcohol amnestic disorder is a deficiency of thiamine, one of the B-complex vitamins, usually induced by years of chronic abuse of alcohol.

Treatment for alcohol amnestic disorder includes an adequate diet and thiamine replacement therapy. Often the disorder can be arrested with some improvement in memory ability.

See also *amnesia*; *organic mental disorders*.

Alcoholics Anonymous (AA): A self-help organization for sufferers from alcoholism established by two persons known as Dr. Bob and Bill W. Starting in Akron, Ohio, the organization has spread to many different countries. If there is an AA group near you, you can probably locate it through your telephone directory.

AA assumes that alcoholism is a disease and that personal recovery from the disease is difficult, if not in some cases impossible, without the help and support of other people. It also assumes that a Higher Power, greater than the sufferer, can restore some semblance of order to a confused existence. These assumptions form the basis of a recovery program called the Twelve Steps.

The families of alcoholic persons can receive help from two related organizations, Al-Anon and Alateen. The alcoholic person's partner goes to Al-Anon meetings. The alcoholic person's son or daughter goes to Alateen meetings.

See also *alcoholism*.

alcoholism: A substance abuse disorder; also known as alcohol dependence. A principal feature of alcoholism is addiction. The alcohol-dependent individual is usually both physiologically and psychologically addicted to alcohol. Withdrawal may produce physical effects such as the "shakes." In extreme cases, there may be delirium tremens. Withdrawal may also produce psychological effects such as depression, anxiety, or resentment toward others.

The fact is that many persons with alcohol dependence "dry out" and get over their physiological addiction for a given time. However, it is a commonplace to "fall off the wagon" and go back to compulsive drinking. The "on the wagon" and "off the wagon" aspect of alcohol dependence suggests the importance of the psychological addiction to alcohol. In brief, the wish to drink remains even though the biological basis for a craving may be gone.

The prevalence of alcoholism is somewhat difficult to estimate because of differing opinions concerning its correct definition. If by alcoholism we mean frequent abuse of alcohol, then perhaps 5% to 10% of adults are involved. If we mean only hard-core compulsive drinking on a regular basis, then the incidence is probably on the order of 1% to 2% of adults. In any event, the abuse of alcohol is a major health problem touching many families. A large percentage of automobile accidents, murders, rapes, assaults, and suicides are associated with alcohol abuse.

Many theories have been advanced in an attempt to explain

alcoholism. There are studies that suggest it is in part related to a genetic factor. It seems more likely, however, that psychological factors are more important. Many abusers of alcohol use the substance as a kind of crutch, a solace for the slings and arrows of outrageous fortune. Almost everyone is familiar with the phrase "drowning your sorrows in a bottle." And there is obviously a lot of truth in it. Alcohol dependence can be looked upon as a habit, a learned pattern of maladaptive behavior. Finally, it is possible to explain some problem drinking in sociocultural terms. The traditions and norms of certain groups encourage excessive use of alcohol.

Alcohol dependence is far from a hopeless condition. Alcoholics Anonymous offers a recovery program. Psychotherapy is often effective.

See also *Alcoholics Anonymous (AA)*; *delirium tremens*; *Korsakoff's psychosis*; *psychoactive substance use disorders (substance use disorders)*.

alexia: An impairment in reading ability associated with brain pathology. Causes of such pathology include strokes (cerebrovascular accidents), brain tumors, and various neurological disorders. Visual ability as such is not necessarily impaired when people suffer from alexia. The extent of brain pathology need not be gross or obvious. The general location of the pathology is usually in the left cerebral hemisphere; this is the general region of the brain used to process language.

An aphasia refers to any deterioration in language functioning. Thus another term for alexia is *visual aphasia*. Alexia, or visual aphasia, can be treated with special reading and writing exercises. These exercises often bring about a substantial improvement. Reading therapists have developed a number of effective ways to help victims of alexia.

See also *aphasia*; *brain pathology*; *cerebrovascular accident (CVA)*; *developmental reading disorder (dyslexia)*.

alienation: A feeling that one does not belong to a given reference group. Thus one can feel alienated from one's family, from one's friends, from one's religion, from one's nation, and so forth. Note that alienation is always alienation *from*. The literal roots of the word *alienation* mean "without ties." An alienated person is, in a sense, not tied to a group he or she was formerly tied to.

It is possible to speak of persons who suffer from a kind of general alienation. They do not really feel that they belong anywhere, that there is no place they can call home. They feel lonely and apart at school, in military service, on the job, and so forth. This kind of alienation may play a significant role in depression and the despair that goes with various kinds of self-destructive behavior, including suicide.

Certain thinkers such as the psychoanalyst Erich Fromm and the psychiatrist R. D. Laing stress the importance of general alienation as a significant process in serious mental disorders. The feeling that one has a proper place in one's society seems to be an important factor in mental health. Both Fromm and Laing argue quite convincingly that the modern world has many alienating influences, making it increasingly difficult for people to feel settled, loved, and secure.

See also *existential neurosis*; *Fromm, Erich*; *Laing, Ronald David*.

alienist: A term with two related meanings. First, an alienist is a physician who specializes in the treatment of mental disorders. This usage makes an alienist synonymous with a psychiatrist and is a correct usage. However, it is somewhat dated.

Second, an alienist is any physician deemed able to testify in a court of law concerning mental competence. Such mental competence may refer to either a party or a witness in a case. Under these circumstances, the physician need not be a psychiatrist to be referred to as an alienist.

See also *legal aspects of mental health*; *psychiatrist*.

Alzheimer's disease: A disease involving degeneration of neurons in the frontal portion of the brain. Characteristic aspects of the degenerative process include tangled nerve fibers and the actual death of a large percentage of neurons.

The disease usually is categorized as a *senile dementia*, one associated with old age. However, Alzheimer's disease sometimes strikes persons in middle age.

It is impossible to tell for sure in a living subject whether or not there is actual degeneration of neurons. This can only be determined by a postmortem examination of the brain. Therefore a diagnosis of Alzheimer's disease is made on the basis of behavioral evidence. Symptoms of Alzheimer's disease include the following: (1) general deterioration of mental abilities; (2) suspicion and distrust; (3) activity without purpose; (4) depression; (5) agitation; (6) confusion; and (7) loss of memory, particularly for recent events.

The causes of Alzheimer's disease are being actively researched, and there is at present no consensus among behavioral scientists concerning causation. Several theories have been advanced. One theory states that the disease is caused by a genetic predisposition. It is possible that a biological clock signals that it is time for the disease to become active. Another theory states that Alzheimer's disease may be caused or aggravated by environmental toxins. Trace amounts of aluminum circulating in the bloodstream have been implicated as possible culprits.

There is no known cure for Alzheimer's disease. The inevitable course is downward, and complications associated with the disease may indeed even cause death. However, the disease can be managed to some extent, thereby diminishing or slowing down the rate of decline. Effective management includes emotional support, understanding, and a simplified environment.

See also *dementia; organic mental syndromes (organic brain syndromes); senile dementia.*

ambivalence: A state in which one thinks or feels two ways about the same stimulus or situation. People sometimes say, "I am of two minds about this." The statement expresses the essence of ambivalence.

Ambivalence manifests itself in many ways: the inability to make a choice, doubt, indecision, confusion, and so forth. When one is in a state of great ambivalence about the pros and cons of marrying someone, about a career option, or something of equal significance, the associated mental conflict can have an adverse effect on one's mental health.

See also *approach–avoidance conflict*.

amnesia: Loss of memory. Of course, all memories are seldom lost. So it perhaps more correct to speak of memory impairment.

Amnesia can be either organic or functional. *Organic amnesia* is amnesia with a clear-cut biological basis. Some of the causes of organic amnesia include Alzheimer's disease, brain tumors, strokes (cerebrovascular accidents), and brain pathology associated with alcohol abuse.

Functional amnesia is believed to be amnesia due to the ego defense mechanism called *repression*. Repression functions in such a way as to protect one's conscious self from threatening memories. A childhood memory associated with shame and/or guilt might be repressed. An action that goes against one's moral code might be conveniently forgotten as time passes. Novels and films have made much of the kind of functional amnesia in which one loses one's sense of identity. Such cases actually do occur. It seems that, in such cases, the individual finds his or her particular existence or personal life situation intolerable in some way. Thus one's name and other personal details are repressed.

See also *Alzheimer's disease*; *fugue*; *repression*.

amotivational syndrome: A pattern of behavior characterized by low achievement motivation and lack of clear-cut goals in life. The person manifesting the amotivational syndrome is seemingly content to merely exist. There is no emphasis in his or her life on growing and the process of becoming a more interesting or accomplished person. The individual seems to live in a kind of eternal present with little ability conceptualize the future.

It has been observed that many abusers of drugs manifest the amotivational syndrome. At first it was believed that drug abuse caused the syndrome. However, it has been suggested since that persons with the syndrome are somewhat more likely to be attracted to drugs. Thus we have a chicken-and-the-egg problem. Cause and effect are too intertwined to separate them in any meaningful way. Causation aside, the amotivational syndrome is a reality. There are people who manifest it. Such people are psychologically "stuck" in their lives. Certain types of psychotherapy may be helpful, particularly somewhat directive therapies such as rational-emotive therapy and reality therapy.

See also *drug addiction*; *rational-emotive therapy*; *reality therapy*.

amphetamines: Drugs that act as potent stimulants of the central nervous system. They temporarily energize behavior and increase alertness. Popular names for amphetamines include *speed*, *pep pills*, *wake-ups*, and *uppers*. Amphetamines are marketed under several trade names, including Benzedrine and Dexedrine.

Amphetamines are often used for recreational purposes. As a consequence, they have often been abused. Some doubt exists concerning their power in terms of physiological addiction. Physical withdrawal symptoms from habitual use may be in some cases quite slight. However, no doubt exists concerning their power in terms of psychological addiction. Frequent users tend to become quite dependent on amphetamines. Withdrawal may produce emotional reactions such as anger, anxiety, or depression. Also, abuse of amphetamines has been known to produce both delusions and hallucination, mimicking psychotic disorders.

Amphetamines have a legitimate place in drug therapy. Hyperkinetic disorder, narcolepsy, and obesity are all problems that may sometimes respond to the prescription of amphetamines.

See also *drug addiction*; *drug therapy*; *hyperkinetic (hyperactive) disorder*; *narcolepsy*; *obesity*.

anaclitic depression: A depressive syndrome associated with infancy, approximately the first 18 months of life. An infant suffering from anaclitic depression is listless and apathetic. Weight loss, poor physical and mental development, and, in some cases, even death have all been associated with anaclitic depression.

The principal cause of anaclitic depression is separation from a parent, usually the mother. The depression is aggravated if the child is isolated, receiving inadequate social stimulation. Even if physical care is quite adequate, the syndrome may appear.

Anaclitic depression is much more common in institutions than it is in a home setting. For this reason, it is sometimes referred to as *hospitalism*. Pioneer investigations conducted in foundling homes by researcher René A. Spitz established the reality of anaclitic depression. The syndrome can, of course, appear in a home setting when there is gross neglect of an infant. Unfortunately, such cases do occur. However, in the vast majority of homes, there is little risk that an infant will develop anaclitic depression.

See also *depression*.

anal character traits: Personality traits assumed in psychoanalytic theory to be caused by fixations of libido in the anal stage of psychosexual development. There are believed to be two principal kinds of anal character traits, and it should be understood that, although they are associated with infantile fixations, these traits manifest themselves in adult behavior. First, persons with an *anal-retentive character* tend to be stingy, inhibited, and withholding of affection. Presumably, such individuals had a traumatic and emotionally difficult time when they were being toilet trained. Possibly they were trained quite young, before they were ready for such training, and their parents were harsh and overcontrolling.

Second, persons with an *anal-expulsive character* tend to be sloppy, stubborn, expansive, and aggressive. Presumably, such individuals obtained during early childhood a great deal of physical pleasure from the expelling of fecal bulk. There is no general consensus among mental health professionals concerning the validity of the idea that adult personality traits are caused by fixations of libido. Traditional psychoanalysts subscribe to the hypothesis. Others have their doubts.

See also *libido*; *psychoanalysis*; *psychosexual development*.

anal stage: The second stage of psychosexual development proposed by Freud. It lasts from approximately 18 months to 3 years of age. It is usually the stage during which the child acquires the voluntary control of bowel movements.

See also *anal character traits*; *psychosexual development*.

analytic psychology (analytical psychology): The name given by Carl Jung to his system of psychology and therapy. The term *analytic psychology* is often used when one wants to make a distinction between Jung's formulations and those of Freud as contained in psychoanalysis.

Here are some important distinctions between Jung's analytic psychology and Freud's psychoanalysis:

1. Freud asserted that all neurotic disorders have their origins in sexual conflicts. Jung argued that neurotic disorders can be caused by all sorts of emotional conflicts as the individual struggles to make adjustments.
2. Freud tended to limit the unconscious mental life to its personal elements. Jung believed in a collective unconscious mind common to all human beings.
3. Freud believed that the symbols in dreams exist for the purpose of disguising forbidden wishes. Jung believed that symbols reveal as much as they conceal; they speak to us in a psychological shorthand.
4. Freud saw therapy primarily as a way of relieving people of their misery, making it possible for them to have at least a tolerable existence. Jung saw therapy in much broader terms. He felt that it could help individuals discover greater joy and meaning in life.

See also *archetypes*; *collective unconscious*; *Jung, Carl Gustav*.

androgens: Male sex hormones produced principally by the testes. Two of these are *testosterone* and *androsterone*. Androgens nurture secondary male characteristics such as facial hair and a deep voice. Varying degrees of these characteristics have an important

• 15 •

effect on masculine self-image and in turn general mental health. A male who feels that he is below average on some important physical male attribute may become anxious or moody.

Testosterone production appears to have something to do with aggressive behavior. Experiments with male monkeys indicate that injections of testosterone can influence some of them to act in a more aggressive and dominant fashion. It is possible that male human beings with very high levels of testosterone production are somewhat more likely than other males to exhibit the kinds of behaviors we associate with certain personality disorders.

Very low levels of androgens may be a cause of, or contributing factor to, erectile insufficiency (i.e., impotence) in males.

See also *erectile disorder (erectile insufficiency)*; *estrogens*; *personality disorders*.

anhedonia: The lack of the ability to experience a normal range of pleasure or pain in one's emotional responses. If a person is suffering from anhedonia, good news will fail to produce any sense of joy or elation. Similarly, bad news will fail to produce any sense of sadness or loss. Anhedonia has approximately the same meaning as *blunted affect*, a flatness of emotional response.

Anhedonia is a common feature of some kinds of schizophrenia and depression.

See also *affect*; *depression*; *schizophrenia*.

anomie: A term with two related meanings. First, if a person is in a state of anomie, he or she feels that the rules, norms, laws, and customs of his or her society are irrelevant to him or her. Second, if a society is in a state of anomie, its rules, norms, laws, and customs are in a rapid state of change or disintegration. It seems clear enough that a state of anomie in the society may in turn produce a state of anomie in some individuals. Those experiencing anomie tend to feel lost, confused, alienated, and depressed. During social upheavals such as wars, depressions, revolutions, and mass migrations, anomie in individuals increases.

The sociologist Emile Durkheim introduced the term *anomie* into behavioral science and used it to explain increases in the suicide rate at times of social crisis.

It has been argued that contemporary industrial society tends to foster anomie in individuals. More than one social commentator has expressed the opinion that our age is one in which many traditions and conventional ideas are no longer taken for granted.

See also *alienation*; *suicide*.

anorexia nervosa: A mental disorder characterized primarily by the refusal to eat enough food for the maintenance of a normal body weight. Although *anorexia* literally means loss of appetite, the individual with anorexia nervosa usually *does* have an appetite. The refusal to eat is just that, a *refusal*; it is an act of will related in most cases to a dread of obesity.

The victim of anorexia nervosa is in the vast majority of cases (about 95%) a female. The high-risk time period for the disorder is adolescence.

Other common symptoms of anorexia nervosa include:

A confused body image. The victim perceives herself as fat even when she is skinny or emaciated. She may look in a mirror and say in disgust, "I'm as fat as a pig."

Amenorrhea. Amenorrhea is a cessation of the menstrual flow. This is an early symptom of anorexia nervosa and often is in evidence prior to substantial weight reduction.

Lanugo. The term *lanugo* is used to describe the growth of a fine covering of hair on the body resembling that of a newborn child.

Psychosexual disturbance. Adolescents with the disorder are often behind others in their sexual development. Adults with the disorder tend to lose interest in sexual activity.

Cooking meals. It is common for the victim to cook meals for others, insisting they eat well.

Anorexia nervosa is a serious mental disorder, one of the few that can be fatal. Its victims may very well die of complications associated with emaciation. The American Psychiatric Association's

Diagnostic and Statistical Manual of Mental Disorders states that the mortality rates for anorexia nervosa may be as high as between 5% and 18%. Therefore, the disorder must be taken very seriously.

Although the disorder has received a great deal of publicity in the popular media, it is fortunately not common. In adolescent females, its incidence is estimated to be under ½ of 1%.

Anorexia nervosa appears to be caused primarily by an interaction of psychosocial factors. Some of these factors are overcontrolling parents, a strong-willed adolescent, an upwardly mobile family, and a culture that overvalues a thin female body. When the adolescent female diets to an extreme, parents often react with stern lectures and warnings. The issue becomes, "Who is in control?" A battle of the wills ensues. Not eating becomes a symbol of the adolescent's ability to exercise autonomy. This analysis is an oversimplification, of course. The psychology of anorexia nervosa is a large subject in itself. However, it is correct that, in broad general terms, a process like the one described here is commonly to be found.

The treatment of anorexia nervosa often requires hospitalization for the medical aspects of the disorder. Sometimes the victim must be force-fed just to keep her alive. This, of course, increases her resentment and makes long-term therapy more difficult. Recovery usually requires both individual psychotherapy with the patient and family therapy. Both the victim of anorexia nervosa and members of her family need to see ways in which they can stop working against each other.

See also *bulimia nervosa*; *compulsive eating*; *obesity*; *Overeaters Anonymous (OA)*.

Antabuse: A drug used to treat alcoholism. Antabuse is the trade name of a drug with the generic name *disulfram*. When alcohol and Antabuse are ingested during the same general time period, a biological process known as the *disulfram reaction* is produced. Pains in the chest, a headache, labored breathing, upset stomach, vomiting, and loss of strength are key features of this reaction. Thus maintenance doses of Antabuse may act as a powerful deterrent to the consumption of alcohol. Because the disulfram reaction can itself be dangerous, Antabuse requires a physician's prescription.

It is clear that the prescription of Antabuse is not in and of itself a cure for alcoholism. Obviously, the patient must cooperate in his or her treatment. Alcoholics Anonymous meetings and/or psychotherapy are usually indicated.

See also *Alcoholics Anonymous (AA)*; *alcoholism*; *drug therapy*.

anterograde amnesia: A kind of amnesia in which there is an impairment of memory for events *following* the beginning of the amnesia. For example, a person has an accident involving a head injury. One year later, he or she cannot recall the events of the accident, and he or she also has no recall of his or her hospitalization the first week after the accident took place. This "lost week" can be described as an anterograde amnesia.

See also *amnesia*; *retrograde amnesia*.

antianxiety drugs: Drugs capable of reducing excessively high levels of anxiety. They are also referred to as *minor tranquilizers*. Such drugs may sometimes be useful in the treatment of anxiety disorders. For example, such a drug may make it possible for a person with disabling anxiety attacks to cope with threatening situations and carry out daily responsibilities.

The drugs can also be useful in other ways. Because of their sedative effect, they are at times prescribed for persons who suffer from psychosomatic disorders (e.g., ulcers). They are on occasion prescribed for seizures and other difficulties associated with the nervous system. They are also prescribed for symptoms of insomnia.

There are two broad general classes of antianxiety drugs: (1) benzodiazepine derivatives and (2) meprobamate drugs. The benzodiazepine derivatives depress the brain's arousal mechanism, and this has a direct effect on anxiety. Two well-known trade names for benzodiazepine are Librium and Valium. The meprobamate drugs induce muscle relaxation, and such relaxation is antagonistic to anxiety. Two well-known trade names for these meprobamate drugs are Equanil and Miltown.

Though the antianxiety drugs have a very appropriate place in the treatment of various disorders, they sometimes have adverse side effects. Because they may impair both alertness and attention, it is often unsafe to drive an automobile or otherwise operate machinery when the drug is active in the body. Also, these drugs have a potential for abuse. Some people become quite dependent on them. They are obviously no substitute for effective coping mechanisms. Life's problems cannot be solved with pills in bottles. If the anxiety agents are thought of as a bridge helping an individual across a difficult transition in life, then they have a proper place in human adjustment. But they should not become a way of life. They are a treatment, not a cure.

See also *anxiety disorders*; *insomnia*; *psychosomatic disorders*.

antidepressant drugs: Drugs used primarily to relieve depression. Depression has been called the "common cold" of mental illness and plays a part in more than one disorder. Sometimes depression is a primary symptom, sometimes a secondary one. In either case, an antidepressant drug may be useful if it is suspected than a particular patient's depression has a biochemical basis.

There are two broad general classes of antidepressant drugs: (1) monoamine oxidase (MAO) inhibitors and (2) tricyclic derivatives. Although the chemical action of the two classes of drugs is somewhat different, both drugs have the same effect: They tend to increase levels of two neurotransmitters in the brain. These two neurotransmitters are *serotonin* and *norepinephrine*, both important chemical messengers. Research on depressive disorders suggests that abnormally low levels of serotonin and norepinephrine may play a significant role in these conditions.

MAO inhibitors are marketed under several trade names including Marplan, Nardil, and Parnate. Tricyclic derivatives are marketed under several trade names including Elavil, Endep, Norpramin, and Aventyl.

These drugs require a prescription and must be taken with prudence. When a person is taking an MAO inhibitor, it is necessary to avoid drinks and foods containing *tyramine*, a body chemical that regulates blood pressure. Red wines, sour cream, salted dried fish, eggplant, and soy sauce are just some of the drinks and foods containing high levels of tyramine. If these substances are ingested with an MAO inhibitor, the blood pressure can rise to dangerously high levels.

See also *depression*; *drug therapy*; *neurotransmitters*.

antihistamines: Drugs that block the action of *histamine*. Histamine is a natural chemical found in the body, and it is released in larger quantities when the body has to cope with foreign substances. Thus antihistamines are often prescribed for allergic reactions and colds. The effect of the antihistamines is to reduce the symptoms associated with these conditions.

One of the principal side effects of antihistamines is that they produce drowsiness by depressing central nervous system arousal. Thus they are sometimes prescribed to treat anxiety or insomnia.

See also *antianxiety drugs*; *insomnia*.

antipsychiatry: A term introduced by the British psychiatrist David Cooper to describe a counterculture movement within the ranks of psychiatry opposed to certain standard psychiatric practices. Antipsychiatry tends to take a rather dim view of many of the usual applications of drug therapy, psychosurgery, and electroconvulsive therapy (ECT). It adopts the position that these treatments are abused and overused. Also, antipsychiatry questions the ethics of imposing confinement and treatment on unwilling patients.

One of the key assumptions of antipsychiatry is that many mental disorders are not really disorders or illnesses at all. They have no organic or biochemical bases. Instead, they are names we assign to problems of living. Alienation, for example, is often at the root of such problems. Thus the mental patient needs to learn more effective ways to cope in his or her social world, not biological interventions.

Although antipsychiatry is identified as a counterculture movement, it can be best understood in the light of a very slow, but very sustained, tendency to respect the human rights of mental patients. Increasingly, laws have been passed restricting the arbitrary powers of persons in power to impose various types of treatments on patients against their wishes.

See also *alienation*; *drug therapy*; *electroconvulsive therapy (ECT)*; *Laing, Ronald David*; *psychosurgery*.

antipsychotic drugs: See *major tranquilizers (antipsychotic drugs)*.

antisocial personality disorder (psychopathic personality; sociopathic personality): A kind of personality disorder characterized by an inadequate set of moral and ethical standards. Such individuals are said to have very little conscience. In Freudian terms, they lack adequate superego development. They can be described as *undersocialized*, meaning they have not accepted the norms and values of their culture.

Although the term *antisocial personality disorder* is applicable only to adults, such adults have usually shown a pattern of misbehavior during adolescence. Common behaviors are truancy, delinquency, running away from home, chronic lying, casual sexual intercourse, abuse of alcohol or drugs, theft, and vandalism.

If we speak of an adult with an antisocial personality disorder, an overall pattern of irresponsibility emerges. Common specific behaviors associated with this pattern are irregular employment, not functioning as an effective parent, lack of respect for the law, difficulty in remaining attached to a single sexual partner, lack of foresight, not meeting financial obligations, and recklessness.

The causes of an antisocial personality disorder are several. An attention deficit disorder (hyperkinetic syndrome) in childhood is in some cases a predisposing cause. Inborn traits of temperament may play a part. Very few researchers would be willing to say that children are "born bad." However, it does seem reasonable to hypothesize that some children might be more difficult to socialize than others. Evidence exists that emotional rejection by parents combines with ineffective or inappropriate discipline to foster the formation of an antisocial personality disorder. Other environmental facts include poverty, not living at home, and the absence of parental role models.

It is estimated that the incidence of antisocial personality disorder in males is about 3%. In females it is somewhat under 1%.

The principal treatment for an antisocial personality disorder is psychotherapy. However, persons with the disorder usually resist treatment. They feel that it is an unfair imposition, that "there is nothing wrong with me." Fairly directive therapies such as rational-emotive therapy or reality therapy are probably the best ones to use with antisocial disorders. The individual must be helped to see the fact that his or her irresponsible behavior will fail to bring him or her any satisfaction in the long run. Such people need to take a longer look into the future and be helped to develop practical goals in life.

See also *attention deficit disorder*; *conduct disorder*; *rational-emotive therapy*; *reality therapy*.

anxiety: A feeling of dread or apprehension lacking a specific well-defined source. The emotional state is similar to fear. There is increased heart rate, rapid breathing, greater muscle tension, and so forth. However, in fear there is an objective stimulus that can be seen or otherwise directly sensed. In the case of anxiety, the stimuli are subjective. They arise from within the individual.

There is more than one kind of anxiety. Freud distinguished three types: (1) objective anxiety, (2) neurotic anxiety, and (3) moral anxiety. *Objective anxiety* (or *realistic anxiety*) is identical in meaning to fear. Such anxiety arises from a clear and present danger. And, as already indicated, in this instance *fear* is the preferred term. *Neurotic anxiety* is anxiety arising from the possibility that one will act on one's forbidden wishes. It is the threat *from within* that one's social inhibitions will crumble. The risk of actually acting on one's repressed sexual and aggressive motives is sometimes a distinct possibility. *Moral anxiety* is anxiety arising from the feeling that one deserves to be punished for real or imagined violations of behavioral standards. Persons with a well-developed superego are the ones most likely to experience moral anxiety.

Sometimes clinicians speak of *free-floating anxiety*. This is simply another name for the kind of anxiety described in the first paragraph of this entry. It is a common symptom in certain kinds of anxiety disorders.

It is also possible to identify *existential anxiety*. This is anxiety about the general quality and direction of one's life. Worries about the future, one's career, one's health, and similar personal concerns are all varieties of existential anxiety. Existential anxiety is normal. However, if the anxiety seems excessive or inappropriate, it is possible to speak of an existential neurosis.

See also *anxiety disorders*; *existential neurosis*.

anxiety disorders: A set of disorders in which anxiety plays a prominent symptomatic role. This can take place in one of two ways. First, the anxiety can be manifest. The troubled person is very aware of the existence of anxiety. For example, in a *panic disorder*, there may be heart palpitations, chest pain, faintness, and the sensation that one is about to die.

Second, anxiety can be latent, buried by neurotic symptoms. For example, in *agoraphobia* anxiety emerges only if the sufferer ventures away from a place perceived to be "safe" such as home. As long as one allows the neurotic symptoms to dictate behavior, anxiety is suppressed.

There are a number of anxiety disorders. These are identified next and discussed elsewhere.

See also *agoraphobia*; *generalized anxiety disorder*; *obsessive-compulsive disorder*; *panic disorder*; *phobia*; *posttraumatic stress disorder (traumatic neurosis)*.

anxiolytics: Drugs used to treat anxiety.
See also *antianxiety drugs*.

apathy: A state of indifference. When a person is apathetic he or she does not care about people or things he or she formerly cared for. Passion, high emotion, and excitement in life are replaced by coolness or boredom. Apathy is associated with more than one adverse mental state. It is often present along with depression. Persons suffering from schizophrenia often display apathy.

Transient apathy is *not* a mental health problem. Most of us go through brief periods of apathy. However, if apathy is chronic, it *is* a sign something is amiss in one's normal life.

See also *affect*; *depression*; *schizophrenia*.

aphasia: Any significant deterioration in the ability to understand or use language. The cause of aphasia is usually some type of brain pathology, including strokes (cerebrovascular accidents), brain tumors, and various neurological disorders.

There is more than one kind of aphasia. *Auditory aphasia* exists when a person has impairment in the ability to comprehend what is being said. *Dysgraphia* exists when thoughts cannot be readily expressed in writing. *Motor aphasia* exists when the person has problems speaking.

Treatment for aphasia usually consists of retraining exercises. These exercises allow the individual to bring into play undamaged areas of the cerebral cortex, and often there is substantial improvement.

See also *alexia*; *brain pathology*; *cerebrovascular accident (CVA)*; *developmental reading disorder (dyslexia)*.

aphonia: Loss of the ability to speak with normal loudness. Instead, the individual is reduced to speaking in a whisper. Aphonia is a symptom of conversion disorder (or hysterical neurosis).

Assuming that there is no hoarseness due to an organic condition, the usual explanation of aphonia is in terms of emotional conflict. For example, assume that one is unconsciously afraid of what one might say to a stern parent. The aphonia reduces the anxiety surrounding the possibility of speaking out of turn.

See also *conversion disorder*.

approach–avoidance conflict: One of the basic kinds of psychological conflicts that people face in life. An approach–avoidance conflict exists when a goal has simultaneously positive and negative aspects. Such a conflict tends to produce indecisive behavior. The goal is at first approached. From a distance, the positive aspects seem more significant than the negative ones. However, when one is close to the goal the negative aspects often seem more significant than the positive ones, and a retreat begins. A mild approach–avoidance conflict may take place when one wants a rich dessert but does not want the calories in it. An intense approach–avoidance conflict may take place when one is in love with a person of a different religion than one's own. Such conflicts can contribute to mental health problems.

See also *ambivalence*; *psychological conflict*.

archetypes: According to the psychiatrist Carl Jung, inborn patterns in the collective unconscious. These patterns are primordial images hypothesized to be derived from the human race's centuries of experience on the face of the earth. Jung and his followers believe that the archetypes reveal the basic nature of humankind.

Some of the archetypes are revealed in legend and folklore. Thus we find in many tales, old and new, such characters as the Hero, the Evil One, the Wise Old Man, and the Great Earth Mother. (Note that the archetypes are capitalized to suggest their important status in the personality.) Although the Hero in a particular story may display superficial differences from a Hero in another tale, the truth is that at root they are the same Hero figure. Robin Hood and James Bond are, in the archetypal sense, the same person.

Other archetypes relate to one's own self. Such archetypes include the Anima and the Animus, the Persona, and the Shadow. The Anima is the female personality in every human being, and the Animus is the male personality. The Persona is the social self, the mask we present to the external world. The Shadow is the undiscovered self, a side of one's personality containing both irrational and creative elements.

Jung believed that mental illnesses, particularly psychotic disorders, result when one is out of touch with the archetypes. A poor understanding of the archetypes and their relation to one's whole personality can lead to serious problems. For example, one can be possessed by the archetype of the Evil One and go on a rampage. Or another person can be so dominated by the

Persona that he or she confuses his or her social reactions with his or her true feelings.

Analytic psychology, Jung's system of psychology and psychotherapy, suggests that we are all on a voyage of self-discovery that challenges us to integrate the archetypes into our conscious life in a meaningful way. This personal voyage Jung called the *individuation process*.

Briefly, Jung suggests that it is not enough for the person to know himself or herself as a particular being. He or she must also know himself or herself as a member of the human race.

See also *analytic psychology (analytical psychology)*; *collective unconscious*; *Jung, Carl Gustav*.

assertiveness training: A systematic training procedure designed to enhance one's social skills. The basic assumption of assertiveness training is that, when people are overly passive in their dealings with others, they tend to eventually feel used and abused. These feelings can be contributing factors aggravating any tendencies the individual has to become either anxious or depressed.

Assertiveness training operates on the premise that it is not necessary to feel better before one acts better. Classical psychoanalysis assumed that improvements in mental health *precede* more effective and realistic action. Assertiveness training, in contrast, operates on behavioral principles. If behavior itself can be *directly* improved, then positive consequences can provide feedback changing one's personality for the better. In keeping with this general philosophy, persons undergoing assertiveness training are taught specific assertiveness skills. These are rehearsed in group settings. The therapist provides a role model, and members of the group acquire the skills in part by observational learning.

Here are some of the assertiveness skills that are recommended:

1. *Feeling talk* requires that one speak with more emotion, more inflection, more conviction, and with sufficient loudness to be heard.
2. *Eye contact* requires that one look directly into another person's eyes when answering a question or making a request.

3. *Broken record* requires one to repeat a request calmly and with conviction until the request is satisfactorily answered.
4. *Fogging* requires that one answer manipulative questions with vague generalizations and indefinite promises.
5. *Saying no* requires that one say "No" to unfair or unreasonable requests firmly and without elaborate explanation.
6. *Using free information* requires that one take note of, and respond to, social cues given by others. These social cues often reveal the other individual's interests or values.
7. *Negative assertion* requires that one gracefully accept criticism offered by others.

If one becomes adept at using assertiveness skills, then one will both feel more comfortable and be more effective in one's dealings with other people.

One of the risks of assertiveness training is that the novice may confuse assertiveness and aggressiveness. Assertiveness requires that one stand up for one's rights. This may in some instances require negotiation and arrival at a working compromise. Aggressive behavior, on the other hand, is hostile and frequently counterproductive.

See also *behavior therapy*; *cognitive-behavior therapy*.

asthma: An illness characterized by chronic breathing problems. Symptoms include coughing, wheezing, a constriction in the chest, and a struggle for adequate amounts of air. The incidence of asthma in the United States population is 3%. Although there is a tendency to associate the illness with children, adults also suffer from asthma.

In the majority of cases, the principal cause of asthma in a given individual is an allergen. House dust, cat fur, airborne spores of certain molds, and pollens are examples of common allergens. An allergic reaction produces spasmodic contractions in the bronchial tubes of the lungs.

The reason that asthma is listed here is because there is a substantial amount of evidence indicating that it is aggravated by emotional factors. It is often thought to be a psychosomatic (i.e., psychophysiologic) disease. In most cases of asthma, this is true only in the limited sense that such states as anxiety or anger might trigger or augment an asthmatic attack. However, it is a mistake to think that the primary cause of most asthma is a set of emotional factors.

There does appear to be evidence that asthmatic children with severe and overcontrolling parents suffer more intensely from their symptoms than do children who live in more comfortable emotional atmospheres. The general conclusion is that sufferers from asthma, aside from taking proper medication, should attempt to lead lives of reduced emotional stress.

See also *psychosomatic disorders*.

attention deficit disorder: A disorder in children characterized by such behavioral problems as seldom completing tasks, not listening, being distracted easily, and problems concentrating on school assignments. These difficulties are summarized in the single word *inattention*. Combined with inattention is an *impulsive pattern*. The child may jump arbitrarily from one activity to another one. Acting without sufficient thought is common.

There are two basic kinds of attention deficit disorders: (1) with hyperactivity and (2) without hyperactivity. If there is hyperactivity, the child will do a lot of running about and climbing on objects. Staying seated will be a problem. Such a child seems to always have his or her "motor" running. Described more formally, there is a chronic high state of arousal.

Although both sexes can suffer from the disorder, boys tend to suffer from it more frequently than girls.

Attention deficit disorder is not to be confused with other problems such as mental retardation, conduct disorder, schizophrenia, or the normal exuberance of childhood.

The disorder usually makes its first appearance before the age of 7 and often continues well into adolescence. It is believed that many adults with a mild form of antisocial personality disorder may have suffered from attention deficit disorder as children. It *is*, however, encouraging to note that both Thomas Alva Edison and Winston Churchill are suspected to have been hyperkinetic as children.

One of the suspected causes of attention deficit disorder is minimal brain dysfunction (MBD). Another factor is heredity; it is suspected that some children are somewhat more prone by temperament to be restless and impulsive. It has also been suggested that some children are allergic to certain food additives, and this may adversely affect their ability to concentrate.

The principal drug treatment for attention deficit disorder is the prescription of a stimulant such as Ritalin. Stimulants normally increase arousal. However, they often have a paradoxical effect on children with attention deficit disorder and often lower arousal. In mild cases, coffee, because it contains the stimulant caffeine, has a therapeutic effect.

The principal psychological treatment for the disorder is behavior modification.

See also *antisocial personality disorder (psychopathic personality; sociopathic personality); behavior modification; drug therapy; methylphenidate; minimal brain dysfunction (MBD).*

aura: A set of sensory, motor, or mood changes that come before an epileptic seizure, migraine headache, or other disturbance of behavior. The aura acts as a warning signal and sometimes gives the afflicted person a little time (i.e., a few seconds to a few minutes) to prepare for an attack.

Prior to a migraine headache, the individual often experiences numbness in an arm or leg, the impression that lights are too bright, ringing sounds, nausea, or emotional upset.

Prior to an epileptic seizure, the individual often feels somewhat confused, that the world has become strange or unreal, or that one is no longer oneself. Light flashes before a seizure are called *visual aura*. Buzzing sounds before a seizure are called *auditory aura*. After a seizure is over, the memory of the aura is frequently retained.

See also *epilepsy; migraine headache.*

autism: Preoccupation with one's own thoughts and feelings. Pathological autism exists when one lives almost entirely in a fantasy world. Some persons suffering from a schizophrenic disorder seem to exhibit autism of this kind. Indeed, the term *autism* was at one time used almost as a synonym for schizophrenia, but this usage is outdated.

Deriving pleasure from a daydream or a fantasy is moderately autistic but is not considered pathological.

See also *autistic disorder (infantile autism)*; *schizophrenia*.

autistic disorder (infantile autism): A very serious developmental disorder characterized by a lack of social interest, mutism or speech problems, and self-destructiveness. This disorder was first identified by the psychiatrist Leo Kanner in 1943. The reason the word *infantile* is sometimes used is because the disorder usually starts in infancy or early childhood. However, it tends to remain a problem as the child matures. *Autism* refers to the fact that these children seem to be living in their own private dream world. They pay attention to themselves and have almost no concern for others.

It is often said that autistic disorder is not a form of mental retardation. Nonetheless, most children with autistic disoder perform very poorly on standardized intelligence tests. It is very difficult to reliably measure their intelligence because they tend to be uncooperative. In fact, it is estimated that about three-fourths of autistic children are mentally retarded.

Autistic disorder tends to be a lifelong problem. It is not easily cured. However, it is treatable. The most effective approach seems to be behavior modification aimed at helping the child live in a family setting. The goal is to avoid years of institutionalization.

It used to be thought that autistic disorder autism was the result of parental coldness (i.e., a rejecting attitude and lack of interest in the infant). Today there is a consensus that it is a *biogenetic disorder*, one that is primarily due to inborn factors. Evidence suggests that the brain of an autistic individual does not process information like most brains.

It is important to discriminate autistic disorder from childhood schizophrenia. At one time, the two disorders were thought to be identical. Children can develop schizophrenia, but it is not autism. Childhood schizophrenia tends to appear after a period of normal development (e.g., at the age of 7), not in infancy or early childhood. Schizophrenic children may have delusions or even sometimes hallucinations. Autistic children do not.

Fortunately infantile autism is a relatively rare disorder. It appears to affect 1 or 2 children per 5,000. Approximately 3 males have the disorder for every female that has it.

See also *autism*; *behavior modification*; *developmental disorders*; *schizophrenia*.

automatic thoughts: Thoughts that appear in consciousness involuntarily, coming and going rapidly. Nonetheless, they are well formulated. The psychiatrist Aaron T. Beck has noted that such thoughts can play a significant role in cases of depression. Certain situations may trigger the individual to think, "I'm no good," or "I'm worthless," or "My life has no meaning."

Automatic thoughts of a negative nature are often illogical. Some of the logical errors include arbitrary inference, magnification, and minimization. An *arbitrary inference* takes place when one jumps to a conclusion on the basis of inadequate information. For example, the individual thinks, "I failed the first test. I'm sure to fail the course." *Magnification* is thinking that a disappointment is of greater importance than it is. For example, the individual thinks, "Oh, this is awful! This is terrible! I don't know what to do! John didn't invite me to the prom!" *Minimization* is thinking that a success is of little importance. For example, the individual thinks, "I got an A in my chemistry course. No big deal. The teacher was an easy grader."

See also *cognitive-behavior therapy*; *depression*.

autonomic nervous system: A nervous system subdivision that regulates involuntary bodily activity such as digestion, breathing, endocrine gland secretions, heart rate, and general arousal. The autonomic nervous system contains two functional divisions: (1) the sympathetic and (2) the parasympathetic. The sympathetic division tends to regulate increases in excitation, and the parasympathetic division tends to regulate decreases in excitation. In a dangerous situation, the sympathetic division prepares the body to fight or flee. Adrenal hormones are released. The muscles become tense. On the other hand, after a large holiday meal, the parasympathetic prepares the body to digest food. Muscles may relax, arousal diminishes, and one sometimes gets sleepy.

The autonomic nervous system plays a significant role in reactions to psychosocial stress. Excessive activation of the sympathetic division plays a significant role in psychosomatic diseases.

See also *psychosomatic disorders*.

autonomy: Self-direction of behavior. Some people have a high need for autonomy. They "want to do their own thing." Others have a low need for autonomy. They are docile and easily led. The psychoanalyst Erik Erikson identifies autonomy as a very important psychosocial need during the preschool years. During the "terrible twos" the child is often quite negative and stubborn. This can be seen as an expression of the child's need for autonomy.

The psychiatrist Eric Berne, father of transactional analysis, saw autonomy as a mental health goal. He believed that well-adjusted persons manifest a high level of control over their own lives. Allowing situations or other people to diminish one's autonomy in turn diminishes one's sense of emotional well-being.

See also *Berne, Eric*; *Erikson, Erik Homburger*; *transactional analysis*.

aversion therapy: A kind of behavior therapy that takes advantage of classical conditioning. A stimulus that brings forth unwanted behavior is presented first. It is then followed by a painful or unpleasant stimulus. For example, a problem drinker takes a shot of whiskey. This is followed by a drug that induces vomiting. Through association, the shot comes to suggest vomiting. Thus the sight of a shotglass full of whiskey may produce nausea, making it somewhat easier for the troubled person to control his or her undesirable behavior.

Aversion therapy has been used to help people with a wide

range of problems. These include drug abuse, sexual deviations, autistic disorder, overeating, and compulsive gambling. Two qualifications must be presented. First, aversion therapy should *not* be imposed on people against their will. Second, the effects of aversion therapy are often quite temporary. Thus the technique is best used in conjunction with other therapies.

See also *behavior therapy*; *classical conditioning*.

avoidant personality disorder: A kind of personality disorder characterized by great fear of personal rejection, an intense desire for acceptance without criticism, withdrawal from others, and low self-esteem. In spite of the withdrawal pattern, the sufferer has an intense wish for affection. He or she dreams of being accepted.

An avoidant personality disorder is not to be confused with everyday shyness, a common problem. The word *shyness* does not suggest a condition as severe as a personality disorder.

An avoidant disorder can be manifest in childhood or adolescence. Symptoms include an exaggerated fear of strangers, an intense wish for family closeness, and inadequate relationships with peers.

See also *personality disorders*; *shyness*.

B

Babinski reflex: The tendency, in infants, of the toes to extend upward when the bottom of the foot is lightly stroked. The greatest extension is displayed by the big toes. The reflex is named after the French neuropathologist Josef Babinski (1857–1932) who first studied its characteristics.

The Babinski reflex disappears after infancy. If it is present in an adult, it is a sign of damage to some of the brain's motor neurons.

See also *neurology*.

barbiturates: Drugs belonging to the general class known as *sedatives*, agents that depress the activity of the central nervous system. Their activity resembles that of alcohol. They have two clinical uses: (1) to reduce tension and (2) to help people sleep. Because of their tendency to reduce tension, they are sometimes prescribed as antianxiety agents. However, the various antianxiety drugs are in most cases preferred agents.

Barbiturates became a part of medical treatment in the 1930s. They have a high potential for abuse because it easy to acquire both a physiological and a psychological dependence upon them.

Excessive usage of barbiturates produces many unwanted side effects such as abrupt emotional changes, poor motor coordination, slurred speech, memory problems, and difficulties in understanding ideas. In general, the thinking is clouded and confused. Personality deterioration is common. Significant abuse can even lead to brain damage.

Withdrawal from barbiturates should be carried out under medical supervision because of the potential dangers associated with physiological responses to the absence of the drug.

See also *antianxiety drugs*; *sedatives*.

battered child syndrome: A pattern of child abuse in which the main feature is physical injury to the child. Battered children are victims of slaps, punches, and burns. Often they are violently thrown against walls or the floor. Injuries frequently include multiple fractures. As many as 5 to 10% of severely battered children die of their injuries. Survivors often suffer impaired intellectual abilities because of central nervous system damage.

The offense is almost always the result of parental loss of self-control. However, this is frequently denied by parents. They say the child had an accident.

Estimates vary, but it is fairly conservative to say that as many as 2 or 3 children per 1,000 under the age of 18 are battered each year.

See also *child abuse*.

bedlam: A deteriorated version of the word *Bethlehem* used in the following name: the priory of St. Mary of Bethlehem, a famous hospital and mental asylum founded in the 1400s in London. The word *bedlam* has acquired these meanings: (1) any event involving a great deal of noise or confused behavior and (2) a madhouse.

See also *Beers, Clifford Whittingham*; *Dix, Dorothea Lynde*.

Beers, Clifford Whittingham (1876–1943): One of the founders of the mental hygiene movement in the United States. As a young adult, Beers was a graduate of Yale University and a person with a professional career in the insurance business. Then he attempted suicide and was hospitalized for depression in 1900. Subsequently, he was diagnosed as suffering from a manic-depressive psychosis.

His direct observations of life in two different mental hospitals convinced him that the treatment of patients was unfeeling and inhumane. Many reforms were needed in administration and treatment. For example, he believed that straitjackets are counterproductive. On the surface, the patient is calmed and stops struggling. But within, the patient becomes increasingly emotionally upset and agitated.

Beers was well enough to return to his career in 1903 and eventually wrote the book *A Mind That Found Itself* (1908). He received encouragement from the eminent William James prior to the book's publication, and eventually the book was very influential. The prominent psychiatrist Adolf Meyer joined forces with Beers, James, and others to stimulate mental hospital reform.

Beers received an award from the National Institute of Social Science for his contributions to human welfare in 1933. He served as the secretary of the National Committee for Mental Hygiene until 1939.

See also *Dix, Dorothea Lynde*; *James, William*; *Mental Health Association*; *Meyer, Adolf*.

behavioral contracting: One of the methods used in behavior therapy. An agreement, oral or written, is made between two or more parties involved in a treatment process. The contract is often between the therapist and the troubled person. If the troubled person is a child, the contract may be between the therapist and one or both parents. In marriage therapy, the contract is sometimes made between the husband and the wife.

The essence of a behavioral contract is that there be a minimum of one specific treatment goal. At least one of the members of the contract is expected to manifest a behavioral change. The other member provides something of value, tangible or intangible, in exchange for the new and more desirable behavior.

Here are some of the advantages of behavioral contracting in contrast to less structured approaches to therapy: (1) The client has a lucid concept of the goal, or goals, of therapy, (2) desirable behavior is reinforced, (3) behavioral changes are expected within a defined time period, and (4) success and failure are defined in behavioral, not abstract, terms.

See also *behavior modification*; *behavior therapy*.

behavioral medicine: The application of psychological principles and methods to the treatment of organic disorders. There are many chronic health problems such as diabetes, ulcers, obesity, hypoglycemia, kidney diseases, high blood pressure, migraine headaches, back pain, and others that are greatly affected by psychological and emotional factors.

People who suffer from these kinds of health difficulties often can benefit from treatment procedures such as biofeedback training, relaxation methods, hypnosis, and suggestions for breaking, or modifying, undesirable habits.

The death rate from chronic diseases has been steadily rising, and there is a rapidly growing interest among health professionals in the methods associated with behavioral medicine.

See also *biofeedback training*; *hypnosis*; *psychosomatic disorders*.

behavior disorder: A disorder characterized by maladaptive behavior. The term *behavior disorder* tends to focus on what is observable in contrast to the more familiar term *mental disorder*. There is, in fact, no formal clinical distinction that can be made between the two terms. Therefore, they are, for all practical purposes, synonyms.

However, it should be noted that some therapists, particularly those who emphasize behavior therapy, prefer "behavior disorder" to "mental disorder." They argue that many troubled persons have no significant mental problems. Their thinking is not grossly disturbed. It is traditional nonetheless to include all behavioral pathology in the general category of *mental disorders*.

See also Diagnostic and Statistical Manual of Mental Disorders; *maladaptive behavior*; *mental disorder*.

behaviorism: A school of psychology based on the point of view that psychology should make its basic subject matter behavior itself, not mental processes. The father of behaviorism is John Watson (1878–1958), and his book *Psychology from the Standpoint of a Behaviorist*, published in 1919, provided the inspiration for many experimental psychologists.

The radical behaviorism advocated by Watson sought to eliminate any discussion of perceptions and thoughts from psychology. However, today's behaviorists, sometimes called *neobehaviorists*, are seldom as stringent as Watson. They are willing to identify perceptions and thoughts as kinds of *cognitive behaviors*.

The importance of behaviorism in the framework of mental health is that it provides the philosophical foundation and the inspiration for behavior modification and behavior therapy.

See also *behavior modification*; *behavior therapy*.

behavior modification: A kind of behavior therapy. Behavior modification is a technique based on principles of operant conditioning, a procedure in which learned behavior is shaped in connection with reinforcers.

The most obvious use of behavior modification is to eliminate maladaptive behavior in a child. Let's say that 3-year-old Barry has the bad habit of screaming at his mother when he wants attention. Inadvertently, she reinforces the habit every time she responds to excessive loudness in his voice. A behavior therapist would advise the mother to be sensitive to Barry's voice level. She should give him prompt attention when his requests are in reasonable tones. This will reinforce desirable behavior. She should ignore as much as possible unreasonable screams. This should eventually produce a decrease in their frequency. Although the theory of behavior modification is quite sound, it is sometimes difficult to put theory into practice.

Behavior modification can be used by parents with essentially normal children to build good habits. For example, Alice can be given 1 point on an index card every time she makes her own bed. The accumulation of 10 points earns her a modest treat such as a comic book or an ice cream cone. This approach not only shapes Alice's behavior in a positive manner, it also helps her build self-esteem because she earns the reinforcer by her own efforts.

It is also possible to think in terms of self-modification of behavior. Ralph wants to smoke less. If he can go 1 hour without a cigarette, he makes a tally mark on a piece of paper in his wallet. He has been wanting to buy a particular golf club and makes an agreement with himself that when he accumulates a total of 40 points he can buy the club.

See also *behavior therapy*; *operant conditioning*.

behavior therapy: A general approach to therapy that focuses primarily on learned aspects of behavior. The general assumption underlying behavior therapy is that much behavior that is termed *sick*, *pathological*, or *maladaptive* is acquired by classical conditioning, operant conditioning, or observational learning.

Broadly speaking, the three basic types of behavior therapies are systematic desensitization, behavior modification, and assertiveness training. If the primary problem involves distressing emotional responses such as chronic anxiety or irrational fears, systematic desensitization is the treatment of choice. If the primary problem involves distressing actions such as excessive smoking, overeating, stuttering, nail biting, overindulgence in alcohol, and compulsive gambling, behavior modification is the treatment of choice. If the distressing behavior involves ineffectiveness in social relations, assertiveness training is the treatment of choice.

It is important to realize that the behavior therapist tends to focus on what people *do* and *how* they can change. The past is usually not explored beyond the minimum requirements necessary to establish a general understanding of the person's problem. Concepts such as *insight*, *self-understanding*, and *unconscious motivation* are not of great importance to the behavior therapist. Instead, concepts such as *conditioning*, *learning*, *change*, and *action* are stressed. The behavior therapist is oriented to the present and what can be done fairly quickly to bring about relief from psychological and emotional distress.

See also *assertiveness training; behavior modification; classical conditioning; operant conditioning; systematic desensitization.*

benzodiazepines: A class of drugs used to treat anxiety, tension, and insomnia. Two well-known trade names are Librium and Valium.

See also *antianxiety drugs.*

Berne, Eric (1910–1970): The father of transactional analysis, a theory of personality and a kind of psychotherapy. Berne was born in Canada and received his M.D. degree there in 1935. He studied psychiatry at the Yale University School of Medicine and continued to reside and work in the United States.

Berne trained to be a psychoanalyst after he became a psychiatrist. However, he broke off an instructional analysis with the famous psychoanalyst Erik Erikson and went on to found his own distinctive approach to therapy. It is evident that transactional analysis owes much to psychoanalysis. In particular, Berne's formulation of the Parent, Adult, and Child ego states bears substantial similarity to Freud's concept of the superego, the ego, and the id. The difference, Berne argued, is that the three ego states are experienced personal realities. In contrast, the agents of the personality identified by psychoanalysis are abstractions.

The really distinctive contribution made by Berne was his focus on the importance of the communication process in human relations. Pathological patterns of communication that repeated themselves over and over and that kept people from becoming emotionally close he called *games.* The principal thrust of transactional analysis was to help people exchange thoughts and feelings in a more effective manner. The psychiatrist Harry Stack Sullivan is usually identified as the principal forerunner of Berne's approach.

Berne had a flair for popular writing, and his ideas came to the attention of the general public. Also, he often gave his concepts colloquial terms in order to give them a striking, memorable quality. Thus a person with low self-esteem was called a *frog*.

A person with high self-esteem was a *prince* or a *princess*. An expression of recognition was a *stroke*. For the reasons cited, Berne was sometimes not taken too seriously by many mental health professionals. However, substantial numbers of psychiatrists, clinical psychologists, and social workers do find merit in Berne's ideas.

Among Berne's books are *Transactional Analysis in Psychotherapy* (1961) and *Games People Play* (1964).

See also *Erikson, Erik Homburger*; *Freud, Sigmund*; *Sullivan, Harry Stack*; *transactional analysis*.

bestiality: In broad general terms, any behavior of a human being that is brutal, gross, or unfeeling. In abnormal psychology, bestiality refers to any sexual contact that a human being has with an animal. It is also known as *zoophilia*, meaning an erotic attraction to animals. Bestiality is classified as one of the sexual deviations.

There are many legends connecting animals to human beings in sexual themes. Zeus took the form of a bull in order to seduce a woman named Europa. Unions between gods (in the form of animals) and human beings produced half-goats (satyrs) and half-horses (centaurs).

How common is bestiality? Based on various sexual surveys, it is estimated that about 2% to 3% of females have had sexual contact with an animal at least once. For males, the estimate is about 6% to 8%. For boys raised on farms the estimate rises to as high as 15% to 17%. However, these figures inflate the true picture of the frequency of bestiality because they include a single contact. Stated differently, it is estimated that bestiality describes less than 1% of the total sexual behavior of human beings.

See also *sexual deviations*; *sodomy*.

Binet, Alfred (1857–1911): The principal author of the first practical intelligence tests. Binet was a French researcher, and, in collaboration with his colleague Theodore Simon (1873–1961), developed at the request of the French government a way of evaluating the intelligence of children. Their collaboration led to the eventual publication of the Binet–Simon Intelligence Scale and the introduction of the concept of mental age.

The concept of intelligence quotient (IQ) was not introduced by Binet and Simon but was suggested instead by Wilhelm Stern (1871–1938), a German psychologist. IQ is based on a comparison of mental age with chronological age.

Prior efforts to test intelligence had failed because the researchers attempted to make direct assessments of biological capacities. For example, the English scientist Sir Francis Galton (1822–1911) thought intelligence might be related to the quickness of one's reflexes. It turns out that it is difficult to show any clear 1 to 1 link between biological measurements and intelligence.

Instead, Binet took the very practical road of measuring a child's actual performance on intellectual tasks. Thus a child was asked to answer questions having to do with vocabulary, arithmetic, comprehension, and recognition of familiar objects. Binet assumed that intelligence *is* as intelligence *does*.

The Binet–Simon scale was adapted in the United States by the Stanford psychologist Lewis Terman and was eventually published as the Stanford–Binet Scale. The Stanford–Binet Scale is generally regarded as the first practical intelligence test used in the United States.

See also *Binet tests*; *intelligence quotient (IQ)*; *mental age (MA)*; *Stanford–Binet Intelligence Scale*; *Terman, Lewis Madison*.

Binet tests: A set of tests in a scale used to measure intelligence. The set is also known as the Stanford–Binet Scale because it was standardized and used for research purposes at Stanford University by the psychologist Lewis Terman.

The Binet tests are the result of the work of Alfred Binet in France (1857–1910). He decided that the intelligence of children could be measured indirectly by testing their performance on various tests. Questions on the tests included items referring to vocabulary, arithmetic, recognition of familiar objects, and comprehension. The more items a child could answer correctly, the higher his or her *mental age*. Later the concept of mental age was incorporated into the now popular concept of an intelligence quotient (IQ).

Terman published an English version of the Binet tests in 1916, and since that time the tests have been widely used. One of their principal mental health uses is to assist in making diagnoses of childhood mental disorders. A clearer picture of almost any pathology in a child is obtained by combining clinical data with an evaluation of the child's intelligence. Also, the Binet tests are helpful in making a diagnosis of mental retardation.

See also *Binet, Alfred*; *intelligence quotient (IQ)*; *mental retardation*; *Wechsler intelligence scales*.

biofeedback training: A method of gaining voluntary control of autonomic responses with the assistance of machines that augment biological signals. It used to be thought that some of the body's processes were completely involuntary. Such processes include the beating of the heart, breathing, the dilation and constriction of blood vessels, muscle tension, and digestion of food. However, with biofeedback training, it is often possible to gain control over these "involuntary" responses.

For example, Leslie has high blood pressure. Using biofeedback training, an electronic monitor gives him a visual display providing moment-to-moment information concerning his diastolic blood pressure. He is instructed by the biofeedback therapist to seek ways to lower his diastolic level. Leslie is free to use any internal technique that works such as thinking relaxing thoughts or invoking pleasant fantasies. The monitor will give him high-quality information (i.e., feedback) concerning the level of success or failure. With practice, he finds he can voluntarily regulate his own blood pressure to some extent. He now is less reliant on blood pressure medication.

As an adjunct to both medical therapy and psychotherapy, biofeedback training is now being used to treat a wide spectrum of chronic health problems including both tension and migraine headaches, high blood pressure, anxiety, and pain. The procedure has moved past the experimental stages and is now of recognized clinical value.

It is possible to think of biofeedback training as belonging to the domain of behavior modification. The procedure is based on principles of operant conditioning. The thought or image that affects an autonomic response is an action with a consequence. It is reinforced by the subject's successes. Positive feedback from the machine (i.e., a successful effort) is perceived as a reinforcer; thus the frequency of the kinds of thoughts and images that diminish hypertension, anxiety, and muscle tension increase in frequency. Thoughts that foster maladaptive responses tend to extinguish.

See also *behavioral medicine*; *behavior modification*; *operant conditioning*; *psychosomatic disorders*.

biomedical viewpoint: The viewpoint in abnormal psychology and psychiatry that mental disorders are caused by problems at a biological level. (This viewpoint is also called the *biomedical model*, the *biological viewpoint*, and the *organic viewpoint*.) It is clear that many mental disorders have an organic basis. Mental retardation, attention deficit disorder, and Alzheimer's disease are examples of disorders that are caused, or complicated, by clear-cut organic pathology.

On the other hand, there are conditions that present greater problems in terms of an explanation. Do anxiety disorders have a constitutional basis? Are some people more prone to "neurosis" than others? Or are anxiety disorders primarily psychogenic in origin? Although Freud believed that negative emotional experiences in early childhood played important roles in neurotic conditions, he also believed that some people were more disposed to neurosis than others. Therefore, he combined a biomedical viewpoint with a psychological one.

Schizophrenia presents a major explanatory problem. Some researchers believe that schizophrenic disorders are due to a genetic predisposition. Others assert that it is due to deficiencies in certain neurotransmitters in the brain. Still others say that poor nutrition throws off the blood chemistry and affects the ability to think lucidly. All of these are versions of the biomedical viewpoint.

If the biomedical viewpoint is accepted as the primary explanation of a mental disorder, this provides a basis for the use of somatic therapies such as drug therapy or electroconvulsive shock therapy. On the other hand if a psychogenic viewpoint is accepted as the primary explanation, this provides a basis for psychotherapy or behavior therapy. Thus the selection of one viewpoint over another is more than a pure theoretical problem.

See also *neurosis*; *psychogenic viewpoint*; *schizophrenia*; *somatic therapy*.

bipolar disorder: A mood disorder with two extremes, mania and depression. (The older term for this disorder was *manic-depressive psychosis*.) There are three basic types of bipolar disorder: (1) depressive, (2) manic, and (3) mixed. In the depressive type, the dominant mood is low. In the manic type, the dominant mood is elevated. In the mixed type, there is frequent alternation of mood. However, in all types, there has been at least one manic episode. (Bipolar disorder is not to be confused with *cyclothymic disorder*, a condition also characterized by mood swings. A basic difference between the two disorders is that in cyclothymic disorder, mood swings are generally neither as extreme nor as severe as they are in bipolar disorder.)

A manic episode is characterized by a set of related behavior patterns. These include excessive excitement, euphoria, rapid mental activity, a great amount of talking, an exaggerated sense of importance, extreme irritability, a sense of great power, and a tendency to sleep very litle. The person's speech often jumps from one subject to another on the basis of chance associations between words. This tendency is termed a *flight of ideas*. Sometimes the thoughts and ideas expressed during a manic episode seem to be beyond all reason. In such a case, the individual is said to be delusional.

A depressive episode is not distinguishable in and of itself from depression in general. Therefore, a person is diagnosed as suffering from bipolar disorder only if, as noted before, there is at least one manic episode. It is typical for the manic episode to appear first. If it eventually gives way to depression, and does not recur, then the diagnosis may still be bipolar disorder but of the depressive type.

Estimates of the incidence of bipolar disorder in the general population suggest that about ½ of 1% to slightly over 1% of adults will suffer from the disorder at least once. Symptoms usually first appear between the ages of 20 and 30. Although depression is twice as common in women as it is in men, bipolar disorder occurs about equally in both sexes.

When bipolar disorder is in an acute phase, the individual is often hospitalized until some regulation can be achieved. The most common form of drug therapy is to prescribe lithium carbonate. This is combined with effective psychotherapy. Many persons with the disorder can and do lead relatively normal lives.

See also *cyclothymic disorder*; *depression*; *lithium carbonate*; *manic-depressive psychosis*; *mood disorders (affective disorders)*.

birth trauma: See *will therapy*.

bisexual behavior: Behavior distinguished by a tendency to engage in sexual activity with members of either sex. A person with bisexual tendencies finds himself or herself aroused in an erotic way by others independent of their gender. Such individuals are often referred to as *bisexuals*.

It is estimated that the incidence of bisexual behavior is fairly large. Research indicates that, among men, about 15% have exhibited bisexual behavior. Among women, the estimate is 10%. However, it should be noted that persons who practice bisexual behavior do, in most cases, prefer members of the opposite sex to their own sex.

It has been noted by a number of researchers that there is some biological basis for bisexual behavior. Males have some female hormones, and women have some male hormones. Freud was one of those who made these kinds of observations. Men, of course, carry both a Y (male) and an X (female) chromosome.

From the psychological viewpoint, many factors may contribute to bisexuality such as gender identity problems and repressed hostility toward members of the opposite sex.

Bisexual behavior is not classified as a mental disorder in the American Psychiatric Association's *Diagnostic and Statistical Manual of Mental Disorders*. Therefore it is not thought of as a condition that requires therapy unless the individual is distressed by his or her bisexual tendencies.

See also *heterosexuality*; *homosexuality*; *sexual deviations*.

Bleuler, Eugen (1857–1939): Introduced the term *schizophrenia* into psychiatry. Bleuler was a Swiss psychiatrist and one of Freud's first advocates. For a period of time, Carl Jung was Bleuler's assistant.

Prior to Bleuler's introduction of the term *schizophrenia*, the name used to label severe thought disorders was *dementia praecox*. This term had been introduced by the German psychiatrist Emil Kraepelin. Kraepelin tended to focus on the importance of early onset, biological factors, and the hopeless quality of thought disorders. Bleuler, instead, wanted to focus on psychological processes and the inner world of mental patients. Also, he believed that many cases were far from hopeless and could respond favorably to treatment.

The literal meaning of schizophrenia is "split mind," and it was chosen by Bleuler to suggest a mind that has departed (i.e., "split") from reality. The aptness of Bleuler's term was evident, and psychiatrists were quick to use it.

Bleuler is responsible for introducing other important terms into psychiatry. For example, he introduced the term *ambivalence*.

Bleuler's general approach to the treatment of schizophrenia was to attempt to understand the disorder in terms of the individual's life experiences and emotions. He believed that too much emphasis on the importance of biological factors was misguided, that it overly limited a psychiatrist's treatment options.

See also *ambivalence*; *dementia praecox*; *Jung, Carl Gustav*; *Kraepelin, Emil*; *schizophrenia*.

body dysmorphic disorder (dysmorphophobia): A somatoform disorder characterized by the idea that one has a significant fault in the face or the body and that this fault makes one unattractive. In order for a person to be diagnosed as suffering from this disorder, the blemish must be more imaginary than real. A slight flaw is perceived as a very large one.

Persons with this disorder may spend excessive amounts of money on unnecessary plastic surgery. They may also suffer from anxiety and depression because of the imagined drawbacks of their imperfection.

The general incidence of body dysmorphic disorder is unknown.

Not a great amount of information exists concerning causal factors in the disorder. However, it is possible to speculate that a developmental history in which one was made to feel ugly or unattractive as a child would contribute to the disorder. Also, feelings of low self-esteem in general would be expected to aggravate the disorder.

The most common treatment for body dysmorphic disorder is insight-oriented psychotherapy. The principal aim is to help the individual develop a more realistic body image.

See also *anorexia nervosa*; *somatoform disorders*.

borderline personality disorder: A disorder that lies on the borderline between mood disorders and personality disorders. Attributes associated with this disorder include (1) impulsive behavior that produces self-defeating consequences, (2) unstable and highly emotional personal relationships, (3) poor self-control over anger or temper, (4) identity and self-image problems, (5) unstable moods alternating between anxiety, anger, and depression, (6) a dislike of being alone for prolonged periods of time, (7) a tendency toward self-injury, and (8) the feeling that life has no meaning. Not all of these attributes need be present. However, if five of the eight are present, the case is strong for the existence of the disorder.

Causes of the disorder are obscure. It is possible that inborn traits of temperament may exist for aggressiveness and mood instability. It is hypothesized that parents who are excessively authoritarian and emotionally rejecting play a role in the psychological history of these disorders.

Drug therapy is seldom the treatment of choice. Psychotherapy can be helpful, particularly if it is the kind that orients the person toward reality and the long-run consequences of his or her maladaptive behavioral tendencies (e.g., reality therapy or cognitive-behavior therapy).

See also *mood disorders (affective disorders)*; *personality disorders*; *reality therapy*.

brain pathology: Any "sickness" of the brain. This includes damage to, and diseases of, the brain. Causes of brain pathology are many and include injuries, infections, cerebrovascular accidents (i.e., strokes), and inherited diseases.

Brain pathology can be a complicating factor in many disorders including Alzheimer's dieases, amnesia, epilepsy, Korsakoff's psychosis, mental retardation, and paresis (see entries).

Brain pathology is involved in many mental disorders but not all. About one-third of first entries into a mental hospital are due to brain pathology. The other two-thirds are classified as functional disorders.

See also *functional disorders*; *organic mental syndromes (organic brain syndromes)*.

brain waves: An informal, but commonly used, name for changes in electrical potential associated with the activity of the brain's neurons. Four well-known waves are these: alpha, beta, delta, and theta. Each one is associated with a specific frequency of cycles per second.

Of the four, *beta waves* are the fastest and have a frequency of about 14 cycles per second. These appear when one is alert and thinking about a problem. *Alpha waves* have a frequency of about 8 to 14 cycles per second. They are identified with a relaxed mental state. *Theta waves* have a frequency of about 4 to 8 cycles per second. They are associated with fantasy and vivid mental images. *Delta waves* have a frequency of about 4 cycles per second. They are associated with deep sleep.

A study of brain waves is useful in making diagnoses of nervous system pathology (e.g., epilepsy and brain damage).

See also *electroencephalogram (EEG)*.

Breuer, Josef (1842–1925): Credited by Freud with being the true discoverer of psychoanalysis. This was a very generous claim on Freud's part, and he held to it consistently. In fact Breuer's contributions to the long-run development of psychoanalysis were small, but it is true that classical psychoanalysis does begin with his work.

Breuer was a highly respected physician in Vienna, about 14 years older than Freud, and already well-established while Freud was still struggling. Breuer sometimes lent Freud small sums of money and referred patients to him.

One of Breuer's patients was a young woman named Bertha Pappenheim, who eventually became immortalized in the annals of psychoanalytic literature as Fraulein Anna O. (She will be henceforth referred to as Anna.) Anna suffered from a number of symptoms of what at that time were called "hysteria." For example, she had trouble with a persistent cough. For a time, she became unable to swallow water. Other symptoms that came and went included a squint, visual problems, and involuntary muscle contractions. Breuer found that under hypnosis the symptoms could be relieved if Anna was allowed to express strong emotions. Anna herself called this general approach "chimney sweeping." It came to be known in psychoanalysis as a *catharsis* (i.e., a cleansing). Thus Breuer had discovered the talking cure.

Breuer told Freud about his discovery, and Freud pressed Breuer to pursue his early lead. However, there was a complication. Anna had developed a great attachment, apparently erotic, to Breuer. (Subsequently Freud referred to this phenomenon as a *transference*.) Breuer was a married man and quite threatened by the implications. He gave up his pursuit of psychoanalysis and retreated to the relative safety of his medical practice.

Freud took up where Breuer broke off and began exploring

the possibilities inherent in psychoanalysis with his own patients. (He never saw Anna.) In good time, Freud pressed Breuer to make Anna's case public for the good of science, and Breuer acceded to Freud's wish. They collaborated on *Studies on Hysteria* (1895), the first book ever published on psychoanalysis. The first case history in the book is the case of Anna O. It is the only case history contributed by Breuer. Freud contributed four case histories. The theoretical portion of the book is written by Breuer, and the section on psychotherapy is written by Freud.

See also *catharsis*; *conversion disorder*; *Freud, Sigmund*; *psychoanalysis*; *transference*.

brief psychotherapy: An approach to psychotherapy that seeks to place a well-defined limit on the total number of sessions required to attain treatment goals. A therapist seeking to do brief psychotherapy often hopes to accomplish good results in as few as 6 or 7 sessions. Past 20 sessions, psychotherapy can no longer be regarded as brief.

Brief psychotherapy is a contemporary movement within the mental health profession in an attempt to avoid having patients "stuck" in psychotherapy for years. The idea is to avoid having psychotherapy become a chronic emotional crutch and a way of life.

At the outset of brief psychotherapy, the therapist and the client negotiate a desirable time span for the therapy. They also define a goal or goals. For example, a goal may be to stop smoking, to eliminate a phobia, to achieve one's first orgasm, or to lose 20 pounds.

Although, in theory, any form of psychotherapy can be brief, in practice it has been behavior therapy that has placed particular emphasis on the value of shortening the length of therapy.

See also *behavior therapy*; *psychotherapy*.

brief reactive psychosis: A kind of psychotic disorder characterized by its sudden onset and short duration. Usually there are no complications following a brief reactive psychosis, and the person returns to the same level of functioning he or she had before the episode.

There is almost always a major psychosocial stressor associated with this kind of psychosis. Examples of such stressors are the death of a spouse, the collapse of a business, or an emotional shock experienced in combat. This disorder is somewhat more likely to appear in adolescents or young adults.

The symptoms of this disorder are similar to those of psychotic disorders in general. If the symptoms last for more than 2 weeks, the disorder can no longer be classified as brief.

See also *psychosocial stressors*; *psychotic disorders*.

Brill, Abraham Arden (1874–1948): Psychoanalyst working in the United States who translated many of Freud's major works into English. Brill was born in Austria, spent his youth in the United States, and returned to Austria as a physician to study psychoanalysis with Freud. He also worked with the influential psychiatrist Eugen Bleuler in Switzerland.

It was Freud who authorized Brill as to become his principal translator into English. The psychoanalytic term *id* was Brill's innovation. Freud, writing in German, simply wrote about the "it" of the personality. Brill took the Latin word for "it," which is "id," and made it a term.

Brill did much to make psychoanalysis an accepted and important form of therapy in the United States. He accomplished more than the translation Freud's works. He applied psychoanalysis to the understanding and therapy of schizophrenia, following the lead of Bleuler, and wrote books of his own. One of his principal publications was *Fundamental Conceptions of Psychoanalysis* (1922).

See also *Bleuler, Eugen*; *Freud, Sigmund*; *id*; *psychoanalysis*.

Briquet's syndrome: An earlier term for what is today called a *somatization disorder*. The original nomenclature was derived from the name of the French psychiatrist Paul Briquet (1796–1881). He was the author of an important work describing what at that time was termed *hysteria*.

See also *hysteria*; *somatization disorder*.

bulimia nervosa: One of the eating disorders. Bulimia nervosa is characterized primarily by binge eating. During the binge, the individual recognizes that his or her behavior is abnormal. There is often present the fear that one will not be able to stop eating at will. After the binge is over, the individual tends to feel depressed and self-critical. In order to qualify as a binge, a large amount of food must be eaten in a well-defined and relatively short time period (e.g., 2 hours).

Here are some of the specific behaviors associated with bulimia nervosa:

1. The eating of high-calorie easy-to-eat foods (e.g., ice cream, candy bars, puddings, and cookies).
2. Sneak eating.
3. Stopping because of a stomach ache, being interrupted, or getting drowsy. Sometimes self-caused vomiting is used to end the binge.
4. A tendency to go on highly restrictive diets.
5. Variations in weight ranging over 10 pounds.

It is not necessary for all five elements to be present. However, if three are present, the term *bulimia nervosa* seems to be applicable to the pattern.

People who suffer from bulimia nervosa are seldom overweight. In fact, they are often slightly below average in weight. Adolescence or young adulthood are the ages usually associated with the disorder. In the vast majority of cases it is females who suffer from bulimia nervosa.

Bulimia nervosa is seldom life-threatening (unlike anorexia nervosa). Nonetheless there can be significant health complications arising from biochemical imbalances and dehydration when vomiting is used to bring an end to a binge.

It is difficult to state with any accuracy the prevalence of bulimia nervosa. A number of surveys report a high frequency, and there is the general opinion that it is fairly common, not a rare disorder at all. However, reliable statistics are not available. It is probably an underreported disorder because, by its very nature, it is a form of hidden behavior.

Causal factors in bulimia nervosa are several. Studies have shown that bulimic patients often have obese parents or siblings.

Thus the binge eater often has a fear of obesity. A culture that stresses the value of being a thin woman has been blamed. The compulsive eating of food is used to satisfy more than one emotional need. If a person has a tendency toward compulsive eating and at the same time has a strong desire to avoid obesity, the unsatisfactory psychological compromise between the two opposing tendencies is bulimia nervosa.

The treatment of choice for bulimia nervosa is psychotherapy. Usually the therapist stresses insight into the unconscious motives for wanting to binge. This approach is combined with behavior modification to help the individual cope with self-defeating habits.

See also *anorexia nervosa*; *compulsive eating*; *eating disorders*.

C

caffeine: A central nervous system stimulant. Coffee, tea, and cola are beverages that contain significant amounts of caffeine. This drug, a somewhat bitter alkaloid, has the effect of increasing alertness and arousal. Thus people often use it to help them overcome feelings of fatigue or to fight off unwanted sleep.

Caffeine is sometimes suggested as a therapeutic drug for attention deficit disorder. A stimulant sometimes has a paradoxical effect on children with this disorder, calming them down instead of increasing their arousal.

It is quite common to acquire a physiological dependence on caffeine. If one stops taking the drug abruptly, there are withdrawal symptoms such as headaches and extreme drowsiness.

See also *caffeine intoxication.*

caffeine intoxication: A transient mental disorder with an organic basis. (This disorder is also known as *caffeinism.*) Its chief features are restless activity, nervous tension, difficulty sleeping, random talk, irregular heartbeat, and agitation. Not every symptom need be present in order for a positive diagnosis to be made.

Some people are overly sensitive to caffeine and may experience severe symptoms from as little as two cups of coffee. Caffeine intoxication can aggravate a peptic ulcer. It can also have adverse effects on heart disease.

Treatment of caffeine intoxication includes withdrawal from, and avoidance of, the drug.

See also *caffeine*.

cannabis: See *marijuana*.

castration anxiety: The unconscious fear, particularly in males, that one may lose one's genital organs. At the conscious level, the anxiety may be expressed as the fear of losing a nose, a finger, a toe, or a limb. According to Freud, as expressed in the formulations of classical psychoanalysis, castration anxiety is due to guilt association with incest wishes during early childhood. A boy, for example, may have a fantasy of sex relations with his mother. He may then develop the fear that his father will punish him by cutting off his testicles or his penis. The fear is repressed to an unconscious level and becomes castration anxiety. Castration anxiety can persist into adulthood.

In the adult, the symbols for the genitals may be more general than in childhood. Thus it is possible to hypothesize that the loss of a business, damage to one's automobile, and similar incidents may aggravate a repressed castration anxiety.

Although it may seem impossible for a female to experience castration anxiety, it can be argued that any threat to self-esteem or anticipated loss of power in life can be interpreted unconsciously by either sex as a danger to the genital organs. In this very general sense, it is possible to speak of castration anxiety in women. However, psychoanalytical theory tends to emphasize male castration anxiety.

Castration anxiety is not a concept accepted by all psychologists and psychiatrists. It is best to associate the concept specifically with psychoanalysis.

See also *Freud, Sigmund*; *psychoanalysis*.

catalepsy: Holding the body in a given position for a prolonged time period. Catalepsy is sometimes a symptom of a schizophrenic disorder, catatonic type, or of conversion disorder. It can also be induced in some subjects by hypnosis.

Three kinds of catalepsy associated primarily with schizophrenic disorder, catatonic type, are catatonic rigidity, catatonic posturing, and waxy flexibility. In *catatonic rigidity*, the patient maintains a given position and resists efforts to move the limbs. In *catatonic posturing*, the patient assumes an odd posture (e.g., a running position or arms outstretched) and stays this way for a long time. In *waxy flexibility*, the patient allows movement of the limbs and then stays the way he or she has been placed.

See also *conversion disorder*; *hypnosis*; *schizophrenia*.

catecholamines: A group of organic compounds produced by the body. Catecholamines include important neurotransmitters such as epinephrine, norepinephrine, and dopamine. Research indicates that deficiencies or imbalances in these substances can play significant causal roles in certain mental disorders.

See also *dopamine*; *epinephrine*; *neurotransmitters*; *norepinephrine (noradrenalin)*.

catharsis: A cleaning out or a purge. In medicine, a laxative provides a catharsis of the alimentary canal. By analogy, in classical psychoanalysis, an emotional catharsis "cleans out" the personality. The patient may confess a sin, express a strong emotion, or cry. The therapeutic effects of catharsis on the personality were discovered early in psychoanalysis by Josef Breuer (1841–1925) working with a patient known as Anna O. Freud made catharsis a part of psychoanalytic technique. The familiar phrase "confession is good for the soul" captures the essence of catharsis. It is used in a general way in many kinds of psychotherapy.

See also *abreaction*; *Breuer, Josef*; *Freud, Sigmund*; *psychoanalysis*.

cathexis: A strong emotional attachment to an object, animal, or person. If a child cries and feels some grief when a pet dies, it can be said that the child had a cathexis for the pet. The experience of being deeply in love is another example of a cathexis.

Freud defined cathexis as the investment of libido (i.e., sexual energy) in the object, animal, or person. However, today's usage, as indicated here, is somewhat more general than Freud's.

Interference with, or frustration of, a cathexis can be a cause of emotional upheavals.

See also *libido*.

central nervous system: One of the two principal divisions of the nervous system. (The other principal division is the peripheral nervous system.) The central nervous system consists of the brain and the spinal cord. The brain, in particular, plays an important role in perception, memory, and thought. These processes are, of course, significant ones in mental health and psychopathology.

Drugs used in psychiatry often affect central nervous system arousal. Stimulants have the effect of increasing arousal. Sedatives, narcotics, and antianxiety drugs have the effect of lowering arousal.

See also *drug therapy*.

cerebrovascular accident (CVA): The breaking or blocking of a large blood vessel in the brain leading to brain damage. Another, somewhat less formal name, for this event is a *major stroke*. An immediate behavioral effect is extreme confusion. Sometimes the victim goes into a coma. The degree of recovery from a CVA depends to a large extent on the amount of brain damage. Many people make very impressive recoveries. Others have significant loss of abilities in functions such as memory, comprehension, or speech.

It is possible to distinguish a CVA from a *small stroke*. In a small stroke, there is breaking or blocking of a minor blood vessel and not as much brain damage. Symptoms of a small stroke include mild confusion, seemingly unreasonable emotional reactions, digestive difficulty, and problems walking.

A principal causal factor in both kinds of stroke is arteriosclerosis, or hardening of the arteries, a very common condition. The incidence of strokes is a function of increasing age. It is estimated that CVAs cause the death of about 200,000 people a year in the United States. Many more are impaired by the effects of strokes.

See also *organic mental syndromes (organic brain syndromes)*.

character disorder: An older and somewhat out-of-date term for what is today called a *personality disorder*. The older term is based on the idea that one's character consists of the distinctive behavioral traits of one's personality. The meaning of the word *character* is thus not identical with the meaning of the word *personality*. Character is best thought of as an *aspect* of one's personality. Thus personality is the more general term.

See also *personality disorders*.

Charcot, Jean Martin (1825–1893): A director of the famous Salpêtrière Hospital in France and widely regarded as the principal founder of neurology. Charcot investigated many aspects of the relationship of organic conditions to both physical and mental disorders.

He was an important influence on Freud. Freud studied under Charcot and became interested in Charcot's investigations of hypnosis as a way of temporarily modifying the symptoms of hysteria (i.e., conversion disorder). Charcot also made the observation that sexual problems were often key causal factors in hysteria, and this impressed Freud greatly.

Charcot did much to establish the credibility of hypnosis in the minds of physicians and demonstrated through its clinical use that symptoms that seem to have organic roots in fact often have their source in psychological conflicts.

At the time of Charcot's investigations, it was thought that hysteria was a disorder exclusively associated with females. This seemed logical because the Greek root *hyster* refers to the uterus, and hysteria was presumably caused by a "wandering" uterus. However, Charcot noted that some males suffered from hysteria, and the problem could not possibly be explained in terms of the female anatomy. Freud expanded on Charcot's observations and presented his conclusions to physicians in Austria. At first the idea of male hysteria was rejected, but, in time, it came to be accepted.

Pierre Janet, a director of the psychological clinic at the Salpêtrière Hospital, was also influenced by Charcot and subsequently made important investigations into unconscious mental processes inspired to some extent by Charcot's lead.

See also *conversion disorder*; *Freud, Sigmund*; *hypnosis*; *hysteria*; *Janet, Pierre Marie Felix*; *neurology*.

child abuse: A pattern of behavior in which the adults in a child's life batter, exploit, molest, or otherwise mistreat the child. As indicated, the pattern of abuse need not be physical. Negligence and insults can also be forms of abuse. Unfortunately, abusers are often parents. There are many causes of abusive behavior. Some of the factors that have been identified in abusive parents are these: youth, low intelligence, mental disorders, criminal background, marriage difficulties, poverty, job instability, and a personal history of having been abused.

Child abuse can have highly adverse effects on both a child's physical and emotional development. Mental health problems in an adult may stem in part from abuse as a child.

Adults who abuse children are subject to criminal prosecution. See also *battered child syndrome*.

chlorpromazine: The generic name of one of the drugs used to treat psychotic disorders. One of the familiar trade names associated with chlorpromazine is Thorazine. Delusions, hallucinations, aggressive behavior, and agitation are all to some degree regulated by chlorpromazine.

One of the significant problems associated with chlorpromazine is a condition known as *tardive dyskinesia*. Some patients who use the drug for extended periods develop problems in the ability to control their muscles. Involuntary extensions of the arm or twitching of the face are examples.

See also *drug therapy*; *tardive dyskinesia*.

chromosomal anomalies: Abnormal unions of chromosomes. Chromosomes normally occur in pairs. Therefore, there are basically two kinds of anomalies: (1) *trisomy*, a set consisting of three chromosomes and (2) *monosomy*, a set consisting of one chromosome.

A familiar example of how a chromosomal anomaly can cause a problem is Down's syndrome that is associated with an extra chromosome on the 21st pair (i.e., trisomy 21). Another example is Turner's syndrome that is associated with a missing X chromosome on the 23rd pair in the female (i.e., monosomy 23).

See also *Down's syndrome; genetic counseling; Turner's syndrome*.

clang associations: Associations produced in speech based on puns or rhymes, not logical concepts. For example, "Yesterday in the woods I saw a butterfly. I was eating pancakes and you should have seen the syrup and butter fly. Then the fly landed on the pancakes and I had to swat it and ruin the pancakes. From now on I'm ordering toast." Or, "I love to look at the stars. That's why I won't buy any new cars. Do you have any candy bars?"

Clang associations are most frequently heard in connection with the verbal behavior of a person suffering from a schizophrenic disorder, and these arbitrary linkings are indicators of underlying irrational thinking. Sometimes such associations are manifest in the manic phase of a bipolar disorder. It should be noted that children, and even some adults, produce clang associations in speech as a form of play. Under these conditions, clang associations are not, of course, symptoms of a disorder.

See also *bipolar disorder; schizophrenia*.

classical conditioning: A kind of conditioning in which a previously neutral stimulus acquires the capacity to elicit a reflex. (This kind of conditioning is also known as *respondent conditioning*, a term suggested by B. F. Skinner.) Classical conditioning is a form of learning because the organism acquires new behavioral patterns through experience.

Classical conditioning was first studied extensively by the Russian physiologist Ivan Pavlov (1849–1936). In a typical experiment, a tone of a given pitch and loudness was sounded. This preceded the feeding of the dog. After a number of pairings of the tone and the food, the tone alone was sounded. The tone, without food, elicited the salivary reflex. Such a reflex is termed a *conditioned reflex*. Essentially, the tone has become a cue, or a signal, informing the organism that food is coming soon. Such a cue is termed a *conditioned stimulus*.

It is believed that the process of living produces many conditioned reflexes in human beings of both a positive and a negative nature. Looking at a photograph of a loved one when one is far from home may produce a pleasant emotional response. The photograph is acting as a conditioned stimulus, and the pleasant emotional response, is, broadly speaking, a conditioned reflex. On the other hand, let's say that 4-year-old Greg has an abusive father. The sounds associated with the father's arrival home from work (e.g., keys in the latch, the front door opening, and footsteps in the entry hall) trigger anxiety. This emotional reaction is a conditioned one. Certainly Greg was not born with this particular response pattern. Conditioned responses underlie many of our adverse emotional reactions such as seemingly irrational anxiety, depression, or anger.

Phobias can also be acquired through classical conditioning. Let's say that Lyn was bitten by a dog when she was 4 years old. Now, at the age of 30 she has an irrational fear of dogs. It is quite possible that she has no conscious memory of the first painful incident. Nonetheless, she is generalizing from the first experience.

Adverse emotional reactions and irrational fears can be extinguished, or modified, by conditioning procedures. Systematic desensitization is a specific kind of therapy based on the principles of classical conditioning.

See also *aversion therapy*; *behavior therapy*; *systematic desensitization*.

claustrophobia: An irrational fear of closed spaces. Examples of such spaces are elevators, telephone booths, public bathrooms, booths in a restaurant, passenger compartments, and so forth. The individual suffering from claustrophobia wants to have control over the exits from such spaces if he or she submits to the confinement at all. Even under these conditions a high level of anxiety is often experienced.

See also *phobia*.

client-centered therapy: A kind of insight-oriented psychotherapy that emphasizes the importance of fostering a troubled person's capacity for personal growth. Client-centered therapy is sometimes called *nondirective therapy*. Although this title is not the preferred one, it does tell us something about the therapy. The therapist *does not* try to direct the client's life or make important decisions. The client is assumed to be the one who is responsible for his or her own future.

Carl Rogers developed client-centered therapy in the 1940s as an alternative to psychoanalysis. Rogers did not believe that it was necessary for a troubled person to recline on a couch, explore unconscious motives, and probe into early childhood. Instead, Rogers felt the client could face the therapist and hold a conversation about consciously held ideas. (This particular idea is not, of course, unique to Rogers. For example, Alfred Adler held a similar viewpoint.)

Note that the word *patient* is being avoided in the preceding discussion. Rogers preferred to use the word *client* in order to call attention to the individual's capacity for psychological health as opposed to pathology. He also wanted to emphasize the *active* role of the client. Psychotherapy is *not* something that is done to the client by the psychotherapist. Instead, it is a cooperative enterprise.

In order to foster the conditions for self-healing, client-centered therapy emphasizes certain attributes and behaviors on the part of the therapist. The therapist should provide unconditional positive regard, empathy, and active listening. *Unconditional positive regard* is uncritical acceptance of the client as a person without regard to moral judgments. *Empathy* is an attempt to fully appreciate the client's thoughts and feelings. *Active listening* is a therapeutic skill requiring the therapist to provide meaningful and thoughtful comments that penetrate somewhat below the surface level of the client's statements. All in all, the therapist must be perceived by the client as a genuine, warm, and caring person.

There is ample research evidence to suggest that client-centered therapy does indeed help a client to develop greater self-esteem. Persons suffering from general feelings of anxiety, self-doubt, and depression seem to be the best candidates for client-centered therapy. On the other hand, highly specific disorders such as phobias require a more focused therapy (e.g., systematic desensitization).

See also *Adler, Alfred; insight therapy; psychotherapy; Rogers, Carl Ransom.*

clinical psychologist: A psychologist who specializes in psychotherapy and psychological testing. Such psychologists often work in mental hospitals, counseling centers, and private practice. Although there are some exceptions, in most cases a clinical psychologist holds a Ph.D degree. Most states now have licensing laws requiring a clinical psychologist to have a high level of academic training combined with many hours of supervised experience.

A clinical psychologist should not be confused with a psychiatrist and a psychoanalyst. A *psychiatrist* has an M.D. degree and can prescribe drugs. A *psychoanalyst* explores a patient's unconscious mental life. Although some clinical psychologists are also psychoanalysts, most are not.

See also *psychiatrist; psychoanalyst.*

clitoris: A female sex organ capable of erectile response. The clitoris is located toward the upper portion of the vulva (i.e., the external portions of the female's sex organs). The clitoris and penis are similar structures. Both consist of a shaft and a sensitive tip called the *glans.*

The clitoris is a very important organ in female sexual response. Research conducted by the sexologists William H. Masters and Virginia E. Johnson indicates that stimulation of the clitoris, either directly or indirectly, is a principal factor in the induction of the female orgasm.

Freud theorized that there are two kinds of female orgasms, clitoral and vaginal. If a female requires additional stimulation of the clitoris prior to, or during, intercourse, Freud believed that this indicated a fixation of libido at an infantile level of sexual development. Today this is believed to be a sexist viewpoint. Contemporary research quite strongly suggests that there is only one kind of female orgasm. The route to the orgasm may vary to some extent from woman to woman. And a female who requires more stimulation than that provided by penile stroking alone is considered to be completely normal sexually.

See also *libido*; *orgasm*.

cocaine: A drug belonging to the general class of stimulants. Cocaine, like all stimulants, acts on the central nervous system in such a way as to temporarily increase alertness and arousal. The substance is a crystalline alkaloid derived from the leaves of the coca plant. "Crack" is the street name for cocaine in a particularly potent form.

At one time, cocaine had some medical uses because of its ability to deaden pain. For example, it was used as a local anesthetic in eye operations. However, it currently is seldom used in medical treatment.

Cocaine is a frequently abused drug primarily because it can produce states of euphoria lasting sometimes for several hours. During a euphoric state, an individual feels content with life and at peace with the world. Other pleasant effects of cocaine include loss of fatigue, greater physical endurance, and stimulation of sexual desire.

Unfortunately, there is price to be paid for the abuse of cocaine. When the pleasant "trip" is over, there is often a "crash" in which the user feels irritable, tired, and depressed. Also, psychiatry identifies a condition called *cocaine intoxication*. Psychological symptoms include random and meaningless movements, an unnatural emotional "high," a feeling that one is very powerful and important, and a great deal of pointless talk. Physical symptoms include rapid heartbeat, constriction of the pupils, an increase in blood pressure, chills, and nausea. In some cases, the abuse of cocaine can have fatal results.

Cocaine addiction is not primarily physiological because the body acquires little or no dependence on the drug. However, it is still considered to be an addictive drug because it is possible for a user to acquire a strong psychological dependence, a dependence that can be very difficult to break.

See also *drug addiction*.

co-dependency: As originally formulated, a process that affects the family of an alcoholic. The process is one in which, in a sense, the whole family becomes "sick." The spouse and children may in various ways support the alcoholic's dependent behavior without being fully aware of how they are doing so. For example, by becoming "strong" and responsible, a child may enable an alcoholic father to "get away" with irresponsible behavior.

Family members are known as *co-dependents*. Co-dependents are less obviously disturbed than the alcoholic but may also be in need of counseling or psychotherapy. To illustrate, the strong child identified before may be foreclosing higher education by taking a job in adolescence. Frustration and repressed anger may be associated with the seemingly mature behavior.

Although the concept of co-dependency has arisen within the context of alcoholism, it obviously can be extended to drug abuse in general and to any family in which a parent is not living up to traditional responsibilities.

See also *alcoholism*; *drug addiction*; *family therapy*.

cognitive-behavior therapy: A kind of behavior therapy that treats thoughts and ideas as learned behavior. (The term *cognitive-behavior modification* is also used to describe this kind of therapy.) The premises of cognitive-behavior therapy are consistent with those of behavior therapy in general. It is argued that maladaptive thoughts, the kinds of thoughts that underlie problems of adjustment, are acquired through the conditioning process. And they can be extinguished or modified like any other learned behavior. A *maladaptive thought* is any thought that precedes undesirable behavior or has negative emotional consequences. If Mary has been told that she should stop smoking by her physician and she still finds herself thinking, "I've just got to have a cigarette," then this is a maladaptive thought. If Richard is prone to anxiety and often finds himself thinking, "Everything's going to go wrong," then this is a maladaptive thought.

Cognitive-behavior therapy emphasizes *training methods*, skills that an individual can acquire to deal with maladaptive thoughts. Donald Meichenbaum, a research psychologist, has explored a number of these methods. An example of such a method is *stress-inoculation training*. In stress-inoculation training, the individual prepares ahead of time to cope with a stressful situation by using explicit strategies.

Let's say that Steven is preparing for a first date with Joanna, a woman he finds very attractive. Unfortunately, Steven suffers from chronic shyness, and he is having problems controlling his anxiety about the date. He keeps thinking, "I'll say something stupid" or "I'll make a fool out of myself." Using stress-inoculation training, it is recommended that Steven do a number of things. He should imagine the outcome of the date in positive terms, seeing it in his mind's eye as a success. He should mentally review his good points as a person. He should rehearse what he is going to say and do on the date. He should stop thinking that he has to get rid of *all* anxiety. He only has to reduce it. These cognitive procedures "inoculate" Steven prior to the date and help to make it more of a success.

See also *behavior therapy*; *cognitive therapy*.

cognitive therapy: An approach to psychotherapy that focuses on replacing maladaptive automatic thoughts with adaptive voluntary ones. The term *cognitive therapy* is usually associated with the work of the psychiatrist Aaron Beck, although it has broad general meaning and can be loosely used to label any cognitive approach to therapy, including cognitive-behavior therapy.

Focusing on Beck's approach, automatic maladaptive thoughts often reside behind depression. People think, "I'm worthless," or "I'm a failure," or "My life has no meaning." In therapy it can be often shown that such thoughts are *cognitive distortions*, ideas that are the result of warped and irrational thought processes. The therapist helps the patient to develop the logical tools necessary to modify the impact of automatic thoughts. Research has shown that, in many cases, cognitive therapy can be an effective way to relieve depression.

Beck has shown that automatic thoughts can be associated with almost any functional mental disorder. Thus cognitive therapy is an approach with a wide spectrum of applications.

See also *automatic thoughts*; *cognitive-behavior therapy*; *rational-emotive therapy*.

collective unconscious: According to Carl Jung, the inborn foundation of the human personality. It is, broadly speaking, a concept that is roughly synonymous with the words *human nature*. Jung believed that the collective unconscious exists at a deeper level than the unconscious level postulated by Freud. Jung referred to Freud's version of unconscious mental functioning as the *personal unconscious*. It is unique to the individual and contains the repressed ideas, motives, and memories of a particular person's life. The *collective unconscious*, on the other hand, is not unique to the individual. We all share essentially the same collective unconscious.

The collective unconscious contains archetypes, inborn patterns. Alienation from the archetypes was considered to be an important factor in mental illnesses. The value of the concept of the collective unconscious in the treatment of mental disorders is an open question. Although Jung was a very influential founding figure in contemporary psychotherapy, particularly on the European continent, his ideas are neither completely accepted nor completely rejected by psychotherapists in general.

See also *analytic psychology (analytical psychology)*; *archetypes*; *Jung, Carl Gustav*.

coma: A pathological state characterized by complete lack of consciousness and the absence of voluntary behavior. Sometimes a coma is described as a *profound stupor*. Some of the causes of a coma are a cerebrovascular accident, a heavy blow to the head, a brain tumor, poisoning, an injury, extreme changes in blood sugar due to diabetes or hypoglycemia, toxicity due to alcohol or other drugs, and similar physical and organic traumata.

Although a coma is in and of itself pathological, there is a form of somatic therapy for mental disorders in which a coma is intentionally induced by a psychiatrist. This kind of therapy is called *insulin coma therapy*.

See also *insulin coma therapy*; *somatic therapy*.

commitment: To place an individual in the custody of an institution such as a prison or a mental hospital. A commitment to a mental hospital is the end result of a legal process requiring *certification*, evidence that the individual in question is either insane or incompetent. This is accomplished in court with due process designed to guarantee the rights of the individual. Although the testimony of friends and relatives is important, expert testimony from mental health professionals is also required.

See also *insanity*; *legal aspects of mental health*.

community mental health center: An outpatient clinic providing drug therapy, individual psychotherapy, group therapy, and general information to mental patients who are well enough to not require hospitalization. Such clinics are usually funded by governmental agencies. However, some are privately operated.

The existence of community mental health centers is part of a larger movement to decentralize the treatment of mental disorders. The basic idea is to return, as much as possible, an individual to a family, a vocation, and a productive life in general. Many mental patients are only partially disabled by their disorders. It is doubtful that it serves them well to spend all of their days many miles from home in a mental hospital.

compensation: A kind of ego defense mechanism characterized by an effort to maximize one's strengths in order to psychologically minimize one's weaknesses. The basic theme of compensation is given by the word *counterbalance*. The individual who is compensating seeks to counterbalance a negative feature of his or her personality with a positive one.

For example, 11-year-old Arthur has poor athletic skills. He may seek to compensate by earning high grades. Or 23-year-old Myra believes she is plain and unattractive. She may seek to compensate by entering a prestigious profession such as law or medicine. Both Arthur and Myra are in essence saying to others, "I'm as good as you are."

The concept of compensation was introduced into the language of psychoanalysis and clinical psychology by Alfred Adler. He presented the idea of compensation in the framework of another concept he introduced, the concept of the inferiority complex (see individual psychology). Adler asserted that people tend to offset real or imagined deficits with behavior designed to restore an equilibrium. He referred to this tendency as the great ability of human beings to turn a minus into a plus.

It is obvious that compensation can be a mechanism that works in the service of mental health. On the other hand, if an individual uses compensation to excess, it may support a neurotic process. For example, persons who appear to have a compulsive need to dominate others may be doing so in an effort to compensate for their own low self-esteem. Unconsciously, they may be seeking to take others down a peg or two.

See also *Adler, Alfred*; *ego defense mechanisms*; *individual psychology*.

complex: In abnormal psychology, a set of related pathological ideas. An individual may have an inferiority complex, an Oedipus complex, or other complex. The complex may express itself in maladaptive behavior and cause problems in living. Insight-oriented therapies seek to make unconscious complexes conscious. Thus the troubled person can gain some measure of voluntary control over behaviors that are induced by the complex.

See also *Oedipus complex*.

compulsion: The urge to act in opposition to one's conscious will or moral standards. The function of a compulsion is to bring relief from a distressing emotional state. In an obsessive-compulsive disorder, carrying out the compulsion brings relief from anxiety. In the case of a rapist or a person with homicidal tendencies, acting out the compulsion may bring relief from intense anger or rage.

Sometimes a person with a schizophrenic disorder, particularly of the paranoid type, hallucinates a voice ordering him or her to carry out a particular action. And the individual may feel under a compulsion to obey the order.

See also *obsessive-compulsive disorder (obsessive-compulsive neurosis)*; *schizophrenia*.

compulsive eating: Eating when it is inappropriate to do so accompanied by the experience that one has little voluntary control over one's behavior. Here are some of the specific behaviors associated with compulsive eating: inability to resist food, inability to stop eating, eating frequently between meals, and bingeing.

One of the factors playing a role in compulsive eating is the ability of food to modulate emotional states. When one is anxious, mildly depressed, or angry, eating often brings a measure of relief. Thus many people have a strong urge to eat not only when they are physiologically hungry but also when they are emotionally distressed.

A second factor playing a role is the tendency of food to be perceived as a symbolic substitute for lacks in a person's life. Thus food may be a substitute for the companionship of friends, romantic love, sex, recognition, or power. Food is often consumed to fill up psychological holes in one's existence.

Factors such as those specified here combine with the learning process to make compulsive eating a habitual pattern. When one obtains gratification from inappropriate eating, the tendency is reinforced and becomes entrenched. Thus the individual finds it harder and harder to resist compulsive eating tendencies.

Compulsive eating plays a significant role in obesity. It also is a primary component in the eating disorders.

See also *eating disorders*; *obesity*; *Overeaters Anonymous (OA)*.

compulsive gambling: Another name for *pathological gambling*. Pathological gambling is classified as a mental disorder in the *Diagnostic and Statistical Manual of Mental Disorders*.

See also *Gamblers Anonymous (GA)*; *pathological gambling*.

compulsive personality disorder: See *obsessive-compulsive personality disorder (compulsive personality disorder)*.

computerized axial tomography (CAT): An X-ray process that provides a detailed image of the structure of a soft organ such as the brain, the heart, or a kidney. The procedure does not require surgery and is therefore described as *noninvasive*. A highly focused X-ray beam is passed through the organ under study 160 to 180 times. A computer program reconstructs the data obtained, giving a complete picture of the organ's internal structure. The final depiction is called a CAT-scan.

In psychiatry and neurology, a CAT-scan is of particular value in detecting abnormalities of the brain. Tumors, damage due to strokes, and atrophy of brain tissue can be seen. The process is of substantial use in diagnosing and evaluating organic mental disorders.

A drawback of CAT is that it reveals only the structure, not the functioning of an organ. However, a similar procedure, positron emission tomography (PET), does do this.

See also *nuclear magnetic resonance (NMR)*; *positron emission tomography (PET)*.

concussion: A shock to one of the body's organs as a result of a blow or an injury. A *brain concussion* results in a temporary loss of functioning producing such symptoms as confusion, dizziness, or unconsciousness. The probable cause of such reactions is a bruising of the brain's neurons. The symptoms are usually temporary because the neurons do heal. Of course, repeated concussions, such as those received by professional boxers, may result in some permanent impairment.

conduct disorder: A disorder of childhood or adolescence characterized by such behaviors as (1) sneak thievery, (2) running away from home, (3) chronic lying, (4) setting fires, and (5) truancy. The oddness and pathology of the behavior is quite beyond the normal impishness and playfulness of childhood.

The *Diagnostic and Statistical Manual of Mental Disorders* distinguishes three kinds of conduct disorders. There are (1) group type, (2) solitary-aggressive type, and (3) undifferentiated type. The *group type* is characterized by pathological behavior in association with friends and peers. The child or adolescent in question "goes along with the gang." The *solitary type* is characterized by pathological behavior on an individual basis without the necessity of group support. The *undifferentiated type* displays characteristics common to the other two types, and no clear clinical picture emerges.

There are many causal factors involved in the conduct disorders. Some of these are a history of attention deficit disorder, emotionally cold parents, too much punishment, absence of a stable home environment, and living in an institution.

The incidence of conduct disorder in child and adolescent males is estimated to be about 9%. In females, the incidence is estimated to be about 2%.

It is impossible to make a general statement about the prognosis for children and adolescents with conduct disorders. On a specific basis, if the behavioral signs are relatively mild, the troubled young person may improve substantially. Treatment consists of counseling and psychotherapy. An approach such as reality therapy in which the troubled child or adolescent is helped to see the adverse long-run consequences of pathological behavior may be helpful.

See also *attention deficit disorder*; *oppositional defiant disorder*; *reality therapy*.

confabulation: A tendency to respond to questions by making up information. The individual may present as a fact something that is completely false. He or she may seem to "remember" an event that never happened. Such individuals do not appear to be consciously lying. Confabulation is an attempt to fill in blanks when there is an organic problem and, as such, is a symptom of a neurological deficit.

See also *organic mental syndromes (organic brain syndromes)*.

congenital defect: A defect that is present at birth. A congenital defect may be due to heredity or a toxic prenatal environment. The use and abuse of certain drugs plays a role in some defects. Disease during pregnancy can also cause a congenital defect. It is estimated that organic imperfections afflict about 5% of infants. Some of these cause mental health problems. The most obvious general variety is mental retardation.

See also *Down's syndrome*; *Huntington's chorea*; *mental retardation*; *phenylketonuria (PKU)*.

conscience: The agent of the personality that makes it possible for the individual to tell right from wrong. In psychoanalytic theory, the conscience is an aspect of the superego, the morality-oriented part of one's personality. Although the conscience is an important feature of the healthy personality, it can cause problems if it is too strict, punitive, and perfectionistic. Such a conscience can make the individual feel miserable, guilty, and depressed over relatively slight matters.

See also *superego*.

controlled drinking therapy: A kind of behavior therapy designed to modify the behavior of the problem drinker. The aim is to help the individual learn how to drink in moderation in social situations. One training method is to reward the person with a second drink if he or she can learn to sip a mixed drink over a

20-minute period. Many heavy drinkers do not sip at all but gulp drinks down too quickly.

Controlled drinking therapy has met with mixed success. Some individuals seem to have responded well to it. Others seem to be unable to use alcohol without abusing it. For these individuals, the only answer seems to be total abstinence from alcohol.

See also *Alcoholics Anonymous (AA)*; *alcoholism*.

conversion disorder: A kind of somatoform disorder characterized by an impairment of physical capacities without an organic basis. (An older term for this disorder was *hysteria*.) The individual may have trouble seeing, hearing, swallowing, talking, or walking. The problem seems to be neurological but is, in fact, a result of emotional conflicts.

In some cases, the symptom may offer a "solution" to a problem in living. A student who faces a threatening examination may develop vision problems. An artist who is anxious about an assignment may develop paralysis in his or her drawing hand.

In most cases, people recover from conversion disorders with the aid of counseling and psychotherapy. Hypnosis is sometimes an effective treatment.

Conversion disorder is of particular historical interest because it is the disorder (i.e., "hysteria") that first interested Freud in psychoanalysis. It was a very common disorder in Freud's day, but it is much less commonly seen by contemporary therapists. It was once thought that conversion disorder afflicts primarily women. (The word *hysteria* is derived from the Greek word *hystera*, meaning uterus.) It is now understood that conversion disorder afflicts both males and females.

See also *hysteria*; *somatoform disorders*.

convulsion: A muscle contraction that is simultaneously violent, pathological, and involuntary. Sometimes convulsions come in a rapid series. *Clonic convulsions* alternate contractions with relaxations. In a *static convulsion*, there is no relaxation phase.

Convulsions can be induced in a variety of ways. Toxic substances, brain disorders, high fevers, electroconvulsive therapy, and epilepsy have all been identified as causal factors in convulsions.

The person having a convulsion needs to be protected against injury, particularly the banging of the head on a hard surface. A pillow or a blanket under the head is helpful.

See also *electroconvulsive therapy (ECT)*; *epilepsy*.

coping strategies: Survival methods used by people to respond to the stresses and strains of everyday living. There are two basic kinds of coping strategies: (1) active and (2) passive. *Active strategies* involve planning ahead for problems, voluntary decision making, and rational thinking. The skills recommended in assertiveness training provide examples of active coping. The techniques for clear thinking suggested by Albert Ellis in rational-emotive therapy provide a second set of examples.

Passive coping, on the other hand, involves behavior that is often ineffective and self-defeating. Ego defense mechanisms such as repression, regression, and fantasy provide examples.

In psychotherapy, individuals are often encouraged to develop active coping strategies.

See also *assertiveness training*; *ego defense mechanisms*; *rational-emotive therapy*.

corpus callosum: A nervous system structure connecting the brain's two cerebral hemispheres. The corpus callosum makes it possible for the two hemispheres to communicate with each other. Sometimes the corpus callosum is surgically severed as a treatment for the relief of chronic epilepsy. Patients who have had the operation have been studied, and the results of split brain research suggest that the two hemispheres have somewhat different, but related, functions. The left hemisphere plays a dominant role in the processing of highly symbolic information. Mathematical computations and language functions appear to take place primarily in this hemisphere.

The right hemisphere plays a dominant role in the processing of highly patterned information. The ability to recognize a photograph or recall the melody of a song appears to take place primarily in this hemisphere. For the prior reasons, the left hemisphere is sometimes called the "logical" hemisphere, and the right hemisphere is called the "romantic" one.

See also *brain pathology*; *epilepsy*.

counseling psychologist: A kind of psychologist specializing in interviewing, guidance, crisis intervention, and vocational testing. Such psychologists most often work in school and college guidance centers. However, they sometimes work in clinics and private practice. Their work is, in fact, very similar to the work of a clinical psychologist. The distinction between the two often blurs in the practical world. However, at a theoretical level, a counseling psychologist works with less severe problems that can be handled at a more or less conscious level. A clinical psychologist deals with more severe mental disorders and may probe deeply into the unconscious mental life of the patient.

See also *clinical psychologist*.

counterconditioning: The conditioning of a response that is antagonistic to an already established conditioned response. The second response thus acquires some ability to extinguish the first response. The purpose of such a procedure is help a person eliminate an unwanted behavior pattern. The technique is one that is used in behavior therapy. For example, 4-year-old Henry has acquired an irrational fear of cats. He might be exposed to cats at a distance while sucking a lollipop sitting in his mother's lap. The relaxation response evoked by sitting safely and eating will be antagonistic to the fear response evoked by the sight of the cat. With repeated exposures, the procedure will almost certainly help Henry feel less afraid of cats.

The behavior therapy technique known as systematic desensitization takes advantage of the counterconditioning principle.

The technique is quite helpful to adults who suffer from phobic disorders.

See also *behavior therapy*; *classical conditioning*; *systematic desensitization*.

counterphobic behavior: Acting in a manner that is diametrically opposed to a fear. Taylor, an adolescent, is walking through a graveyard at night. He wants to break his stride and run. Instead, he saunters along slowly and whistles. He is trying to prove to himself that he is not afraid. Sometimes counterphobic behavior can be quite dramatic. A person may scale the exterior of a building as a way of saying to the world, "I have no fear of heights!" A certain amount of daredevilish and death-defying behavior, seemingly irrational, can be explained in terms of the counterphobic principle.

See also *phobia*.

countertransference: In psychoanalytic theory, the development toward the patient of feelings in the therapist representing the therapist's unconscious projection. The patient is used as a substitute figure for another person in the therapist's life. Perhaps the patient may remind the therapist of a long-lost sweetheart. The therapist may find himself or herself falling in love with the patient. Of course, such "love" is synthetic love. It has no substance. It is an artifact arising from the mechanism, already noted, of unconscious projection.

The phenomenon being described here includes the word *counter* because it is often in response to a transference by the patient. The patient may fantasize that he or she is in love with the analyst. This is *transference*. If the feeling is returned in some way by the analyst, this is *countertransference*.

Although erotic feelings often form a basis for transference phenomena, it is possible for transference and countertransference to involve other emotional reactions, particularly hostility.

See also *projection*; *transference*.

couple counseling: Counseling sessions with both partners of a relationship present. Most of the time, couple counseling refers to a heterosexual married couple. However, it is possible to speak of unmarried couples and homosexual couples. The basic idea of couple counseling, in contrast to individual psychotherapy, is that emotional problems are often the result of the interplay between two people. For example, even if only one member of a couple is depressed, this can be a reactive depression. The depressed person may feel mistreated and discounted. The "well" person needs counseling as much as the "sick" person in order to learn more effective and constructive ways of relating to the "sick" person.

See also *Berne, Eric*; *Sullivan, Harry Stack*; *transactional analysis*.

crack: See *cocaine*.

cretinism: A form of brain damage caused by low thyroid secretion during the prenatal period or infancy. If a mother suffers from a thyroid problem during her pregnancy, the infant can be born with cretinism. Or, if an infant has a malfunctioning thyroid gland, cretinism can develop in early childhood. In either event, the child with cretinism is mentally retarded and greatly stunted in growth. Victims of this disease tend to have short legs, a wide nose, wiry hair, a large abdomen, and dry skin. Their metabolic rate is low, and they are very sluggish in their actions.

The most common cause of a thyroid deficiency is inadequate amounts of iodine in the diet. Infections and genetic factors can also cause thyroid disease and, in turn, cretinism. At one time, cretinism was fairly common in Switzerland and the Great Lakes area in the United States because of small quantities of iodine in the soil. In the United States, with the use of iodized salt and the treatment of thyroid problems with thyroid extract, cretinism is at present relatively rare.

See also *mental retardation*.

crisis intervention: Counseling offered to individuals when their inability to adapt to life situations reaches a point of emotional emergency. Such acute states include overdoses of drugs, attempts at suicide, extreme depression, food binges, drunken episodes, being beaten by a spouse, inability to cope with a child or adolescent, and so forth. The troubled person is encouraged to call a *crisis intervention center*, a unit staffed by volunteers trained to offer guidance and emotional support. There are many such centers in local communities, and they usually have hotlines listed in the telephone directory.

cunnilingus: A form of oral-genital contact in which the tongue and the lips are used to stimulate the external sexual organs of the female. Quite commonly, the tongue is used to stimulate the clitoris as a means of increasing sexual excitement or inducing an orgasm. At one time, cunnilingus was thought to be a form of sexual perversion. However, recent sexual surveys indicate that more than half of couples use cunnilingus in premarital sexual foreplay. Today's sexologists regard cunnilingus as a normal and desirable behavior if it is enjoyed by both participants.

See also *clitoris*; *fellatio*; *orgasm*.

Cushing's syndrome: An endocrine disorder involving excessive production of adrenal hormones. Physical symptoms of Cushing's syndrome include weakness, low sex drive, obesity, cessation of menstruation in women, and excessive hair growth. Psychological symptoms include depression, anxiety, agitation, and irritability. In a few cases, thinking becomes quite disordered.

Cushing's syndrome is associated with the malfunctioning of either an adrenal gland or the pituitary gland, a gland that regulates the action of the adrenal glands. The malfunctioning itself can be due to a tumor in an adrenal gland, the pituitary gland, or other endocrine pathology. Sometimes excessive administration of the drug cortisone can induce Cushing's syndrome. The discoverer of the disease was Harvey Cushing (1869–1939), a pioneer neurosurgeon.

The victim of Cushing's syndrome can often be treated with substantial success by a combination of endocrine therapy and surgery.

See also *endocrine system.*

cyclothymic disorder: A mood disorder characterized by alternating periods of elation and depression. (This disorder is also sometimes called *cyclic disorder.*) Obviously, cyclothymic disorder bears a great resemblance to bipolar disorder (i.e., manic-depressive disorder).

The difference between cyclothymic disorder and bipolar disorder is primarily one of degree. Indeed, some clinicians think of cyclothymic disorder as a mild form of bipolar disorder. The elevated phase of cyclothymic disorder is distinguished by symptoms such as little need for sleep, an inflated self-concept, excessive talk, and very high sex drive. The depressive phase of the disorder is distinguished by such symptoms as a poor self-concept, withdrawal from people, decreased sex drive, and a negative attitude toward goals. In neither case are there delusions or hallucinations. So this is not a psychotic disorder.

Causal factors are difficult to specify. However, they may include a disturbed period of development in childhood, a currently difficult life situation, physical illness, and a predisposing temperament.

Cyclothymic disorder is associated with young adulthood, is fairly common, and women tend to suffer from it more often than do males. Also, it tends to be a long-lasting condition. In some cases, it is treated with drugs. However, psychotherapy is probably of greater value with cyclothymic disorder than with bipolar disorder. The individual's reality contact is basically intact, and he or she can respond intelligently to ideas. In the broad sense, cyclothymic disorder can be thought of as having a neurotic component. Thus insight and self-understanding may ameliorate the individual's suffering.

See also *bipolar disorder; mood disorders (affective disorders).*

D

death anxiety: A general fear of the loss of personal existence. A certain amount of death anxiety is normal. In existential thought, death anxiety is built into the human condition. However, if death anxiety becomes excessive, it may have neurotic roots. Under such circumstances, death anxiety may be a reaction formation against self-destructive impulses. The conscious fear of death is used to help the individual avoid situations in which he or she may engage in suicidal actions.

See also *existential therapy*; *reaction formation*.

death instinct: According to Freud, an inborn impulse toward both destruction of others and self-destruction. Freud gave this instinct the name *Thanatos*, the Greek god of death. In youth, Thanatos is suppressed by Eros, the Greek god of love. Thus in the early years of one's life, the death instinct seems to lack much force. However, when one ages, Thanatos eventually gains ascendancy over Eros and eventually brings about the individual's end.

In deeply troubled persons, Thanatos may make an early appearance. Thus we witness many acts of destruction toward others such as murders, rapes, and assaults. Freud believed that World War I was an outbreak of the death instinct, and it made him pessimistic about the human race in general.

In some troubled persons, Thanatos may be turned toward the self. Thus alcohol and drug abuse, unnecessary risk taking, compulsive eating, and suicide are seen in classical psychoanalysis as premature expressions of the death instinct.

Although it is not possible to rid human existence of the death instinct, Freud believed that it is possible to minimize its effects through psychoanalysis. Freud's concept of Thanatos is a part of classical psychoanalytical theory. However, there is no general consensus among therapists concerning the value of the concept. Many clinicians consider it unnecessary. They explain destructive behavior in terms of aggression as a built-in response to frustration.

See also *frustration–aggression hypothesis*; *suicide*.

defense mechanisms: See *ego defense mechanisms*.

deinstitutionalization: The decentralization of mental health care. In recent times, there has been a movement toward reducing the patient populations of large state mental hospitals. The idea is to return the disturbed person to the community as an outpatient. The general motive is a humanistic one. The logic is that mental patients are more likely to improve in "normal" environments than in the confines of a hospital. Their outpatient care is provided through community health centers.

Advocates of deinstitutionalization agree with the reasoning indicated here. Opponents of deinstitutionalization argue that many mental patients are being released who are too sick to be on their own. They become homeless and neglect themselves.

See also *community mental health center*.

delinquency: In general, any failure to live up to an obligation or a responsibility. In the context abnormal behavior, *juvenile delinquency* is primarily a legal term. It refers to the transgressions, either antisocial or immoral, of minors. Juvenile courts thus exist, and they mete out punishment or indicate the necessity for corrective action. Such courts handle about two million cases a year.

Juvenile delinquency has been on the increase in recent years.

In the past decade the frequency of recorded delinquent acts has more than doubled. About one-third of robberies are committed by juveniles.

Causal factors in juvenile delinquency are many. Some that have been identified are personal adjustment problems, distressed family relationships, portrayals of violence on television, undesirable companions, and overcrowding in cities. Speaking in broad sociocultural terms, it appears that large-scale changes in traditional values and family life have contributed to feelings of alienation and confusion in many minors.

Correctional institutions, probation programs, and personal counseling are all ways that society has developed in an attempt to cope with the problem of juvenile delinquency in a constructive manner.

See also *conduct disorder*; *legal aspects of mental health*.

delirium: A type of organic mental syndrome characterized by a clouding of consciousness. Clear thinking is impaired. Some of the specific symptoms of a delirium are inability to pay attention, difficulty in concentration, confusion, impairment of memory, and perceptual errors. Sometimes delusions and hallucinations are present. Dementia frequently exists along with delirium but is not to be confused with it.

There are numerous causal factors that can play a role in deliriums including head injuries, withdrawal from drugs, infections, low blood sugar, lack of oxygen, high fever, shock, and inadequate blood supply to the brain. Most deliriums represent acute states and are of short duration. The individual suffering from a delirium needs protection from self-injury due to psychomotor agitation. Also, he or she needs adequate medical care. In some cases, a delirium may precede a coma and death.

See also *delirium tremens*; *dementia*; *organic mental syndromes (organic brain syndromes)*.

delirium tremens: A kind of delirium cased by withdrawal from the heavy use of alcohol. (This state is also called *alcohol withdrawal* *delirium*. The slang term for delirium tremens is the DTs.) Psychological symptoms associated with delirium tremens include delusions, hallucinations, excitement, and agitation. Physical symptoms include rapid heart and breathing rate, heavy perspiration, high blood pressure, trembling of the body, seizures, and fever.

The condition is dangerous and without proper medical supervision can result in death. Such supervision consists of bed rest, drug and vitamin therapy, emotional reassurance, protection against self-injury, and a well-balanced diet. If properly treated, the acute phase of delirium tremens is over in a few days.

See also *alcoholism*; *delirium*.

delusion: A belief that most members of an individual's family or culture regard as irrational or false. Facts offered by a spouse, a friend, or a therapist have little effect on delusions. Delusions often refer to the self and are associated primarily with psychotic disorders.

There are many kinds of delusions. Three varieties are bizarre delusions, nihilistic delusions, and delusions of being controlled. *Bizarre delusions* are those that seem preposterous to most observers. For example, Nathaniel insists that his eyeballs are attached to his brain by incandescent wires implanted by Thomas Alva Edison. *Nihilistic delusions* are characterized by thoughts of death or decay. For example, Barbara says that her arms are withering like old leaves and will soon drop from her body. *Delusions of being controlled* are distinguished by the helpless feeling that one's thought processes and actions are under the influence of external agents. Lillian believes that the aliens from the planet Anteres IV direct her actions by telepathic hypnosis.

See also *hallucination*; *psychotic disorders*.

delusional (paranoid) disorder: A disorder characterized by delusions that lack the outlandish and grotesque character of schizophrenic delusions. The delusions associated with this disorder have a superficial plausibility and can be quite convincing. The types of delusional disorder include erotomanic, grandiose, jealous, persecutory, and somatic.

A common delusions associated with the *erotomanic type* is "He [or she] is in love with me." Common delusions associated with the *grandiose type* are "I am a great person" or "I have created a marvelous invention." A common delusion associated with the *jealous type* is "My spouse [or lover] is cheating on me." Common delusions associated with the *persecutory type* are "Someone is plotting against me" or "Someone is poisoning my food." Common delusions associated with the *somatic type* are "I smell terrible" or "A disease inside of me is eating me alive."

The incidence of delusional disorder is low. It is estimated that less than one in a thousand people are afflicted with the disorder. A few more females than males appear to suffer from the disorder. Delusional disorder is a problem of adult life and may have an adverse effect on important relationships such as marriage. However, in many respects, the individual may continue to function quite effectively. Persons with the disorder seldom seek help because they do not see themselves as ill. The disorder itself in essence says that there is something wrong with *him*, or *her*, or *them*, not *me*.

It does not seem that delusional disorder is caused by biological factors such as a genetic predisposition or a biochemical imbalance. The principal causal factors appear to be the developmental history and recent psychosocial stressors. It is possible to speculate that parents who failed to adequately meet a child's emotional needs may have fostered an underlying sense of mistrust. There is an unspoken lack of confidence in others and the world in general. An example of a psychosocial stressor that can trigger a delusional disorder is deafness. It is relatively easy to project on others the idea that "they are plotting against me." Another example of a psychosocial stressor that can trigger a delusional disorder is recent arrival in the United States from a foreign country. Any condition in which one feels alien, an outsider, can aggravate a tendency toward paranoid thought.

The treatment for a delusional disorder often consists of antipsychotic medication combined with psychotherapy. Frequently family therapy is recommended, and sessions may be conducted on a group basis. This approach helps the patient overcome the isolation and loneliness associated with delusional disorder.

See also *drug therapy*; *family therapy*; *folie à deux*; *major tranquilizers (antipsychotic drugs)*; *paranoid personality disorder*; *psychotic disorders*; *schizophrenia*.

dementia: A type of organic mental syndrome characterized by a deterioration in functional intelligence. The individual's higher thought processes such as abstract reasoning, memory, mathematical abilities, verbal fluency, and so forth are greatly impaired. Pathological changes in the victim's personality may also be manifest. A significant dementia will interfere with vocational performance.

dementia praecox: An outdated term for schizophrenia. The familiar word *precocious*, suggesting advanced or premature development, is derived from the Latin word *praecox*. Thus *dementia praecox* has a literal meaning indicating "an early onset of mental decline." The German psychiatrist Emil Kraepelin (1856–1926) favored the term because schizophrenic disorders often make their first appearance in adolescence or young adulthood. The Swiss psychiatrist Eugen Bleuler (1857–1939) introduced the term *schizophrenia* in the early 1900s, and it has remained the preferred usage since that time.

See also *Bleuler, Eugen*; *Kraepelin, Emil*; *schizophrenia*.

demonology: Within the framework of abnormal psychology, the explanation of mental disorders in terms of possession by an evil spirit or a devil. Contemporary mental health professionals tend to look upon demonology as representative of a prescientific world view. Thus demonology is not taken seriously as an actual cause of mental disorders. However, it must be noted that throughout much of human history some version of demonology has been a prime way of explaining odd or deviant behavior. Also, even today, in many underdeveloped countries, demonology is a popular explanation of aberrant behavior.

denial of reality: An ego defense mechanism characterized by a refusal to face unpleasant facts. Tina is on a long motor trip and notices that the needle of the gas gauge is on empty. There isn't a gas station within 25 miles. She thinks, "I'll make it. I've got plenty of gas." Upton's wife tells him that she no longer loves him and wants a divorce. He thinks, "She doesn't mean it. I know she really loves me. This is a test of some sort."

It should be noted that denial of reality is an unconscious mechanism. It is an unwilled mental act.

See also *ego defense mechanisms*.

dependent personality disorder: A personality disorder characterized by an impairment of autonomy in human relations. Persons with this disorder are too passive in their dealings with significant other people such as a spouse or a parent. For example, Leah, a married woman, allows her husband to dictate where they will live, who their friends will be, what she wears, how the house is decorated, and where they will go on vacation. Traits associated with this disorder include lack of self-confidence, a fear of asking too much of others, and a tolerance of physical or verbal abuse.

Causal factors in this disorder cannot be clearly specified. It is possible to speculate that a childhood in which one was dominated and made to feel stupid by overcontrolling parents may be a contributing factor. A learning history in which one was rewarded for being agreeable is perhaps another contributing factor.

A dependent personality disorder interferes with one's competence and effectiveness. Although the impairment may superficially seem to be mild, it can be very distressing. Therefore this disorder is also often associated with depression. A fairly common disorder, women tend to suffer from it somewhat more often than do men.

Psychotherapy is the treatment of choice for this disorder. In particular, assertiveness training may be of value.

See also *assertiveness training*; *personality disorders*.

depersonalization disorder: A type of dissociative disorder characterized by distortions in the perception of self. (An older term for this disorder was *depersonalization neurosis*.) Such distortions may include the feeling that one has become unreal, that one is walking outside of one's body, that arms or legs have either shrunken or expanded, that one has become strangely tiny, that movements are robotlike, and that one is living in a fantasy world. Associated distortions may include the feeling that other people are dead and that things such as chairs and ashtrays have become weirdly unfamiliar.

There is a tendency for a depersonalization disorder to make its first appearance rather suddenly. Recovery is an on–off process over a time period. When the subject feels worried or depressed, the symptoms often return.

If an individual has a tendency toward depersonalization disorder, the first incident usually appears during adolescence or young adulthood.

It is important to realize that a person suffering from a depersonalization disorder is not psychotic. The individual is usually aware that the distortions of perception do not conform to external facts. On the whole, the person has not lost touch with reality as most of us know it. For this reason, depersonalization disorder is broadly conceived of as an essentially neurotic condition.

It is very difficult to specify the deep causal factors underlying depersonalization disorder. It can be hypothesized that a set of childhood experiences in which one was excessively abused or punished plays a contributing role. It is, however, possible to specify a number of "triggers" of the disorder. These include being very tired, withdrawing from a drug, great pain, extreme worry, and emotionally disturbing events. It should be noted that it is possible to induce experiences similar to those associated with depersonalization disorder through the use of hypnotic and meditative techniques. However, a person having such experiences under these conditions is not a victim of the disorder.

Psychotherapy is the treatment of choice for depersonalization disorder. Because the disorder is thought to have neurotic roots, the therapist will often attempt to have the patient explore childhood experiences and connect them to present thoughts and perceptions. The insight gained may bring about some relief from the symptoms.

See also *dissociative disorders*.

depression: A negative emotional state characterized by sadness, self-doubt, and a loss of interest in daily living. Depression plays a part in a number of mental disorders, particularly the mood disorders. Along with anxiety, depression is one of the most frequent complaints heard by therapists. It has been called "the common cold of mental illness." Statistical surveys suggest that during any given time period, about 4% of the adult population is suffering from some degree of depression. The portrait of depression can be greatly enriched by listing some of the symptoms often associated with it. These include dejection, poor self-image, crying, inability to laugh, pessimism, suicidal impulses, loss of interest in sexual activity, and fatigue.

A first way to classify depression is as endogenous or exogenous. *Endogenous depression* is depression that arises from within. It has no known external cause in present circumstances. Such depression may be biological in nature (i.e., genetic or biochemical). Or it may be due to psychological factors with roots in negative childhood experiences. *Exogenous depression* is depression that arises from without. It is sometimes called *reactive depression*. It has a known external cause in present circumstances such as a divorce, the loss of a job, or the death of a loved one. If it is mild in severity, it is thought of as normal.

A second way to classify depression is as neurotic or psychotic. In *neurotic depression*, the individual maintains contact with reality. He or she maintains stable perceptions of time, space, and the external world. In *psychotic depression*, the individual has impaired reality contact. There is great mental confusion, and there may be delusions. (Do not identify the word neurotic with mild. Neurotic depression can be severe, and can in some cases lead to suicide.)

A third way to classify depression is in terms of severity. The range is from mild to moderate to severe. In *mild depression*, the person may complain that life is not fun any longer, that a marriage is not rewarding, that he or she needs a lot of rest, and so forth. Although the depression is irritating, the individual is able to continue functioning and carries out major responsibilities without too much difficulty. In *moderate depression*, the person may feel that life has become very boring and lost much of its meaning. There is a lack of interest in other people, good grooming becomes unimportant, and there may be suicidal fantasies. The person can usually meet major responsibilities but with a great effort of will. In *severe depression*, the person may be convinced that nothing makes any sense at all, that life is totally without meaning, and that he or she is not loved or lovable. There is great apathy about almost everything, and there may be suicidal attempts.

Explanations of depression tend to fall into three major categories. These are biological, psychological, and existential. The *biological explanation* states that depression is caused by genetic or biochemical factors. It is hypothesized that some people are predisposed to depression in terms of their inborn temperament. There is evidence, for example, to suggest that, in bipolar disorder, genetic factors probably play a role. A biochemical deficit such as a lack of normal levels of the neurotransmitter norepinephrine may contribute to depression. Biological explanations are used primarily to help us understand endogenous depressions.

The *psychological explanation* states that depression has its roots in the individual's developmental history. Classical psychoanalysis suggests two principal factors play a role. First, the "good little boy" or "good little girl" is taught to repress aggressive responses. They are not "nice." Second, such a child may also acquire a very moral and high-minded outlook on life. In Freudian terms, this means the individual has a very strict superego. Thus whenever, even as an adult, normal aggressive responses want to surface, they are repressed by the superego. The inability to express real feelings, particularly aggressive ones, in a normal way leads to depression. In brief, psychoanalysis looks upon depression as bottled-up anger.

It should be noted that the psychological explanation does not end with psychoanalysis. Another major psychological explanation is the one offered by learning theory. Learning theory states that depression is an acquired response pattern, a kind of emotional habit. For example, a child raised in a household with a depressed parent may, through the process of observational learning, imitate and acquire depression as a maladaptive way of coping with the stress of life. Another possibility is a phenomenon known as *learned helplessness*. A series of failure experience may lead a person to generalize and believe that he or she is helpless in situations where this is not in fact so.

The *existential explanation* states that depression is inescapable. It is a part of life. We all know that we may have losses, experience illnesses, and eventually die. Any person of normal intelligence who profoundly contemplates the nature of existence can hardly escape some feelings of depression. However, existential therapists help a person to minimize the impact of existential depression by developing an attitude of courage toward the very real hardships of life.

Depression can be treated with drugs or psychotherapy. If it is believed that the depression is both biological and endogenous in nature, then drug therapy is the treatment of choice. If these two conditions are not met, then the treatment of choice is psychotherapy.

See also *bipolar disorder*; *dysthymic disorder (depressive neurosis)*; *learned helplessness*; *major depression (unipolar disorder)*; *mood disorders (affective disorders)*.

desensitization therapy: A type of behavior therapy designed to help a troubled person adapt to stimuli that produce maladaptive emotional reactions. The father of desensitization therapy is the psychiatrist Joseph Wolpe, and he based the approach on well-known principles of classical conditioning. Essentially, a counterconditioning approach is used in which relaxation is pitted against the unwanted emotional reaction.

For example, Alcott has an irrational fear of spiders. In therapy, he is given suggestions that bring about deep muscle relaxation. Then the therapist induces fantasies in Alcott involving spiders. At first, these fantasies are mild. A spider is seen from a distance constructing a web. Whenever Alcott's anxiety rises to an uncomfortable level, the therapist switches back to the relaxation suggestions. Gradually, it is possible to increase the intensity of the fantasies. Eventually, Alcott might be able to fantasize a harmless spider crawling in his hand without anxiety. When he can do this, he is essentially over his phobia.

It is possible to do desensitization therapy without the use of fantasies. The therapist in the preceding example could have used pictures of spiders, spiders in a bottle, and visits to a museum as the fearful stimuli. This approach is known as *in vivo* desensitization. However, it is more time-consuming and cumbersome than the fantasy technique. And research indicates that the fantasy method tends to be quite effective in the motivated subject.

Although, in theory, desensitization therapy can be used to reduce the effects of almost any unwanted emotional reaction, in practice, it has been used mainly to treat the anxiety associated with phobic disorders. It is generally regarded as one of the most effective and reliable techniques available to therapists.

See also *behavior therapy*; *classical conditioning*; *counterconditioning*; *phobia*; *Wolpe, Joseph*.

determinism: A philosophical viewpoint underlying most of the work that is done in psychology and psychiatry. Determinism asserts that all behavior is caused, that it can be explained. The human being is an organism in the world. And all of the laws of nature apply to us and our behavior as much as they do to the atoms, the plants, and the animals. Thus, whenever a person thinks, acts, or feels, there is some factor or set of factors causing the behavioral event. These factors may be genetic, biochemical, or psychological. But they are there. As a consequence, human behavior can be explained and, to some extent, predicted. If some order can be found in behavior, it makes sense to treat abnormal behavior with drugs or psychotherapy. Sigmund Freud, John Watson, and B. F. Skinner are among the advocates of determinism.

The philosophical viewpoint opposed to determinism is known as *voluntarism*. Voluntarism asserts that we have a free will. Our choices are our own. We must take responsibility for our behavior. This doctrine is associated with the teachings of both Catholic theology and existentialism. St. Thomas Aquinas, the philosopher Jean-Paul Sartre, and Abraham Maslow are among the advocates of voluntarism.

As already indicated, determinism underlies most of the work done in psychology and psychiatry. This, however, does not mean that determinism is "true" in any profound sense. It is simply taken as a working hypothesis, a useful fiction, for daily work. The ultimate truth of the two viewpoints is still debated and discussed in philosophical circles.

See also *Freud, Sigmund*; *Maslow, Abraham Harold*; *Skinner, Burrhus Frederic*; *Watson, John Broadus*.

detoxification: A set of treatment procedures that assist the body in ridding itself of excessive amounts of alcohol or other drugs. Usually medical care is implied in which the patient receives plenty of rest, medicines if necessary, good nutrition, and ample fluids.

See also *delirium tremens*; *drug addiction*.

developmental disorders: Disorders of infancy, childhood, or adolescence characterized by impairment of the maturation process. There are two broad ways to categorize such disorders. These are pervasive developmental disorders and specific developmental disorders. *Pervasive developmental disorders* affect all aspects of the child's functioning in a profound way. Thinking, perception, social skills, and motor control are all affected. *Autistic disorder* is the principal pervasive developmental disorder, and it is distinguished by an absence of normal interest in other people.

Specific developmental disorders affect a given area of a child's functioning. In *developmental reading disorder*, there are substantial problems in the child's ability to comprehend written words and sentences. The term *dyslexia* is sometimes applied to this disorder. In *developmental arithmetic disorder*, there are substantial problems in the child's ability to grasp basic concepts of number and the processes of addition, subtraction, multiplication, and division. In *developmental language disorder*, there are substantial problems in the child's ability to comprehend what is said and to express thoughts in speech.

It is believed that the principal causal factors in the pervasive disorders are biological in nature. There may be a genetic predisposition, or the child may have some degree of mental retardation complicating the developmental picture. In the case of the specific disorders, it is believed that environment plays a more significant role. Ineffective parenting involving such behaviors as abuse, neglect, overcontrol, or emotional coldness may contribute to the formation of these disorders.

Behavior therapy has been shown to be of some value in the treatment of pervasive developmental disorders. Various training and educational procedures are of value in treating the specific developmental disorders.

See also *autistic disorder (infantile autism)*; *developmental reading disorder (dyslexia)*; *mental retardation*.

developmental reading disorder (dyslexia): In the context of child development, difficulties in acquiring the ability to read with facility. A developmental reading disorder does *not* suggest mental retardation or gross organic brain damage. On the contrary, the child's reading level is usually below what might be expected in terms of the child's IQ score.

A child suffering from a developmental reading disorder will display such behaviors as hesitant oral reading, leaving out words, modifying words, not recognizing words, reversing the perception or reproduction of letters, and general lack of reading comprehension. Frequently, children with this disorder also suffer from attention deficit disorder. The disorder is more common in males than in females.

Reading instruction using special techniques can benefit the child with developmental reading disorder. Often the child seems to have what has been described as a *word blindness*, an inability to perceive words correctly. Thus a technique such as having the child trace his or her finger over sandpaper letters glued to blocks of wood can be helpful. While tracing the letter, the child can also say the letter aloud. The child thus sees the letter while, at the same time, making motor movements (i.e., moving the hand and speaking). Thus an improved sensorimotor connection may form between seeing letters (and words) and their reproduction by the child in speech or writing.

Parents who have a child suffering from a developmental reading disorder should take heart. Much improvement can result if the child has the right kind of instruction.

Sometimes developmental reading disorder is called *dyslexia*. The literal meaning of the term is a "defective understanding of words."

See also *attention deficit disorder*; *developmental disorders*.

deviant behavior: Any behavior that is odd or unusual. The person who engages in such behavior is sometimes called a *deviate*. In order for behavior to be deviant, it must be significantly different from some standard or norm held by a social group such as the family or a given culture. If all of the people in a particular family take daily showers, then if one of them begins to take showers once a week, he or she is exhibiting a mild form of deviant behavior in terms of that family. There is really no essential difference between the terms *deviant behavior* and *abnormal behavior*. The two can be used synonymously.

See also *abnormal behavior*; *sexual deviations*.

dexedrine: The trade name of one of the amphetamine drugs.
See also *amphetamines*.

diagnosis: In the context of abnormal psychology and psychiatry, the act of deciding that a given set of symptoms or behavioral signs suggest the presence of a particular mental disorder. Reliable diagnosis of a mental disorder is difficult and should not be undertaken lightly. As a consequence, clinical psychologists and psychiatrists use standardized psychological tests, interviews with the troubled person, family interviews, and the guidelines set forth in the American Psychiatric Association's *Diagnostic and Statistical Manual of Mental Disorders* when they make a diagnosis.

See also Diagnostic and Statistical Manual of Mental Disorders.

Diagnostic and Statistical Manual of Mental Disorders: A manual published by the American Psychiatric Association to aid mental health professionals such as psychiatrists and clinical psychologists in making reliable diagnoses of mental disorders. The manual has undergone a number of revisions, and at the time of this writing is in its revised third edition. The various mental disorders identified in this encyclopedia are in agreement with those specified in the manual.

The *Diagnostic and Statistical Manual of Mental Disorders* evaluates mental disorders on five axes (i.e., dimensions or aspects). *Axis I* is an evaluation of a patient's primary clinical syndrome such as mental retardation, alcohol abuse, a schizophrenic disorder, or an anxiety disorder. *Axis II* is an evaluation of developmental problems (in children) or personality problems (in adults). *Axis III* is an evaluation of organic difficulties or medical problems the patient may have. These often affect the progress of a mental disorder. *Axis IV* is an evaluation of the severity of psychosocial stressors in a patient's life. Deaths of friends or relatives, changes in careers, sexual abuse, and divorces are examples of psychosocial stressors that can aggravate the symptoms of a mental disorder. *Axis V* is an evaluation of a patient's level of functioning during the past 12 months. Serious problems in a person's social relations or vocational effectiveness may also aggravate the symptoms of a mental disorder.

In addition to providing diagnostic criteria for the various mental disorders, the *Diagnostic and Statistical Manual of Mental Dis-*

orders also provides a certain amount of information about the disorders. Areas of interest include average age at onset, probable course, amount of impairment, complications, predisposing factors, prevalence, sex ratio, and family pattern.

It should be noted that *neurosis* does not form a diagnostic category. It was one in the first and second editions of the manual. However, for more precision in diagnosis, neurotic conditions are now included in five categories: mood disorders, anxiety disorders, somatoform disorders, dissociative disorders, and sexual disorders. It is still acceptable to use the word *neurosis* in a descriptive way or to specify a kind of psychological process. However, it is not a mental disorder for diagnostic or statistical purposes.

See also *diagnosis*; International Classification of Diseases *(ICD)*; *neurosis*.

diathesis: An inherited predisposition to develop a given disease. The word *diathesis* is from Greek roots with the literal meaning "in order to take place."

See also *diathesis-stress viewpoint*.

diathesis-stress viewpoint: The viewpoint that a disease or disorder develops in a given individual as a result of two factors: (1) a diathesis, or inherited predisposition, and (2) stress. For example, a good deal of research suggests that a diathesis may play a role in schizophrenic disorders. However, a given individual with the diathesis may not develop the disorder unless there is a psychosocial stressor of sufficient magnitude to trigger a schizophrenic episode. Under these circumstances, the diathesis is seen as a *necessary* condition for the disorder. Stress provides the *sufficient* condition. Thus the diathesis-stress viewpoint gives importance to both inborn and environmental factors in the explanation of mental disorders.

See also *psychosocial stressors*; *stress*.

diazepam: One of the minor tranquilizers. Diazepam is prescribed primarily to treat anxiety, nervousness, tension, muscle spasm, and convulsive disorders. It is marketed under several trade names. The most well known is Valium. Some other trade names are Novodipam, Rival, and Vivol. Diazepam is often prescribed to alleviate the symptoms of anxiety disorders. One of the most popular drugs in human history, it is estimated that as many as 50,000,000 prescriptions a year are written for it.

The most common side effects of diazepam are clumsiness, drowsiness, and dizziness. This is because diazepam is classified as a sedative-hypnotic agent, one that depresses central nervous system arousal. Contrary to popular opinion, a "tranquilizer" does not necessarily allow a person to remain completely clearheaded. Thus persons taking diazepam should be careful when operating an automobile or other machinery.

The addictive potential of diazepam has been frequently discussed. Physiological dependence on the drug tends to be slight. Psychological dependence is often substantial. Thus withdrawal from the drug should be gradual and under medical or psychiatric supervision.

Users of diazepam are warned not to combine it with alcohol. The two drugs interact in such a way as to produce a very great sedation effect. The same is true when diazepam is combined with marijuana. On the other hand, diazepam is less effective when combined with cocaine or tobacco.

Although diazepam is a very useful drug, it is subject to abuse. It is available only by prescription and should be taken strictly in accordance with instructions.

See also *antianxiety drugs*; *drug therapy*.

Dilantin: A well-known trade name for the drug phenytoin.
See also *phenytoin*.

directive therapy: Therapy in which the therapist gives direct advice, guidance, instructions, or evaluations. The therapist accepts quite a bit of responsibility because he or she is willing to judge the patient's thoughts, emotions, and actions. For instance, certain ideas might be targeted as irrational or unrealistic. Examples of therapies that tend to be somewhat directive are cognitive therapy, rational-emotive therapy, and reality therapy.

Two traditional therapies that are *not* directive are psychoanalysis and client-centered therapy.

A therapist uses a directive approach under certain conditions. Two principal conditions are when the time available for therapy is brief and when the patient is emotionally immature.

See also *client-centered therapy*; *cognitive therapy*; *psychoanalysis*; *rational-emotive therapy*; *reality therapy*.

disaster syndrome: A set of pathological emotional and behavioral reactions experienced by the survivors of a disaster such as a flood, a tornado, an earthquake, a fire, being confined to a concentration camp, a boat sinking, or an airplane crash. A disaster can be divided into an impact period and a poststress period. During the *impact period*, the disaster is actually taking place, and its victims often become very bewildered, fearful, and excited. The *poststress* period follows the disaster, and many survivors suffer from nightmares, lack of joy in existence, impaired human relationships, fear of abrupt death, and a feeling that life has no meaning.

The general treatment of choice for disaster syndrome is psychotherapy, particularly a type of psychotherapy that focuses on questions revolving around the meaning of life. Logotherapy, developed by the psychiatrist Viktor Frankl, is an example of such a therapy.

See also *Frankl, Viktor*; *logotherapy*; *posttraumatic stress disorder (traumatic neurosis)*.

disorientation: A psychological state characterized by confusion. The disoriented person has lost his or her bearings and may be mixed up about time, place, events, or the self. For instance, the individual may think it is 5:00 A.M. when in fact it is 2:00 P.M. Disorientation is not a specific mental disorder but is a condition associated with various traumata, diseases, and disorders such as

Alzheimer's disease, intoxication, delirium tremens, concussion, emotional shock, and schizophrenic disorders.

See also *dementia*.

displacement: A defense mechanism in which the ego is protected by directing toward a second source an emotional reaction that correctly should have been directed toward a first source. The most common kind of displacement is *displacement of aggression*. For example, Stewart, owner of a business, is criticized by his wife during breakfast. He acts a bit grumpy but avoids a fight and confrontation. Later he gives an employee a tongue lashing for a minor error. The hostility that Stewart displays is clearly excessive in terms of the offense.

See also *ego defense mechanisms*.

dissociation: A pathological mental state in which given mental processes are isolated or cut off from the person's personality. The mental processes may have to do with memory, emotions, or identity. In dissociation, the processes acquire a sort of autonomy or life of their own. They "take over" and "run the show." For example, a person may "snap" and act out rage. Later, he or she says, "I wasn't myself. I don't know what came over me." Sometimes there is a loss of memory for the critical events, a kind of psychological blackout. In some instances the process of dissociation may be the central one in a given mental disorder.

See also *dissociative disorders*.

dissociative disorders: Disorders in which the usual integrity of memory, action, or personality is significantly disturbed. The principal dissociative disorders are psychogenic amnesia, fugue, multiple personality, and depersonalization disorder. Sleepwalking disorder, usually beginning in childhood, is also essentially a dissociative disorder.

See also *depersonalization disorder*; *fugue*; *multiple personality disorder*; *sleepwalking disorder (somnambulism)*.

distress: In general, any psychological or emotional state in which the person is experiencing worry, pressure, harassment, pain, or other suffering. In the context of stress research, Hans Selye made a distinction between two kinds of stress: eustress and distress. *Eustress* is "good" stress. It is the kind of stress we experience when we face an exciting challenge to our abilities. It is *distress* or "bad" stress that does organic and psychological damage.

See also *eustress*; *Selye, Hans*; *stress*.

disulfram: See *Antabuse*.

Dix, Dorothea Lynde (1802–1887): An early crusader in the fight to gain a generally more humane treatment for mental patients. When Dix began her battle against antiquated attitudes, mental patients were often treated somewhat like animals. For example, it was widely believed that people who were mad were unable to feel pain. Therefore it was considered justifiable to neglect to heat their quarters in the winter.

Dix visited many institutions such as almshouses and prisons and found that mentally ill persons were often randomly mixed in with poor persons and prisoners. She found conditions to be deplorable in general in all institutions and documented her findings by careful observation. The first official recognition of her work came when the state legislature of Massachusetts passed a bill designed to reduce adverse conditions in the Worcester State Lunatic Hospital.

In her long career as a reformer, Dix was directly responsible for both the improvement and construction of over 30 mental hospitals in the United States. She extended her work to Europe and was involved in reforms in countries ranging from Scotland to Italy. A needed mental hospital was built in Rome as a result of her intervention.

Dix also served as the Superintendent of Women Nurses during the Civil War.

See also *Beers, Clifford Whittingham*; *Pinel, Phillipe*.

dopamine: One of the neurotransmitters. Dopamine is of particular importance because of the dopamine hypothesis. The *dopamine hypothesis* states that one of the causal factors in schizophrenic disorders is excessive activity of dopamine. Excessive activity may be caused by overproduction of dopamine or hypersensitivity to dopamine by receptor neurons.

A substantial body of research supports the credibility of the dopamine hypothesis. For example, Parkinson's disease is associated with a deficiency of dopamine. And Parkinson's disease is almost never associated with a schizophrenic disorder. Also, physiological researchers have studied the neurons in the brains of deceased schizophrenic patients. And they have found direct evidence that there are more receptor sites for dopamine on such neurons than on the neurons of nonschizophrenic persons.

See also *neurotransmitters*; *Parkinson's disease*; *schizophrenia*.

double-bind communication: A communication pattern in which Person 1 creates an insolvable psychological problem for Person 2. No matter what Person 2 does, he or she cannot win. The anthropologist Gregory Bateson believed that such a communication pattern is a causal factor in schizophrenia. For example, a mother expresses to her daughter in both words and actions, "You're not a very affectionate child. You should love mother. You should be more demonstrative." When the daughter responds by moving emotionally toward the mother, the mother reacts, paradoxically, with cold and distant behavior. The daughter is bewildered and confused, particularly if these events are taking place during childhood.

Double-bind communications experienced in childhood are almost certainly not the principal causal villains in schizophrenia. But it is certainly reasonable to think of pathological communications as secondary, or contributing, causes.

See also *Laing, Ronald David*; *schizophrenia*; *transactional analysis*.

Down's syndrome: A set of related symptoms, both mental and organic, caused by an extra chromosome in the twenty-first pair (i.e., Trisomy 21). An older name for Down's syndrome was *mongolism* because the person with the syndrome has almond-shaped eyes and flattened features. Because of overtones of racial bias, the more neutral term *Down's syndrome* is the preferred one. The syndrome was originally studied by Langdon Down in the 1880s.

A principal feature of Down's syndrome is mental retardation. The range of retardation is usually from moderate to severe; this is an IQ range from about 20 to 49. The incidence of Down's syndrome is 1 in every 600 infants. This translates into somewhat over 400,000 people with the syndrome in the United States. It has long been known that the risk of having an infant with Down's syndrome increases with the mother's age. Contemporary studies also suggests the father's age may be a factor.

Children with Down's syndrome tend to respond well to instruction. They can learn to help themselves in many ways and often develop quite remarkable social skills. On the whole, they are affectionate and oriented toward people.

In addition to the almond-shaped eyes, a constellation of physical features are signs of Down's syndrome. These include short fingers, a fold of skin on the inner side of the eye, a very small amount of hair on the face and body, a large tongue, a short neck, and a curved little finger. Cataracts are common in children with Down's syndrome. The life expectancy for an infant with Down's syndrome is 16 years. Compare this with the general expectancy of 73 years, and one sees that Down's syndrome is associated with significant health problems.

Genetic counseling is one way to reduce the risk of having an infant with Down's syndrome. Another way is for parents to be relatively young. If an infant is born with the syndrome, treatment consists of good medical care, parental affection, and special training for retarded persons.

See also *genetic counseling*; *mental retardation*.

dream analysis: Any process by which an individual attempts to discover the meaning of a dream. Humankind has attempted to translate dreams since the dawn of history. The ancient Egyptians had an elaborate system of symbols with unique meanings. Using these symbols, it was presumably possible to decode the dream and discover its message.

A well-known kind of dream analysis is the one recommended by Freud in one of his most influential books, *The Interpretation of Dreams*, first published in 1900. Freud suggested that every dream contains an unconscious wish. This is called the *latent content* of the dream and is its true meaning. On the surface, there are a set of symbols. This set is called the *manifest content*, and it masks the true meaning. The aim of the masking is to aid the ego in repression of the wish. The reason the wish is repressed is because it represents something forbidden (i.e., an incest wish or an aggressive impulse toward a loved one). The unconscious wish is discovered in therapy through the technique of free association.

Although Freud's formulation is not accepted in its specific details by all therapists, many tend to favor its broad conceptual outline. There is a common assumption that dreams do signify something important about the person's concerns in life. And this is often cast in a sort of picture language that requires some sort of translation.

Jung used a method of dream analysis in which the patient was required to provide elaborations of the symbols in the dream. This can be done through creative imagination; one can write poems, stories, songs, and make drawings inspired by the dream. These amplifications may provide additional insights into the dream's basic message.

The purpose of dream analysis is therapeutic. It is assumed that greater self-understanding leads in the direction of greater mental health.

See also *free association*; *Freud, Sigmund*; *Jung, Carl Gustav*; *latent dream content*; *manifest dream content*.

drug addiction: A physiological or psychological dependence on a drug. In the case of physiological addiction, withdrawal from the drug will produce organic symptoms. Depending on the drug in question, examples of such symptoms are rapid heartbeat, changes in body temperature, perspiration, cramping of muscles, and changes in breathing rate. Such withdrawal symptoms are unpleasant, and, in some cases, extreme withdrawal symptoms may suggest a state of shock and danger of death.

In the case of psychological addiction, withdrawal from the drug will produce emotional reactions such as crying, anger, anxiety, and depression. Amphetamines, cocaine, marijuana, and lysergic acid diethylamide-25 (LSD) are habit-forming in the psychological sense. However, physiological withdrawal symptoms are often mild.

On the other hand, alcohol, barbiturates, opium, morphine, codeine, and heroin are very habit-forming in both the psychological *and* physiological sense.

It is important to make a clear distinction between drug use and drug abuse. Persons who experiment with drugs, even illegal ones, as a way of modifying moods cannot necessarily be classified as addicts. The term *addict* should only be used if the individual is (1) abusing and (2) dependent on a given drug. However, it should be noted that it is impossible to become an addict unless one is first a drug user. Thus drug use is the first step toward drug addiction.

It used to be believed that there is a characteristic addictive personality. There does not appear to be a single pattern. However, it can be asserted that individuals prone to anxiety and depression are at somewhat greater risk of becoming addicted to a drug. The same can be said of persons with extremely low self-esteem. However, these are very general statements, and their predictive power is low.

It is impossible to estimate the number of persons addicted to drugs in the United States because there are so many drugs available. And it must be remembered that some people are addicted to both legal drugs and prescription drugs. The popular picture of the addict as a "fiend" who breaks the law fits only a small percentage of addicted individuals. If one includes all types of drugs, even caffeine and nicotine, it is obvious that millions of persons are addicted to drugs.

Treatment for drug addiction involves many modalities: self-help groups (e.g., Alcoholics Anonymous), psychotherapy, drug therapy (e.g., methadone used as a substitute for a narcotic), and medical supervision. There is hope for people addicted to drugs. Many people have broken free from an addiction through a combination of desire and outside assistance.

See also *addiction*; *alcoholism*; *barbiturates*; *methadone*; *narcotic drugs*; *stimulants*.

drug therapy: In general, the use of drugs to treat any kind of organic or mental pathology. In the context of abnormal psychology, drug therapy refers to the use of drugs to treat mental disorders. In fact, psychiatry has undergone a drug revolution in the past two decades, and today a wide spectrum of prescription drugs are available to treat mental disorders. These tend to fall into distinct classes.

Antianxiety drugs or *minor tranquilizers* (e.g., diazepam) are used to treat anxiety disorders, tension, convulsive conditions, and insomnia.

Antipsychotic drugs or *major tranquilizers* (e.g., chlorpromazine) are used to treat the symptoms of psychotic disorders. They are of particular value in treating the delusions and hallucinations associated with schizophrenic disorders.

Antidepressant drugs (e.g., monamine oxidase inhibitors) are used to treat unipolar disorder and other depressive conditions.

There is a single *antimanic drug*. The generic name of this drug is *lithium carbonate*, and it is used to treat manic episodes associated with bipolar disorder.

Stimulants (e.g., amphetamines) are used to treat attention deficit disorder, narcolepsy, and obesity.

See also *antianxiety drugs*; *antidepressant drugs*; *major tranquilizers (antipsychotic drugs)*; *lithium carbonate*; *sedatives*; *stimulants*.

Durham rule: A legal rule put forth in 1954 that established a general principle stating that persons with mental disorders are not necessarily responsible when they break the law. Specifically, the rule states that "an accused is not criminally responsible if his unlawful act was the product of mental disease or mental defect."

The Durham rule has been augmented by an American Law Institute formulation adopted by courts in the District of Columbia in both 1966 and 1972. The new formulation sets forth the basic concept of the Durham rule in somewhat more precise language.

The important point is that the Durham rule and the American Law Institute formulation can be used by an accused to buttress an insanity defense.

See also *insanity defense*.

dyslexia: See *developmental reading disorder (dyslexia)*.

dysmorphophobia: See *body dysmorphic disorder (dysmorphophobia)*.

dyspareunia: A sexual difficulty characterized by pain during sexual intercourse. Although dyspareunia can affect either a male or a female, it is more common in females. Organic causes of dyspareunia include infections and abnormally formed sex organs. Psychological causes of dyspareunia in females include lack of lubrication due to insufficient arousal and a condition known as vaginismus.

See also *frigidity*; *sexual therapy*; *vaginismus*.

dysrhythmias: In the context of brain activity, irregular electroencephalographic patterns. Irregular, or abnormal, patterns sometimes are useful in diagnosing pathological conditions such as epilepsy, narcolepsy, and minimal brain dysfunction.

See also *brain waves*; *epilepsy*; *minimal brain dysfunction (MBD)*; *narcolepsy*.

dysthymic disorder (depressive neurosis): A mood disorder characterized primarily by depression. Secondary symptoms include sleeping problems, fatigue, loss of self-confidence, loss of interest in friends and family, and a generally negative outlook on life.

In the case of dysthymic disorder, the depression does not stem from an obvious organic cause. Instead, it seems to be caused by primarily psychological factors such as emotional conflict and personal loss. (For a discussion of the causes of depression, see its entry.)

The treatment of choice for dysthymic disorder is psychotherapy, particularly one that orients the individual toward modifying the kinds of thoughts that produce depression. Examples of such therapies are cognitive therapy and rational-emotive therapy.

See also *cognitive therapy*; *depression*; *rational-emotive therapy*.

E

eating disorders: A set of related disorders distinguished by abnormal eating behavior. There are four principal eating disorders.

Anorexia nervosa is characterized by a fear of becoming fat and a tendency toward self-imposed eating restrictions.

Bulimia nervosa is characterized by binges and purges.

Pica is characterized by the eating of substances without nutritional value such as clay or paint.

Rumination disorder of infancy is characterized by bringing back into the mouth previously swallowed food.

These disorders can have quite serious consequences such as biochemical imbalances, emaciation from undereating, obesity from overeating, and death from self-imposed starvation.

Eating disorders are usually treated with psychotherapy. In the case of adolescents and adults, the approach is usually two-pronged. First, the individual is helped to understand *why* he or she abuses food. Second, the individual is aided with behavior modification strategies revealing *how* eating behavior can become more normal. Infants and children are helped primarily with behavior therapy.

See also *anorexia nervosa*; *bulimia nervosa*; *compulsive eating*; *obesity*; *pica*; *rumination disorder of infancy*.

echolalia: A tendency of one person to repeat portions of the statements of a second person. Thus the first person "echoes" the second person. Repetitions are sometimes described as *parrotlike*, suggesting that they are meaningless imitation. A nurse says to a patient, "I just received a phone call from your mother. She is going to come and visit you this afternoon." And the patient says, in a seemingly mocking voice, "Come and visit, come and visit." No sensible response is given to the nurse's comment.

In some cases, echolalia can be caused by a neurological defect. Echolalia sometimes appears in cases where the individual is suffering from an organic mental syndrome. However, in other cases, it is probably due to the lowering of functional intelligence associated with such mental disorders as autistic disorder and schizophrenic disorders.

See also *autistic disorder (infantile autism)*; *organic mental syndromes (organic brain syndromes)*; *schizophrenia*.

echopraxia: A tendency of one person to mimic or copy the movements of a second person in a meaningless or reptitive fashion. This behavior is sometimes observed in schizophrenic disorders of the catatonic type.

See also *schizophrenia*.

ego: The "I" of the personality. (The Latin word for *I* is *ego*.) In psychoanalytic theory, the ego is one of the three principal parts of the personality; the other two are the id and the superego. The ego was conceptualized by Freud as reality-oriented. It is the ego that takes on the difficult task of mediating differences between the emotional demands of the id and the moralistic supervision of the superego. When the ego is not up to its job, when there is inadequate ego strength, symptoms of mental disorders may appear.

Sometimes the word *ego* is used as a synonym for the word *self*. Although this usage is common, it blurs the conceptual distinction between the ego and the whole personality. It is probably best to say that the ego is the *conscious self*. This suggests that the ego is at the center of the personality and that the whole self revolves around it.

The term *ego* is often used as a prefix, and, immediately following this entry, there are seven entries where this is the case. See also *Freud, Sigmund*; *id*; *psychoanalysis*; *superego*.

egocentric: A way of orienting toward the external world such that it seems to revolve around one's ego. A person with an egocentric attitude tends to see the whole world, including other people, revolving around him or her. The general viewpoint underlying an egocentric orientation is called *egocentrism*.

Egocentrism is not to be confused with *egotism*, a tendency toward boastfulness, conceit, and self-preoccupation. A preschool child, for example, can be egocentric without being egotistical.

It is, indeed, natural for children between the ages of about 2 and 7 to be egocentric. They perceive themselves as being at the center of the universe, and it is very difficult for them to imagine any viewpoint but their own. This natural orientation was described by Jean Piaget (1896–1980), a scientist who made extensive studies of how children think.

When an adult displays an excessive amount of egocentrism, it is considered pathological. Egocentrism is a component in many mental disorders including organic mental disorders, paranoid disorders, schizophrenic disorders, and personality disorders. Very troubled persons often have a very constricted view of existence in which only they and their problems seem to exist.

ego defense mechanisms: A set of involuntary psychological processes that protect the individual against the harsher aspects of reality. Defense mechanisms, arranged unconsciously by the ego, provide a buffer between unpleasant facts and threats to the integrity of the personality.

Defense mechanisms play a significant role in psychoanalytic theory. If used to a moderate degree, they are seen as normal and useful in maintaining the health of the personality. If they are used excessively, they contribute to neurotic tendencies and personality disorders. If they stop functioning, the person is left without protection, and there may be a collapse of the personality. Schizophrenic disorders can be conceptualized in this way.

The ego defense mechanisms were first identified and described by Freud. Later they were studied more extensively by his daughter, Anna Freud.

See also *fantasy*; *Freud, Sigmund*; *narcissism*; *projection*; *rationalization*; *reaction formation*; *regression*; *repression*; *sublimation*.

ego-dystonic homosexuality: See *homosexuality*.

ego ideal: An aspect of the superego that sets for the individual a level of aspiration. The ego ideal points the person in the direction of the future and paints a fantasy picture of what life can become if certain efforts are made. In our culture, a young person who dreams of becoming well-educated with an honorable vocation may be thought of as having a high ego ideal.

In psychoanalytic theory, the ego ideal is seen as coming primarily from the wishes and dreams of a child's parents. These wishes and dreams often become a part of the child's personality.

An individual's natural tendencies may be at odds with the ego ideal. If so, an emotional conflict may result. And this can be a basis for personal distress. (Natural tendencies are represented by Maslow's concept of *self-actualization*.)

See also *conscience*; *Maslow, Abraham Harold*; *self-actualization*; *superego*.

ego psychology: In general, an approach to psychology that focuses on the functions of the ego. These include will, memory, perception, language, and other mental processes that orient us toward reality. In psychoanalytic theory, stressing the importance of the role that the ego plays in adjustment and personal growth.

ego strength: In psychoanalytic theory, an ego that is able to avail itself of ample amounts of psychological energy (i.e., libido) is one with strength. Thus individuals who have ego strength are able to make decisions fairly readily, act on their dreams, and, on the whole, function effectively. Individuals who lack ego strength are often immobilized, insecure, or unable to move forward in life.

The terms *strong ego* and *weak ego* are sometimes used to suggest differences in ego strength.

See also *ego*; *libido*.

ego-syntonic homosexuality: See *homosexuality*.

ejaculatory incompetence: See *inhibited male orgasm (ejaculatory incompetence or retarded ejaculation)*.

Electra complex: Another name for the *Oedipus complex*. The term *Electra complex* is sometimes used when this particular complex refers to females. However, it is correct to use the single term *Oedipus complex* when referring to either males or females.

The name *Electra complex* is derived from an ancient Greek tragedy by Sophocles in which Electra urges her brother to kill their mother.

See also *Oedipus complex*.

electroconvulsive therapy (ECT): A kind of somatic therapy in which a brief, low-intensity electrical current is passed through the frontal part of the brain. (This kind of therapy is also sometimes called *electroshock therapy*.) The current induces a seizure that is similar to the kind associated with grand mal epilepsy.

ECT was introduced in 1937 by two Italian psychiatrists, Ugo Cerletti and Lucia Bini. For many years, ECT was used to treat all types of psychotic disorders, including schizophrenic ones. Today, however, its principal value appears to be in the treatment of major depression.

The reason that ECT is sometimes a useful therapy for depression is that it stimulates the central nervous system to produce greater quantities of the neurotransmitter norepinephrine. It has been shown that norepinephrine levels are often below normal in severely depressed individuals.

A great deal of controversy surrounds the use of ECT. Advocates say that it is one of the best treatments for depression, that it has few side effects, that it is obviously not habit forming, and that it does almost no long-term damage to the nervous system. Opponents say that it is inhumane, that it does significant damage to the brain's cortex, and that it impairs memory. Perhaps because of the controversy, the use of ECT has diminished. Nonetheless, it is still a treatment that exists and is sometimes prescribed.

See also *grand mal epilepsy*; *major depression (unipolar disorder)*; *norepinephrine (noradrenalin)*; *somatic therapy*.

electroencephalogram (EEG): A record over a given time period of changing electrical potentials in the brain. The art and science of making such a record is known as *encephalography*. Electrodes attached to the skull pick up weak signals from neurons as they depolarize (i.e., "fire"). The signals are amplified greatly in order to make the recording. An EEG is helpful in making a diagnosis of nervous system pathology such as epilepsy or minimal brain damage.

See also *brain waves*.

Ellis, Albert (1913–): The principal founder of rational-emotive therapy. Ellis is a New York psychotherapist and received his early training in the psychoanalytic mold. When he began to practice psychotherapy, he found himself discontent with the slow pace of therapy and the tendency of the analytic method to focus on the past. Ellis recognized that the important thing was change and the principal function of therapy was to dislodge the patient from old and ineffective ways of coping with life.

Ellis discovered that the conscious level of the personality provided much readier access than did the unconscious level. He could work directly with a patient's conscious thoughts. Thus Ellis began to encourage patients to examine their conscious thoughts, root out their irrational elements, and make a systematic effort to think more clearly.

Ellis has made a sustained effort over the years to bring rational-emotive therapy to the attention of psychotherapists, and he has succeeded. Today it is recognized as an important treatment approach.

Ellis has written a number of books. One of the best introductions to his general line of reasoning is *A New Guide to Rational Living* (1976) by Ellis and Robert A. Harper.

See also *cognitive-behavior therapy*; *cognitive therapy*; *rational-emotive therapy*.

Ellis, Henry Havelock (1859–1939): An English author and pioneer sexologist. Ellis explored sexual behavior from the biological, psychological, and anthropological aspects. Great Britain has the reputation of having been sexually very strait-laced during the reign of Queen Victoria (1819–1901). Ellis was working toward the end of, and shortly after, the Victorian period. Therefore his work is seen as a breakthrough, an early attempt to view sexual behavior in scientific terms.

Studies in the Psychology of Sex was published in seven volumes over a period of time ranging from 1897 to 1928 and helped to make the study of such subjects as reproduction, love, and eroticism respectable.

Ellis is also noted for investigations into the meaning of dreams and states of consciousness.

See also *Krafft-Ebing, Richard von*; *paraphilias*; *sexual deviations*; *sexual disorders (psychosexual disorders)*; *sexual therapy*.

emotion: A positive or negative change in physiological arousal accompanied by the perception that the change is either pleasant or unpleasant. As the definition indicates, there are two dimensions to an emotion. The first dimension is the *arousal* dimension. The extreme ends of this dimension are *excitement* and *calm*. The second dimension is the *hedonic tone* dimension. The extreme ends of this dimension are *pleasant* and *unpleasant*. Thus every emotion, or emotional state, is some combination of points on these two dimensions. *Anger* represents a high level of excitement combined with an unpleasant sensation. *Ecstasy* represents a high level of excitement combined with a pleasant sensation. *Depression* represents a low level of arousal with an unpleasant sensation. And *tranquillity* represents a low level of arousal with a pleasant sensation. Similar statements can be made about other emotions such as fear, anxiety, and so forth.

Human beings seem to be so constituted that life without emotions is meaningless. Most people would be loath to give up such experiences as joy and love. However, a price must be paid. We laugh and sing. But we also mourn and wail.

An important concept in abnormal psychology is *emotional conflict* in which two emotions are at odds. Thus is it possible to feel both hostility and affection toward the same person. Mental health problems can follow if the antagonistic feelings are intense and difficult to resolve.

See also *emotional blunting*; *emotional insulation*.

emotional blunting: An emotional reaction of low and inappropriate intensity. For example, Naomi, a woman suffering from a schizophrenic disorder receives the news that her mother is very ill. She says in a flat tone of voice, "That's too bad. Well, that's life. Do you think we're going to have spaghetti for dinner tonight? I like it a lot."

emotional disorders: Another term for mood disorders.
See also *mood disorders (affective disorders)*.

emotional insulation: An ego defense mechanism characterized by withdrawal and a lack of ability to experience a given emotion. For example, Theodore's father dies suddenly and tragically. Father and son were very close. In the days following the death, Theodore is dry-eyed and amazingly free of depression or grief.

He is almost certainly repressing these emotions at the moment because they are associated with almost unbearable pain. It is quite possible that he will be able to cry and experience grief after a time period has elapsed.

empathy: Having a sensitive appreciation for the thoughts, attitudes, and feelings of another person. The informal phrase "being on the same wavelength" captures the idea of empathy.

According to Carl Rogers, the ability to establish empathic communication is one of the arts and skills of an effective psychotherapist. It is important that the client, the troubled person, feel that the therapist has a deep understanding of his or her world of experience.

See also *client-centered therapy*; *Rogers, Carl Ransom*.

encephalitis: An inflammation of either the brain or the thin tissue covering it. (Popular names for encephalitis are *sleeping sickness* and *brain fever*.) Common causes of the condition include bacterial infections, viral infections, and the action of parasites. Encephalitis sometimes results in association with mumps, smallpox, and measles.

Early symptoms of encephalitis are lethargy and drowsiness. Treatment consists of medical care for the infection. After recovery from the condition itself, there is often some neurological damage. This can produce significant changes in the individual's thought and behavior, often of a pathological nature.

See also *brain pathology*.

encopresis: Involuntary expulsion of fecal bulk. The term is usually used to describe the behavior of children who have not learned either adequate or appropriate control of their bowel movements. For example, a 4-year-old child who defecates while sleeping or playing with friends may be said to be suffering from encopresis.

Organic encopresis has a biological basis and requires medical treatment. *Functional encopresis* has an emotional or psychological basis and is the type discussed next.

Causal factors include inadequate toilet-training procedures and hostility toward the parents. The problem of encopresis is similar in nature to the problem of enuresis. Treatment consists of psychotherapy aimed at helping the child resolve emotional conflicts. This is combined with training procedures designed to help the child gain greater voluntary control of the anal sphincter.

See also *enuresis*.

encounter group: A group that meets with the principal aim of fostering human potential. The word *encounter* is used to suggest a real meeting of selves at a profound level in contrast to a social meeting at a superficial level. Thus, in encounter groups, people talk about their hopes, their fears, the meaning of life, their sexual attitudes, their talents, and so forth. The group interaction is intended to foster self-actualization.

The encounter group movement reached its zenith in the 1960s when there were many growth centers. Now the movement has lost its vogue. Nonetheless, encounter groups still exist and can be found in many settings including schools, clubs, university extension classes, and churches.

It is important to recognize that the activity of an encounter group is not the same process as group therapy. Group therapy is aimed at helping distressed people experience relief from their depression, anxiety, or maladaptive behavior patterns. Encounter groups assume that the person is, on the whole, well. The purpose is to achieve high-level wellness as opposed to just getting by, or just existing.

See also *group therapy*; *Maslow, Abraham Harold*; *self-actualization*.

endocrine system: An interacting set of ductless glands that secrete hormones directly into the bloodstream. Hormones can have a profound effect on emotions and actions. Therefore, a knowledge of the endocrine system contributes to an understanding of human behavior, including behavioral pathology.

Principal glands affecting emotions and behavior are the pineal, the pituitary, the thyroid, the adrenals, the pancreas, and the gonads.

The *pineal gland* regulates circadian rhythms such as the sleep and menstrual cycles. It is involved in such reactions as jet lag and premenstrual syndrome.

The *pituitary gland* is the master gland of the body. It regulates growth and sends messenger hormones to other endocrine glands. During stressful periods, it activates the adrenal glands to secrete their hormones.

The *thyroid gland* regulates metabolism. A sluggish thyroid gland can contribute to feelings of apathy or depression.

The *adrenal glands* play an important role in the body's capacity to handle stress.

The *pancreas gland* secretes insulin and is important in the regulation of blood sugar. Chronic low blood sugar (i.e., hypoglycemia) can contribute to feelings of fatigue, anxiety, and depression.

The *gonads* secrete hormones that stimulate sexual drive. These hormones also are involved in the development of secondary sexual characteristics such as a beard in males and breasts in females.

An individual suspecting that he or she is suffering from a problem caused by the incorrect functioning of an endocrine gland should consult a physician specializing in the treatment of such conditions, an *endocrinologist*.

See also *adrenal glands*; *gonads*; *hypoglycemia*; *premenstrual syndrome (PMS)*.

endogenous depression: Depression that originates from an internal source. The source can be biological such as a deficiency of the neurotransmitter norepinephrine. Or the source can be psychological such as an emotional conflict.

See also *depression; exogenous depression*.

endorphins: Naturally occurring morphinelike substances with the capacity to relieve pain. (The word *endorphin* is a contraction of the two words *endogenous* and *morphine*.) The brain and the pituitary gland appear to produce endorphins in response to fear, anxiety, exercise, and challenging situations. They help us to cope with psychosocial stressors. Research suggests that endorphins belong to the general class *neurotransmitters*.

It is possible that the *placebo effect*, the capacity of an inert substance or a sham treatment to relieve pain, may be in part due to the capacity of a placebo to induce increased endorphin production.

Within limits, the kind of moderate stress induced by a challenging vocation, exercise, and novel experiences (i.e., eustress) can help the body to produce optimal levels of endorphins. These optimal levels help a person maintain a sense of well-being and emotional health.

See also *eustress*; *neurotransmitters*; *placebo effect*.

enuresis: A disorder characterized by the uncontrolled release of urine. It is possible to discriminate organic enuresis from functional enuresis. *Organic enuresis* is due to pathology at a biological level and requires medical treatment. *Functional enuresis* is basically psychological in nature and is the type that is discussed next.

If enuresis occurs in the day, it is known as *diurnal enuresis*. If enuresis takes place during sleep, it is known as *nocturnal enuresis* and is the most common kind. Nocturnal enuresis usually takes place during deep sleep. (The popular term for nocturnal enuresis is *bed-wetting*.)

Enuresis is more common in children than in adults. About 7% of boys and 3% of girls 5 years of age suffer from the disorder. In adults, functional enuresis is very rare.

The disorder tends to run in families. Thus it is possible to hypothesize the existence of at least some genetic predisposition toward it. Research with identical twins tends to support this hypothesis. On the other hand, emotional factors and maladaptive habits also appear to be causative. For example, unconscious hostility toward a parent may aggravate the condition.

Several modes of treatment exist for enuresis. The antidepressant drug imipramine sometimes relieves symptoms. Psychotherapy aimed at helping a child resolve emotional conflicts can be of value. A pad that is wired to sound a bell when the pad is wet with urine has been found to be very useful. The pad–bell method is based on conditioning principles and was developed by O. Hobart Mowrer, a former president of the American Psychological Association.

See also *encopresis*.

epilepsy: A disorder in which pathological functioning of the brain causes a variety of symptoms such as seizures, odd actions, and altered states of consciousness. It is a neurologic disorder, not a mental one. About 1,500,000 people in the United States suffer from epilepsy. General causes of epilepsy include damage to the brain and nervous system at time of birth, the toxic effects of alcohol or other drugs, head wounds, infections of the central nervous system, and tumors in the brain. However, the cause of epilepsy in a given individual is often obscure. In *idiopathic epilepsy*, there is no distinct organic basis for the symptoms. In *symptomatic epilepsy*, there is an identifiable organic brain pathology. Only 25% of cases fall in this category.

Perhaps because of its capacity to produce altered states of consciousness, epilepsy has, in folklore, been called a "gift from the gods." The great writer Fyodor Dostoevsky, author of *Crime and Punishment* and *The Brothers Karamozov*, suffered from epilepsy and may have been inspired by ideas generated in association with his convulsive seizures. However, epilepsy is no gift from the gods. It is a pathological condition, distressing to both the individual and his or her family, and one that requires treatment.

In addition to the distinction made previously between idiopathic and symptomatic epilepsy, four basic kinds of epilepsy are identified: grand mal, petit mal, Jacksonian, and psychomotor.

Grand mal (major) epilepsy is characterized by severe convulsive seizures.

Petit mal (minor) epilepsy is characterized by a lapse in consciousness. The individual seems to be unaware of what is happening or seems somewhat confused. This state is termed a *nonconvulsive seizure*. Petit mal epilepsy is more likely to affect children than adults.

Jacksonian epilepsy is characterized by involuntary movements of the body such as twitches and spasms without the loss of consciousness. Jacksonian epilepsy was identified and described by J. Hughlings Jackson (1835–1911), a neurologist.

Psychomotor epilepsy is characterized by actions that do not seem to fit the individual's normal personality. (This kind of epilepsy is also called *temporal-lobe epilepsy*.) A usually soft-spoken person may become loud and aggressive. Or an individual may begin to laugh uncontrollably without apparent cause.

(It should be noted that *narcolepsy*, a tendency to fall suddenly and involuntarily asleep, is not usually listed as a form of epilepsy.)

In most cases, epilepsy is incurable. However, it is treatable and controllable with anticonvulsant medication. With adequate medical supervision, the life of a person suffering from epilepsy can be free, or almost free, from seizures. Depending on a given state's laws, persons with epilepsy who have been free of symptoms for a given time period are eligible for a driver's license.

See also *brain waves*; *electroencephalogram (EEG)*; *grand mal epilepsy*; *narcolepsy*; *neurology*.

epinephrine: A hormone produced by the medulla of an adrenal gland. (Epinephrine is also known as *adrenalin*, but this is not the preferred term.) Epinephrine helps the body to prepare for action.
See also *adrenal glands*.

erectile disorder (erectile insufficiency): A type of sexual dysfunction in which the male is either unable to attain an erection or sustain one adequate for sexual intercourse. (Erectile disorder is also more popularly known as *impotence*, which suggests lack of power. However, this is an older, no longer preferred, term.)

A distinction is sometimes made between primary and secondary erectile dysfunctions. A *primary* dysfunction suggests the male has never had an erection adequate for sexual intercourse. A *secondary* dysfunction suggests that he has had an erection adequate for intercourse at least once.

Causes of erectile disorder can be either biological or psychological. Among biological causes are blockage of penile arteries, neurological problems, and side effects of antihypertensive medication. Among psychological causes are repressed hostility toward the partner, lack of appropriate responses from the partner, underlying depression, anxiety over ability to perform adequately, and an Oedipus complex.

Erectile disorder is a common problem, and it is correlated to some extent with age. For men in their 30's, the incidence of the problem is only 2%. For men in their 50's, the incidence is 10%. For men in their 70's, the incidence is 50%.

Medical treatment often helps the male who suffers from erectile disorder for biological reasons. Psychotherapy, including sexual therapy, can often be useful in helping the individual who suffers from erectile disorder for psychological reasons.

See also *impotence*; *Oedipus complex*; *sexual disorders (psychosexual disorders)*; *sexual therapy*.

Erikson, Erik Homburger (1902–): Developed the concept of psychosocial stages as a logical extension of Freud's psychosexual stages. Erikson was born in Germany, studied under Freud, became a psychoanalyst, emigrated to the United States, and did research in association with Harvard University.

Erikson's investigations suggest that we move through eight stages of development from birth to death. The first stage is trust versus mistrust, and the last is ego integrity versus despair. Each stage presents a developmental task, and life challenges us to develop the positive attribute associated with the stage (e.g., trust or ego integrity).

It was Erikson who coined the now-famous term *identity crisis*. An identity crisis is associated with the fifth stage of psychosocial development, identity versus role confusion.

Erikson's work has done much to further our understanding of the causal factors involved in the formation of both the healthy and the pathological personality. Two of Erikson's books are *Childhood and Society* (1963) and *Identity: Youth and Crisis* (1968).

See also *Freud, Sigmund*; *identity crisis*; *psychosexual development*.

erogenous zones: Regions of the body that are particularly involved in the induction of sexual excitement. The name is derived from Eros, the Greek god of love. The three principal erogenous zones are the oral, anal, and phallic. The focus of the phallic zone in women is the clitoris, and, in men, it is the penis.

Freud placed great emphasis on the role played by the erogenous zones in psychosexual development.

See also *clitoris*; *psychosexual development*.

essential hypertension: Chronic high blood pressure lacking a clear-cut organic basis. The unadorned term *hypertension* can suggest high blood pressure due to either organic or functional causes. Although high blood pressure can be caused by known organic conditions such as atherosclerosis, tumors on an adrenal gland, and kidney disease, the vast majority of hypertension does not fall into this category. Essential hypertension is much more common. A very common disorder, about 5% of adults suffer from hypertension. It is called the "silent killer" because its symptoms often go unnoticed. For this reason, all adults should have their blood pressure checked with some frequency.

Hypertension, whatever the origin, is a complicating factor in cerebrovascular accidents (i.e., strokes), heart attacks, kidney disease, and other diseases.

Essential hypertension can be classified as a psychophysiologic, or psychosomatic, disease. Psychological factors such as emotional conflicts, psychosocial stressors, or Type A behavior seem to induce the disease.

Treatment of essential hypertension can be with antihypertensive drugs, psychotherapy, or both in combination. Treatment is usually effective and can be life-saving.

See also *psychosomatic disorders; Type A behavior.*

estrogens: A set of hormones produced primarily by the ovaries. Estrogens are also produced by the adrenal glands. Although estrogen production is usually identified with the female, in the male, a modest amount is produced by the testes.

Sexual maturation is to some degree regulated by estrogen production. After puberty, estrogen levels increase, and the female develops mature genital organs and breasts. Estrogens also dictate that body fat in the adult female be deposited on a different basis than in the child. These alterations in the form and appearance of the adult are called *secondary sexual characteristics.* (*Primary sexual characteristics* are, of course, present at birth, allowing for the distinction of males from females.)

Sexual drive in females is to some degree mediated by estrogen levels. When levels are high, just prior to ovulation, there is a tendency for desire to also be high. This helps increase the likelihood of impregnation. However, it should be noted that sexual behavior is complex and is certainly affected by psychological factors as well.

Estrogen levels also seem to have some effect on mood and temperament. Irregularities in estrogens may play a role in conditions such as premenstrual syndrome.

See also *endocrine system*; *gonads*; *premenstrual syndrome (PMS).*

etiology: The study of the causes, reasons, or explanations of a given event. In the context of abnormal psychology, the study of the causes of mental disorders. Etiology can be general or specific. Research can be done, for example, to find the general causes of schizophrenic disorders. Or the case history of a particular patient can be taken in an effort to explore the unique reasons he or she has developed a schizophrenic disorder. The same is true of all mental disorders and pathological conditions.

See also *biomedical viewpoint*; *diathesis-stress viewpoint*; *psychogenic viewpoint*.

euphoria: An emotional state characterized by a high level of arousal and extremely pleasant sensations. When one is *euphoric*, one feels very good, "on top of the world." Euphoria is often produced by specific experiences such as seeing an old friend, attaining an important goal, hearing a certain song, looking at a sunset, or having an orgasm. Abraham Maslow referred to such experiences as *peak experiences* and believed they contributed to mental health.

On the other hand, euphoria can be pathological. When it is seen in association with the manic phase of a bipolar disorder, it does not "ring true." It seems to be a sham euphoria in contrast to an authentic euphoria. And it is expected that the individual will subsequently pay a price in the form of depression.

See also *bipolar disorder*; *Maslow, Abraham Harold*; *peak experience*.

eustress: Stress with positive qualities. Eustress is "good" stress. It is experienced as a challenge and contributes to a sense of well-being and mental health. Examples of situations that might produce eustress for some individuals are running in a race, passing a difficult examination, making a sale, getting married, taking a moderate risk, and so forth.

The stress researcher Hans Selye distinguished between distress (i.e., stress with negative qualities) and eustress. He noted that eustress adds zest to life, suggesting that not all stress is to be avoided.

See also *distress*; *Selye, Hans*; *stress*.

exhibitionism: A sexual disorder characterized by male self-exposure of the genitals to an unknown female. A desire to shock and surprise are often elements of the act, and no attempt is made at sexual intercourse. However, the individual suffering from exhibitionism does obtain sexual excitement. Sometimes he masturbates while engaged in self-display. Exhibitionism is most common in young adults.

General causal factors in exhibitionism may include a poor masculine self-image, hostility toward females, erectile insufficiency, and fixations of libido at the phallic stage.

The usual treatment for exhibitionism is psychotherapy. However, the condition is frequently very resistant to change, and the course of psychotherapy is often very slow and difficult. Sometimes antiandrogenic drugs (i.e., drugs that lower sexual arousal) are prescribed. However, this approach is considered to be a last resort.

See also *sexual disorders (psychosexual disorders)*.

existential neurosis: A condition characterized by such feelings as chronic anxiety, depression, demoralization, and emptiness revolving around questions concerning the nature of life and being. Although not listed as a formal mental disorder in either the American Psychiatric Association's *Diagnostic and Statistical Manual of Mental Disorders* or the World Health Organization's *International Classification of Diseases*, existential neurosis is widely recognized by psychotherapists as a common problem.

The concept of an existential neurosis is derived from the tradition of existentialism on the European continent. *Existentialism* is the point of view that the starting point for explaining being and consciousness is the inner world of experience, not the outer world of facts. Some key figures in the history of existentialism are the philosophers Søren Kierkegaard, Martin Heidegger, and Jean-Paul Sartre.

Examples of existential questions are: Who am I? Where am I going? What is the meaning of life? What is the meaning of *my* life? Although it is normal to ask, and attempt to answer such questions, sometimes the individual feels unable to respond adequately to the challenge they offer. Then the anxiety and other mood states associated with the questions become exaggerated, and an existential neurosis exists.

An existential neurosis can be a very serious condition and is sometimes a factor in suicidal impulses. Fortunately, the condition is treatable with existential therapy.

See also *existential therapy*.

existential therapy: An approach to therapy that focuses on the nature of one's unique life as it is both lived and experienced. The therapist helps the individual resolve *existential questions*, questions pertaining to one's identity and the meaning of life. It is not the therapist's aim to present ready-made answers to such questions. However, a therapist can help a troubled person discover personal answers through in-depth discussions.

Two of the most well-known kinds of existential therapy are Daseinsanalysis and logotherapy. *Daseinsanalysis* was developed by the European psychiatrist Ludwig Binswanger and is inspired by the work of the German philosopher Martin Heidegger. In Heidegger's philosophy, the concept of Dasein plays a significant role. Dasein is usually translated as Being-in-the-world. It is how each individual experiences the world in light of his or her own unique consciousness. The point is that one's Being-in-the-world can seem marvelous and full of opportunities. Or it can seem to be empty and constricted. The Daseinsanalyst helps the individual explore possibilities and open doors to a richer psychological world.

Logotherapy was developed by the Austrian psychiatrist Viktor Frankl and is discussed elsewhere in this encyclopedia.

There are other approaches to therapy that might be broadly classified as existential in tone. Client-centered therapy, Gestalt therapy, and individual psychology all fit in this category.

See also *client-centered therapy*; *Frankl, Viktor*; *Gestalt therapy*; *individual psychology*; *logotherapy*.

exogenous depression: Depression that originates from an external source. Psychosocial stressors, including negative life changes, are the principal external sources. Examples are death of a loved one, divorce, the end of a romantic relationship, the loss of a job, and so forth. Exogenous depression is sometimes called *reactive depression* to suggest that it exists in response to a real situation.

Exogenous depression is a natural reaction to loss and is not in and of itself pathological. However, if the individual has a tendency toward endogenous depression, this tendency can interact with exogenous depression and greatly increase its severity.

See also *depression*; *endogenous depression*; *life change units (LCUs)*; *psychosocial stressors*.

exorcism: A ritual involving prayers and incantations designed to cast out demons or other evil spirits. Exorcisms are used by a number of religions. They are also used by *shamans*, tribal medicine men or magicians in underdeveloped countries. Although contemporary clinical psychology and psychiatry tend to reject demon possession as an objective explanation of mental disorders, it is widely recognized that the *belief* in evil spirits can aggravate behavior pathology. Therefore, mental health professionals usually seek to work *with* the practitioners of exorcism, not against them.

See also *demonology*.

experimental neurosis: In the framework of the research on conditioning conducted by Ivan Pavlov, an experimental neurosis is a state of great agitation and confusion caused by the inability of a dog to make a meaningful choice between two similar stimuli. Pavlov taught dogs to discriminate between a circle and an ellipse. When this discrimination was established, he gradually made the ellipse more and more circular. At a certain point the dogs began to howl, urinate, and stopped giving predictable responses. They resisted being returned to the experiment on subsequent days. These were dogs that had previously been docile and stable, quite capable of learning.

The important point about an experimental neurosis is that it demonstrates that a pathological condition in an organism can be induced by experience alone. Biological pathology (e.g., a genetic predisposition, biochemical imbalances, a brain tumor) does not need to be present. This suggests, of course, that human neurosis, and other behavioral disorders, may often be caused primarily by psychological factors, not biological ones.

See also *classical conditioning*; *neurosis*; *Pavlov, Ivan Petrovich*.

explosive disorder: See *intermittent explosive disorder (explosive disorder)*.

extinction: The process by which the frequency of a given category of behavior is reduced. Informally, it can be thought of as the unlearning, or breaking of, a habit. There are various ways to bring about extinction. Two of the most reliable ways are withholding reinforcement and counterconditioning. (A reinforcer is similar but not identical to a reward.)

Extinction is an important concept in behavior therapy because it is the avenue by which the troubled person is helped to give up maladaptive behavior. Systematic desensitization, for example, is a counterconditioning procedure designed to facilitate extinction of useless anxiety. Much of our contemporary understanding of extinction is derived from the original work of Ivan Pavlov with classical conditioning and B. F. Skinner with operant conditioning.

See also *classical conditioning*; *counterconditioning*; *desensitization therapy*; *operant conditioning*; *Pavlov, Ivan Petrovich*; *Skinner, Burrhus Frederic*.

extraversion: As originally conceived by Carl Jung, an attitude characterized by the flow of libido, or psychological energy, toward the outer world. Thus it is through the attitude of extraversion that we are interested in meeting people, learning how things work, and exploring the environment. The opposite attitude is *introversion*.

Both attitudes coexist in most people. However, there is often a tendency for one attitude to be dominant. Thus if extraversion is dominant, the individual is sometimes called an *extravert*.

Descriptively, the extravert tends to meet people easily, is inclined to action, and is not particularly interested in passive thinking.

Pathology of the personality exists when (1) one of the attitudes almost completely eclipses the other one and (2) the individual is unstable. Thus a person who is highly extraverted and simultaneously unstable could be described with words such as *touchy, aggressive, excitable,* and *changeable.* The approach being described here was developed by the research psychologist Hans J. Eysenck.

See also *Eysenck, Hans Jurgen; introversion; Jung, Carl Gustav; libido.*

Eysenck, Hans Jurgen (1916–): Experimental psychologist known for his investigations into the structure of personality and for his contributions to behavior therapy. Eysenck was born in Germany, received his doctorate from the University of London, and works in England.

One of Eysenck's important areas of investigation has been to relate Jung's concepts of extraversion and introversion to the general concept of emotional stability.

Eysenck was an early critic of the effectiveness of Freudian psychoanalysis. His investigations suggested that psychoanalysis was often of dubious value for personal problems and that the criteria used to evaluate improvement of patients were not sufficiently objective.

Eysenck suggests that behavior therapy is more effective than psychoanalysis because behavior therapy has well-defined objectives, employs clearly defined principles of learning, tends to be brief in duration, and offers objective criteria useful in evaluating the outcome of therapy.

See also *behavior therapy; extraversion; introversion.*

F

fabrication: As a sign of behavioral pathology, a story or falsehood made up by a troubled person. The aim of the fabrication can be to rationalize illogical behavior, to make sense of events, to fill in gaps, to maintain self-esteem, and so forth. As suggested here, the principal purpose is not to deceive others. Indeed, usually the patient is not fully aware that he or she is fabricating. Patients with organic problems are more likely to fabricate than are other patients.

Fabrication and *confabulation* are essentially synonyms.

See also *confabulation*; *organic mental syndromes (organic brain syndromes)*.

factitious disorders: A class of mental disorders characterized by false symptoms, symptoms that are not valid signs of the pathologies they seem to point to. In a *factitious disorder with psychological symptoms*, a patient may present complaints such as depression, chronic anxiety, hearing voices, or terrible fears when none of these are actually present in the patient's experience. In a *factitious disorder with physical symptoms*, a patient may present complaints such as severe joint pains, chronic backaches, disabling headaches, and stomach distress when none of these is actually present in the patient's experience. Some patients with physical symptoms are masochistic and wound themselves or seek surgery. Factitious disorders are relatively rare.

These disorders are not to be understood in terms of malingering. When a person malingers, he or she is usually attempting to avoid some unpleasant responsibility. In the case of factitious disorders, the motivation seems to be different. The individual wants to be cast in the role of a patient. Behind this aim, there is often an unusually strong need for nurturance, a wish to be cared for in a loving way. In the case of self-destructive, or masochistic, individuals there often exist guilt feelings and the desire for punishment to alleviate the intensity of these feelings.

The treatment of choice for factitious disorders is psychotherapy aimed at fostering self-understanding. In psychotherapy, it is of particular importance to focus on the kinds of emotional needs identified here. Somatic therapies such as drug therapy or electroconvulsive shock are of little or no value in treating factitious disorders.

See also *malingering*; *masochism*.

familial mental retardation: A kind of mental retardation without definite organic basis. It appears to be essentially functional in nature and is probably caused by a highly disadvantaged home environment. Often the parents are mentally retarded themselves and do not provide the child with sufficient stimulation of the right kind for adequate cognitive development in the early years.

Sometimes this kind of mental retardation is called *cultural-familial mental retardation* to suggest that the family itself may exist in a socially deprived setting.

Familial mental retardation accounts for the majority of mental retardation in the United States. It is hoped that, in the future, much retardation can be prevented by enriching the environments of deprived children. Training programs can be of great value for individuals who are already mentally retarded.

See also *mental retardation*.

family therapy: An approach to therapy in which the family unit is seen as the troubled entity, not a single individual within the family. It is, of course, possible that only one person is displaying symptoms of behavioral pathology. Nonetheless, all members of the family meet in therapy sessions to assess ways in which patterns of communication may be fostering the maladaptive behavior.

Family therapy is not tied to one approach such as psychoanalysis or behavioral psychology. Nonetheless, because interactions between people are involved, some theoretical orientations tend to be more readily adopted by family therapists than others. Thus, approaches such as existential therapy and transactional analysis are particularly suited to family therapy. Transactional analysis provides a way to understand patterns of communication within the family. Existential therapy emphasizes authentic living and encounters between people.

See also *Berne, Eric*; *existential therapy*; *transactional analysis*.

fantasy: In general, a set of mental images inspired by imagination and owing no allegiance to reality. A daydream is such a fantasy. In psychoanalysis, fantasy is an ego defense mechanism. Its purpose is to protect the ego against facts that threaten its integrity. Within limits, fantasy is a normal mechanism, and is often used to bolster sagging self-esteem. Thus, after being criticized by a supervisor, an employee may have a fantasy in which he or she cleverly insults the supervisor with a display of wit.

Fantasy can become excessive. Thus some people may spend a great deal of time daydreaming without constructive action. Fantasy is an important process in schizophrenic disorders. The troubled schizophrenic patient is often more in touch with a fantasy world than the one most of us agree is the real one.

See also *ego defense mechanisms*; *schizophrenia*.

fellatio: A form of oral-genital contact in which the mouth and tongue are used to stimulate the penis. The male orgasm can often be induced by fellatio alone. At one time, fellatio was thought to be a form of sexual perversion and/or an activity engaged in primarily by male homosexuals. However, recent sexual surveys indicate that between 50% and 70% of couples use fellatio in premarital sexual foreplay. Today's sexologists regard fellatio as a normal and desirable behavior if it is enjoyed by both participants. See also *cunnilingus*; *orgasm*; *sexual deviations*.

fetal alcohol syndrome: Abnormal development of the fetus during pregnancy due to excessive intake of alcohol by the mother. The toxic effects of too much alcohol can interfere with growth and development. Some of the problems in infants associated with fetal alcohol syndrome are poorly formed limbs, microcephaly, mental retardation, skeletal malformations, heart problems, and neurological problems. Fetal alcohol syndrome is the third principal cause of birth defects. (Down's syndrome and spina bifida, malformation of the base of the spine, are the two principal causes.)

How much is "too much" alcohol? This is difficult to say with any precision. However, it is estimated that more than two mixed drinks, two cans of beer, or 8 ounces of dry wine cross the line between moderate and immoderate drinking during pregnancy. The American Medical Association advises pregnant women to not drink at all during pregnancy if possible. Even modest amounts of alcohol can have an adverse effect on the fetus' development.

See also *alcoholism*; *Down's syndrome*; *microcephaly*.

fetishism: In general, the worship of an inanimate object such as a statue or a large stone. In abnormal psychology, fetishism is the obtaining of sexual arousal by an object of stimulation (i.e., a fetish) not commonly thought to be particularly erotic such as a pair of shoes or other article of clothing. A common practice is for the individual to masturbate while looking at, or contacting, the object.

It is also possible to make a fetish out of a particular part of a partner's body such as the ears, the breasts, or the feet. If this is the case, looking at, caressing, or kissing these body parts may be a requisite for sexual excitement.

Fetishism can be thought of as a sexual disorder only if the individual is much more interested in the object than in another person. Some individuals prefer contact with the fetish than contact with a human being.

Often fetishism is a part of sexual activity with a partner. For example, Fairfax finds that he is aroused during sexual intercourse only if his wife wears silk stockings and high-heeled shoes. Does Fairfax suffer from fetishism? This is a borderline case, and no categorical answer is possible. If Fairfax and his wife both enjoy sex under the conditions described, it seems to be a minor problem.

If fetishism presents a difficulty in one's life or in a relationship, psychotherapy aimed at uncovering the roots of the problem is usually the treatment of choice. If one's partner is disturbed by the fetish, sexual therapy should be considered.

See also *paraphilias*; *sexual deviations*; *sexual therapy*; *transvestic fetishism (transvestism)*.

fixation: In general terms, a preoccupation or an obsession. A miser might be said to have a money fixation. Or a man with an Oedipus complex might be said to have a mother fixation. In psychoanalysis, a fixation is the excessive attachment of libido to an erogenous zone associated with pregenital development. Thus individuals can have oral fixations, anal fixations, or phallic fixations. Such fixations may play a complicating role in certain kinds of maladaptive behaviors. For example, oral fixations may play a role in compulsive eating.

See also *erogenous zones*; *libido*; *Oedipus complex*; *psychosexual development*.

flashback: The involuntary reappearance of an experience induced by prior drug use. Usually the experience is both a hallucination and unpleasant such as seeing a monster or hearing a blood-curdling scream. The drug most frequently mentioned in association with flashbacks is lysergic acid diethylamide-25 (LSD). However, flashbacks have been reported in connection with marijuana and other drugs.

The intensity of flashbacks tends to fade with time. However, reports exist of flashbacks after 2 years without taking LSD.

The biology and psychology of flashbacks are somewhat confusing. Research indicates that flashbacks *can* occur even if the body has been completely cleared of the drug in question. They *do* seem to occur more often in unstable persons. Thus it would appear that psychological processes play a significant role in flashbacks.

See also *hallucination*; *lysergic acid diethylamide-25 (LSD)*; *marijuana*; *psychedelic drugs*.

flight of ideas: A rapid and steady flow of half-formed ideas based on superficial and arbitrary associations such as rhymes or double meanings. Such a flight of ideas is sometimes displayed in the speech of patients suffering from (1) the manic phase of a bipolar disorder, (2) schizophrenic disorders, and (3) organic mental disorders. Here is an example of flight of ideas: "My mother is very good looking. Have you ever caught yourself looking in a looking glass? There is a lot of glass in a church when they say mass. Mass times the speed of light squared is equal to energy according to Einstein."

See also *bipolar disorder*; *clang associations*; *organic mental disorders*; *schizophrenia*.

flooding: The deliberate raising of a patient's anxiety to an intense level for a therapeutic purpose. Flooding can be accomplished by the use of vivid fantasies or actual situations and is a specific technique used in connection with implosive therapy. For example, a patient suffering from a snake phobia might be asked to imagine that hundreds of snakes are crawling all over his or her nude body. Tolerance to such a fantasy often builds rapidly and often reduces the severity of a phobic disorder. Of course, not all patients are good candidates for implosive therapy. It is important that the patient have a high level of emotional stability and be free of psychotic symptoms.

If flooding does not seem to be appropriate in a particular case, the slower procedure of systematic desensitization is the alternative.

See also *desensitization therapy*; *implosive therapy*; *phobia*.

folie à deux: A French term meaning "a madness shared by a couple." A *folie à deux* exists when two intimates share the same delusion, usually a delusion of persecution. For example, a husband may believe that Martians are listening in on his thoughts and plan to take him to Mars for their zoo. He convinces his wife that this is the case, and now there is a shared delusion. Usually this particular kind of pathology is seen only in two people who share a high level of emotional closeness. Married couples, a parent and child, and siblings are the most common pairs observed.

Folie à deux is also termed *shared delusional (paranoid) disorder*.

See also *delusional (paranoid) disorder*.

forensic psychiatry and psychology: Fields of psychiatry and psychology having to do with the law. *Forensic psychiatry* tends to be somewhat more specific and directly applied than forensic psychology. Thus forensic psychiatry attempts to answer questions such as: Is this person insane? Should this person be involuntarily committed to a psychiatric treatment program? Does this individual have diminished responsibility for his or her actions? Can this person stand trial?

Forensic psychology is usually thought of as being somewhat more broadly based and theoretical than forensic psychiatry. It deals with all aspects of psychology and the law. Thus forensic psychology attempts to answer questions such as: Under what conditions can the memory of an eyewitness to a crime be trusted? How do attitudes affect testimony in court? When is evidence reliable? What are the factors involved in diminished responsibility? What are the rights of a person with a mental disorder? Do mental patients have a right to refuse treatment?

In actual practice, any formal distinction between forensic psychiatry and forensic psychology blurs. For example, psychiatrists and clinical psychologists often are called as expert witnesses in court cases. In such instances, they function in approximately the same manner and call on the same general body of knowledge.

See also *commitment*; *Durham rule*; *insanity*; *insanity defense*; *legal aspects of mental health*; *M'Naghten rule*.

Frankl, Viktor (1905–): The father of logotherapy, a kind of psychotherapy based on existential and humanistic principles. Frankl is a European psychiatrist, and has been a frequent lecturer in the United States.

Frankl was confined to the concentration camps of Auschwitz and Dachau during World War II and had a number of dehumanizing experiences. He noted that although most human beings became demoralized in the camps, some were able to retain a sense of hope and their human dignity. He concluded from his observations that we have the power of free will, that we can take a stand against adverse conditions, and that we can usually discover meaning in life.

Frankl has applied the insights of logotherapy with good results to many patients having a broad range of mental health problems. His most influential book, a book that has sold more than two million copies to people in all walks of life, is *Man's Search for Meaning* (1959).

See also *existential neurosis*; *existential therapy*; *humanistic therapy*; *logotherapy*.

free association: A technique used in psychoanalysis to explore the unconscious aspects of mental life. Free association was developed by Freud. He instructed individual patients in analysis to recline on a couch and relate to him anything and everything that came to mind without regard to logic. The patients generally looked at a wall and Freud sat behind them. If something that produced a feeling of shame or guilt was thought of, the patients were not to edit or hold back the information. Freud told patients to compare free association to being on a railroad journey looking out the window of a coach. They were simply to be observers and relate to him anything that presented itself to consciousness.

The assumption behind free association is that if the attention is allowed to wander about at random it will sometimes escape or avoid the censorship imposed on many memories and desires by the ego. Thus the technique provides access to repressed memories and wishes.

See also *ego*; *Freud, Sigmund*; *psychoanalysis*; *repression*; *unconscious mental life*.

Freud, Anna (1895–1982): Made major contributions to techniques of child psychotherapy, the theory of the ego defense mechanisms, and methods of preventing mental disorders. Anna Freud was the daughter of Sigmund Freud and was his only child to become a psychoanalyst. She left Austria with her father in 1938 and continued her professional career in England. In 1947, she was appointed the director of the London Hampstead Child-Therapy Clinic and served in that position for more than 25 years.

Two of Anna Freud's books are *The Ego and the Mechanisms of Defense* (1936) and *Normality and Pathology in Childhood* (1965).

See also *ego defense mechanisms*; *Freud, Sigmund*; *psychoanalysis*.

Freud, Sigmund (1856–1939): Father of psychoanalysis, a major school of psychology. Psychoanalysis is at once a personality theory and a method of psychotherapy. Psychoanalysis was the first of the contemporary psychotherapies and, as such, has exerted an enormous amount of influence. Its influence is rivaled only by behaviorism, on which behavior therapy is based.

Freud was born in the Austro-Hungarian empire and spent the majority of his professional career working in Vienna, Austria. His early training was in biology, and his initial ambition was to pursue a career as a professor of biology. However, he was advised by his major professor, Ernest Brücke, that his future as an academician would be limited because he was Jewish. Freud then decided on a career in medicine and earned an M.D. degree when he was 25 years of age.

Shortly after Freud's graduation, he obtained a financial grant that enabled him to study neurology under Jean Martin Charcot in France. Freud was impressed by Charcot's repeated demonstrations that the symptoms of hysteria (i.e., conversion disorder) could be temporarily removed through hypnotic suggestion. Charcot's work with hypnosis confirmed for Freud that there was a deep unconscious level to mental processes, a level that could cause pathological symptoms. Charcot's observation that sexual problems were often important causal factors in hysteria was also an important influence on Freud's thinking.

When Freud returned to Austria, he set up a private practice and married his fiancée of several years, Martha Bernays, and eventually became the father of six children. One of his children, Anna Freud, became a psychoanalyst.

In his early years of medical practice, Freud was assisted with loans and patient referrals by Josef Breuer, an eminent physician. Josef Breuer told Freud about a case of hysteria he was treating with hypnosis and his own innovative methods. This case eventually became known as the case of Anna O. and is considered the first psychoanalytic case. Freud consistently gave Breuer credit for discovering psychoanalysis or the "talking cure." Breuer discontinued his investigations, but they became a jumping-off place for Freud.

Freud developed psychoanalysis over a period of years in "splendid isolation." All of its fundamental assumptions and basic concepts were developed without the assistance of colleagues. This period of time lasted about 15 years and culminated in the publication of the highly influential book *The Interpretation of Dreams* in 1900. This book brought followers to Freud, among them Carl Jung and Alfred Adler.

Little by little, psychoanalysis gathered momentum and influence, and in 1909 Freud was invited to give a series of lectures in the United States at Clark University. This marked the transition of psychoanalysis as a development of local Austrian interest to one of much greater status. In 1910, The International Psychoanalytic Association was formed.

The Nazi government gave Freud permission to emigrate from Austria in 1938, and he died in London in 1939.

The history of the psychoanalytic movement under Freud's guidance was turbulent. He had a number of loyal followers who always saw him as the "master." Others became impatient with Freud and defected from the ranks after a few years to form their own splinter movements. Today Freud is regarded as the most influential single psychologist who ever lived. There is continuing debate over the value of his theories and his methods of therapy. He still has many followers—and many detractors.

The first book published in psychoanalysis was *Studies on Hysteria* (1895), written in collaboration with Josef Breuer. Among Freud's influential books are *The Interpretation of Dreams* (1900), *The Psychopathology of Everyday Life* (1901), and *The Ego and the Id* (1923).

See also *Adler, Alfred*; *Breuer, Josef*; *Charcot, Jean-Martin*; *conversion disorder*; *hypnosis*; *hysteria*; *Jung, Carl Gustav*; *psychoanalysis*.

frigidity: A very general term suggesting that the person is "cold" toward sex. Most commonly, it indicates either lack of interest in sex or inability to become excited by erotic stimuli. Sometimes it refers to difficulty in reaching an orgasm. The term is somewhat out of date. It tends to have sexist overtones because it is almost always used to describe the behavior of women, not men. Also, as indicated, it is not specific enough. *Hypoactive sexual desire disorder* is a term that takes the place of frigidity, and it can be applied to both males and females.

See also *erectile disorder (erectile insufficiency)*; *hypoactive sexual desire disorder (inhibited sexual excitement)*; *orgasm*; *sexual disorders (psychosexual disorders)*.

Fromm, Erich (1900–1980): A psychoanalyst and major revisionist of Freud's theories. Fromm earned his Ph.D. degree in Germany, was associated with the Berlin Psychoanalytic Institute, and eventually emigrated to the United States. He ended his career as the director of the Mexican Psychoanalytic Institute in Mexico City.

Fromm accepted the importance of the unconscious level of mental life as outlined by Freud but was convinced that Freud put too much emphasis on the sexual drive and not enough emphasis on the role of culture in the shaping of personality. Although Fromm is often identified as a neo-Freudian, this is a somewhat restricted view of Fromm. He was an innovative thinker in his own right and can be credited with making major contributions to humanistic therapy.

Fromm focused his attention on such themes as loneliness, alienation, and how the conditions of modern existence often undermine mental health. He was also very concerned with the role played by aggressiveness in human relationships.

Among his books are *Escape from Freedom* (1941), *The Art of Loving* (1946), and *The Anatomy of Human Destructiveness* (1973).

See also *alienation*; *humanistic therapy*; *neo-Freudian*.

frustration: Frustration has two principal meanings. The first meaning refers to a *situation,* and the second meaning refers to a *state.* First, frustration consists of either a physical or psychological barrier blocking a motivated person from approaching a positive goal or avoiding a negative one. Here are two examples of frustrating situations. Wade proposes marriage to Carla and is turned down. Ingrid tries to leave a boring party and is unable to do so.

Second, frustration can refer to an emotional state. Thus one can "feel frustrated." Emotional states can act as motives. Thus a feeling of frustration may intensify a person's efforts to remove the obstacle producing the frustration. If frustration is moderate, it can help a person gather the required impetus to meet a challenge. If frustration is excessive, it may lead to depression, despair, and demoralization.

See also *frustration–aggression hypothesis*.

frustration–aggression hypothesis: A hypothesis advanced by the research psychologists Neal Miller and John Dollard in the 1950s stating that frustration always generates a certain amount of aggression. The aggression may be expressed. For example, the frustrated individual may engage in a verbal attack, break something, hit someone, and so forth. Or if the individual feels guilty about expressing aggression, it may be turned inward. Then the individual becomes self-destructive. Such repressed aggression may play a role in mental problems such as depression. Psychoanalytic theory suggests that depression is often a result of unexpressed rage. One can here see the frustration–aggression hypothesis and psychoanalysis taking the same general approach.

It is often asserted that the frustration–aggression hypothesis is circular in its reasoning. For example, why is this person acting in aggressive manner? Because he or she is frustrated. How do you know he or she is frustrated? Because he or she is acting in an aggressive manner. In spite of the assertion of circularity, experiments with both animals and human beings indicate that frustration and aggression are associated.

However, aggression is not the only consequence of frustration. Frustration can lead a person to act in rigid and stereotyped ways. For example, if a person cannot solve a problem in life, he or she may nonetheless keep resorting to the same useless approach to the problem over and over again. Or frustration can induce regression, and a person may begin acting childish. Or extreme frustration may be a causal factor in depression and despair.

See also *depression*; *frustration*; *regression*.

fugue: A dissociative disorder characterized by leaving home or a familiar territory combined with loss of personal memories. The individual suffering from fugue essentially combines flight with amnesia. He or she sometimes begins a different life and adopts a new identity. (The word *fugue* means "flight" in Latin. And one can see the same root in the familiar word *fugitive*.)

The kind of fugue being described here is assumed to be without organic basis. Thus its more complete name is *psychogenic fugue*, which suggests its explanation resides in the psychological domain. There is often a background of alcohol abuse in people who develop fugue. A fugue is usually triggered by highly stressful situations or events such as marital problems, vocational difficulties, a great disappointment, or a disaster (e.g., an earthquake or a flood). In essence, the fugue state says, "I want to be somebody else somewhere else."

Recovery from fugue is often spontaneous. However, if treatment is required, a useful approach is psychotherapy aimed at helping the individual understand how the symptoms of fugue are being used to meet emotional needs. The patient is also helped to find more effective ways to meet the same needs. Relapses after recovery are uncommon.

See also *amnesia*; *dissociative disorders*.

functional disorders: Disorders without a clear-cut organic basis. It is assumed that some mental disorders are caused primarily by psychological, or emotional, factors. In psychological factors, one should include the learning history of the person. Maladaptive mental and emotional habits also contribute to mental disorders. In the case of a functional disorder, it is not the "equipment" (e.g., the brain or the nervous system) that is defective but the way the equipment is being used.

Some disorders are primarily functional, and others are primarily organic. Still others seem to be a complex mixture of functional and organic factors and are difficult to classify. Examples of functional disorders are anxiety disorders, somatoform disorders, dissociative disorders, personality disorders, and sexual disorders. (These disorders are loosely classified as "neurotic.") Examples of organic disorders are organic mental syndromes, Down's syndrome, and Alzheimer's disease. Examples of difficult-to-classify disorders are schizophrenic disorders and mood disorders.

It should be understood that few, if any, disorders are purely functional or organic. Biology and psychology almost always interact in a complex way to produce behavior.

See also *organic mental disorders*.

future shock: A term coined by the author Alvin Toffler to indicate that stress reactions can take place in people when change in a society is rapid. It is assumed that such cultural change is a psychosocial stressor and may contribute to mental health problems such as anxiety, depression, suicide, and alienation. Toffler's concept is very similar to the earlier concept of *anomie* proposed by the sociologist Emile Durkheim in the nineteenth century.

See also *alienation*; *anomie*; *suicide*.

G

Galton, Francis (1822–1911): Made contributions to the study of genetics and the measurement of human abilities. Galton was a man with a broad range of interests and explored many regions of science. One of his inventions was the Galton whistle, known by many as the "dog" whistle, capable of producing frequencies inaudible to the human ear. Three years before he died he was knighted in recognition of his discoveries, and he became Sir Francis Galton.

Galton believed that genetic factors make a paramount contribution to human behavior, and he conducted studies that he believed supported this point of view. He was one of the first researchers to study twins in an effort to explore the role of genetic factors in behavior.

Galton attempted to measure intelligence through the use of the *biometric method*, a method that employs a direct measurement of human abilities such as quickness of reflex or strength of grip. His efforts met with very little success, and it remained for Alfred Binet in France to discover a practical method of measuring intelligence.

From today's vantage point, Galton can be seen as a forerunner of the contemporary interest in such subjects as genetic counseling and genetic predisposition.

Two of Galton's principal books are *Hereditary Genius* (1869) and *Inquiries into the Human Faculty and Its Development* (1883). See also *Binet, Alfred*; *genetic counseling*; *genetic predisposition*; *intelligence*.

Gamblers Anonymous (GA): A self-help organization for sufferers from pathological gambling. GA came into existence in 1957 in Los Angeles. Its founders were two individuals who found compulsive gambling to be a chronic personal problem. Many GA groups have been formed throughout the United States.

GA is based on principles pioneered by Alcoholics Anonymous and has a recovery program based on AA guidelines. In the program, pathological gamblers receive emotional support and encouragement from recovering gamblers to change their self-destructive gambling habits.

If there is a GA group near you, you can locate it through your telephone directory.

See also *Alcoholics Anonymous (AA)*; *compulsive gambling*; *pathological gambling*.

gay: An informal term used to describe a homosexual orientation. It can be applied to either males or females. The word *gay* has been adopted by members of the homosexual community in order to suggest the idea that they are happy with their sexual orientation, that they do not perceive it as "sick" or pathological. In consequence, "gay" actually is highly similar in meaning to the term *ego-syntonic homosexuality*, a clinical term sometimes used in the mental health professions.

See also *homosexuality*.

gender identity disorder of childhood: A kind of sexual disorder in children characterized by the intense wish to be a member of the opposite sex. Often, in a gender identity disorder of childhood, a boy denies that he is a boy, or a girl denies that she is a girl. Children suffering from this disorder tend to reject their own genitals, finding it difficult to identify with them. Instead, they fantasize that they have different sexual organs. The disorder begins before adolescence, and it is fairly rare.

Gender identity disorder of childhood does not appear to have a biological basis but is probably explained primarily in psychological terms. Excessive identification of a boy with his mother or of a girl with her father may play a role in causing this disorder. This kind of identification may be fostered by a relationship between parent and child in infancy or in early childhood that has been called *symbiotic*, meaning one in which two individuals are overly dependent on each other.

Many children with this disorder improve without treatment as they mature. If professional help is required, the principal treatment for gender identity disorder of childhood is psychotherapy. The focus of the therapy is on helping the child become less dependent on the parent of the opposite sex. Also, the child needs to be helped to develop his or her own sense of identity and autonomy.

See also *gender identity disorders*; *transsexualism*.

gender identity disorders: Kinds of sexual disorders characterized by unhappiness with one's biological gender. The person with a gender identity disorder wishes that he or she could have the genitals and social role of the opposite sex.

In spite of the publicity that these disorders have received, they are fairly rare.

There are two principal gender identity disorders. These are *transsexualism* and *gender identity disorder of childhood*. *Transvestic fetishism*, a tendency toward cross-dressing, is not a gender identity disorder. It belongs to the class of disorders known as *paraphilias*.

See also *gender identity disorder of childhood*; *paraphilias*; *transsexualism*; *transvestic fetishism (transvestism)*.

general adaptation syndrome: A predictable three-stage stress response pattern. The concept of the general adaptation syndrome was introduced by the physiologist Hans Selye. The first stage is the *alarm reaction*. During the alarm reaction, the individual's capacity to resist stress increases. The adrenal glands respond by increasing their output of key hormones. The second stage is the *stage of resistance*. During this stage, the individual seems to be doing quite well. He or she seems to be coping and adapting to the sources of stress. However, the body is being heavily taxed. The third and final stage is the *stage of exhaustion*. The body is unable to continue to pay the price. Serious illness or even death can be associated with this stage.

Selye studied the physiology of the general adaptation syndrome in animals under many conditions. It is clear that human beings also display the general adaptation syndrome and pay the price for unremitting stress in the form of chronic illnesses and susceptibility to infection. Sources of stress in human life include psychosocial stressors, significant life changes, and one's own habitual behavior patterns (e.g., *Type A behavior*).

See also *adrenal glands; life change units (LCUs); psychosocial stressors; Selye, Hans; Type A behavior*.

generalized anxiety disorder: A kind of anxiety disorder characterized primarily by the constant feeling that some sort of unfortunate or terrible event is about to take place. The term *free-floating anxiety* is often used to describe the emotional state because the apprehension does not have a specific source. The individual may imagine, for no obvious reason, that he or she will have a heart attack, catch a deadly disease, go crazy, and so forth. Related symptoms include muscle tension, increased pulse, and being constantly "on guard." Sometimes the anxiety refers to family members such as a spouse or children. They, not the person with the disorder, are in danger. There is the fear that some disaster will befall one of them. The overall state is captured with the words *chronic dread*. In informal terms, persons with this disorder are called "worrywarts."

A generalized anxiety disorder should not be confused with a phobic disorder. In a phobic disorder, there is a specific source of the irrational fear (e.g., high places, closed rooms, dogs, etc.).

The classic psychoanalytic explanation of a generalized anxiety disorder is that the id (i.e., a set of biological impulses) is in conflict with the superego (i.e., moral training). There is the possibility that one will not be able to contain one's forbidden wishes, and this possibility produces anxiety. The anxiety is vague because the conflict is to a large extent fought at the unconscious level. Dread of the external world is thought to be due to a projection of the unconscious conflict.

Other explanations include generalized conditioned fears. One may have had traumatic experiences at some earlier period. Objects and events that are roughly similar to those associated with the original trauma may elicit anxiety. Again, the anxiety is vague because the similarity between the first set of stimuli and the second set may not be directly perceived.

Biological explanations are seldom used to explain generalized anxiety disorder. It is thought of as primarily functional in nature, not organic.

There are several approaches to treatment. Antianxiety drugs are often prescribed. A very common treatment is psychotherapy aimed at uncovering the emotional roots of the disorder. Less common treatments include biofeedback training, relaxation techniques, and meditation.

See also *antianxiety drugs*; *anxiety*; *anxiety disorders*; *phobia*; *projection*.

general paresis: An organic disorder caused by syphilis. General paresis is characterized by paralysis and dementia. The brain and central nervous system are gradually destroyed by the action of the syphilis spirochete, a corkscrew-shaped bacterium.

In the 1970s, general paresis accounted for about 1% of admissions to mental hospitals. Its incidence has declined to some extent since that time due to both prevention and early detection of the disease. However, syphilis continues to be a major public health problem. About 5% of persons with untreated syphilis will develop general paresis.

The primary ways to prevent syphilis are to avoid promiscuous sexual contacts and to use condoms. The principal class of drugs used to treat syphilis are the antibiotics.

See also *dementia*.

genetic counseling: Counseling in which an assessment is made of the likelihood that a particular couple will produce offspring with an inherited disease. An individual can be personally free of a given recessive genetic disorder and, nonetheless, be a carrier of that disorder. If both members of a couple are carriers, the statistical expectation is that one-fourth of their children will actually have the disease associated with the recessive genetic disorder. Couples with a family history of inherited diseases might consider genetic counseling. Such counseling is available at a number of clinics and medical centers.

Examples of inherited diseases are Huntington's chorea, phenylketonuria (PKU), and Tay-Sach's disease (a relatively rare metabolic disorder). All three of these diseases are associated with mental retardation. Although Down's syndrome is caused by a genetic defect, it is *not* due to two recessive genes.

See also *Down's syndrome*; *Huntington's chorea*; *phenylketonuria (PKU)*.

genetic predisposition: A tendency to manifest either a certain kind of behavior or a particular mental disorder because of one's genes. There is a good deal of evidence to suggest that certain traits of temperament (e.g., reserved versus outgoing, emotionally unstable versus emotionally stable, and humble versus assertive) are due in some part to one's genetic predisposition. There is also evidence that suggests a proneness to certain mental disorders (e.g., schizophrenic disorders and bipolar disorder) have a genetic basis. The existence of genetic predispositions has led to a field of study known as *behavioral genetics*, the study of how genes play a role in determining temperament, talents, and mental disorders.

It is important to warn that the existence of genetic predispositions sometimes offers a too facile explanation of either personality or mental disorders. One should not oversimplify by saying, "Oh, it's all inherited," or "It's just in the genes." The individual's developmental history must also be considered in explaining behavior.

See also *bipolar disorder*; *schizophrenia*.

genital stage: According to Freud, the last stage of psychosexual development. The genital stage begins at puberty (around 12 or 13 years of age) and continues throughout adolescence and adulthood. In psychoanalytic theory, if development is normal, during the genital stage the individual will both desire and enjoy sexual relations with members of the opposite sex. If, on the other hand, libido has become fixated at an earlier stage of development, there may be sexual dysfunction or desire for a member of the same sex.

See also *Freud, Sigmund*; *homosexuality*; *libido*; *psychosexual development*.

geriatrics: A field of medicine that deals with problems associated with the aging process. Many mental health problems are linked to this process. *Senile dementia* is an example of one such problem. *Alzheimer's disease* is also associated with aging. *Organic mental syndromes* are often complicated by the advanced age of the patient. In general, pathological organic changes in the brain and nervous system linked to aging may produce changes in personality and behavior.

Geriatrics is actually the medical sector of a much larger field of study called *gerontology*, the science of aging. Gerontology takes as its domain all aspects of the aging process such as its psychological, social, and legal ones. In view of the fact that people are living longer than in the past, both geriatrics and gerontology are becoming increasingly important fields of study.

See also *Alzheimer's disease*; *organic mental syndromes (organic brain syndromes)*; *senile dementia*.

Gestalt therapy: A method of psychotherapy pioneered by Frederick ("Fritz") S. Perls (1893–1970). The German word *Gestalt* can be translated as "organized whole." Thus Gestalt therapy aims to help the troubled person make an organized whole out of a fragmented and self-alienated personality. For example, Perls made a distinction between what he called the *top dog* in the personality and the *underdog*. He called these two agents the "two clowns of the personality." They are always tripping each other. Top dog tries to make the person be responsible. And underdog, like a brat, whines or rebels. For instance, top dog says, "You must go on a diet and lose weight." Underdog says, "I won't! I don't have to." In order to move in the direction of mental health, these two opposing agents must reach some sort of working compromise. (It should be noted that the top dog is very similar to Freud's concept of the superego. And the underdog is very similar to Freud's concept of the id. Perls was trained as a psychoanalyst.)

In order to bring about wholeness in the personality, Gestalt therapy uses a set of techniques. A patient in therapy can alternately role-play top dog and underdog, engaging them in a dialogue. Or a patient can be encouraged to focus on the here and the now, becoming more aware of pathological thoughts and feelings.

Perls was a very creative and innovative therapist, and many of the concepts and methods of Gestalt therapy have been incorporated into psychotherapy in general.

See also *id*; *psychotherapy*; *superego*.

glove anesthesia: A lack of feeling in the hand following the general outline of a glove. In view of the fact that the loss of sensation follows boundaries dictated by clothing, not by known nerve pathways, it is clear that a glove anesthesia is psychological in nature, not organic. It is the patient's imagination that defines the region of anesthesia. And most patients are more familiar with articles of clothing than the structure of the nervous system. Thus a glove anesthesia is a symptom of a conversion disorder. Similar conditions in other regions of the body are a *hat* *anesthesia*, a *belt anesthesia*, a *stocking anesthesia*, and a *shoe anesthesia*.

See also *conversion disorder*.

gonads: The sex glands of either sex. In the male, the gonads are called the *testes*, and, in the female, the gonads are called the *ovaries*. Sperm are produced by the testes; ova are produced by the ovaries. The gonads are also endocrine glands and produce important hormones affecting mood and behavior. One of the important hormones produced by the testes is *testosterone*. One of the important group of hormones produced by the ovaries are the *estrogens*.

See also *androgens*; *endocrine system*; *estrogens*.

grandiosity: An excessive sense of self-importance, talent, or position. For example, a person of mediocre musical talent may be convinced that he or she is a virtuoso. Or a person who has written an amateurish first novel is convinced that it is a great work of art destined to become a classic of literature. Grandiosity can be a symptom of a mental disorder, particularly of the manic phase of a bipolar disorder.

See also *bipolar disorder*; *mania*.

grand mal epilepsy: A kind of epilepsy characterized by severe convulsive seizures. This kind of epilepsy is also known as *major epilepsy*. (The words *grand mal* in French mean "great sickness.") One of the distinguishing features of grand mal seizures is loss of consciousness. Somewhat more than one-half of epilepsy is of the grand mal type. A large percentage of persons with the disorder receive a brief warning that an attack is coming in the form of gastric upset, odd odors, loss of feeling in limbs, light flashes, and muscle spasms. The warning is called an *aura* and sometimes offers an opportunity to sit down or recline before the onset of the seizure.

A grand mal seizure has two principal phases. During the first phase of a grand mal seizure, the muscles contract, respirations halt temporarily, the pupils of the eyes expand, and sometimes the individual involuntarily urinates. This is called the *tonic phase*. During the second phase, a series of convulsions make their appearance; these consist of involuntary contractions of the large muscles of the body. This is called the *clonic phase*. Usually the convulsions are over in a few minutes. It is important to protect the person against self-injury (particularly of the head) during a grand mal seizure. After the tonic phase is over, some individuals quickly regain consciousness. Others sleep soundly for an hour or more.

Individuals who suffer from grand mal epilepsy are advised to wear a medic-alert bracelet.

See also *epilepsy*.

grief work: The natural and spontaneous process of accommodating to a personal loss. The most obvious loss is the death of a loved one or a close friend. However, one can experience grief over the loss of a pet, a career, a limb, and so forth. Grief is a natural reaction to loss and is to be distinguished from depression that may have other causes. As one does one's grief work, one finds personal ways to cope with the loss. When one finds the strength to carry on with some degree of confidence and a minimum of suffering, the grief work is complete. It is important to recognize that grief needs to be confronted and that grief work is a health-giving process.

See also *depression*.

group therapy: Psychotherapy conducted in a setting with two or more people. In practice, group therapy is seldom done with only two people. Groups of five to nine are common sizes. Group therapy first came into its own as a result of World War II. Psychiatrists and clinical psychologists needed to treat many combat personnel, and they found themselves unable to offer each patient prolonged individual psychotherapy. Therapy in groups started as a practical solution to the heavy case load and was found to be surprisingly effective. In many instances, the group interaction acted as a therapeutic agent. Ever since the 1940s, group therapy has been a mainstay of clinical practice.

The term *group therapy* does not identify any particular approach to therapy. Therefore it is possible to do, for example, psychoanalytically oriented therapy, behavior therapy, rational-emotive therapy, client-centered therapy, and transactional analysis in groups.

See also *encounter group*; *psychotherapy*.

growth motivation: According to Abraham Maslow, the motivational principle underlying self-actualization. The inborn tendency of the individual to develop, to mature, to reach the limits of his or her potential has at its core growth motivation. Maslow distinguished between two kinds of motivations, deficiency motivation and growth motivation. Deficiency motivation helps us meet our needs for food, water, safety, belongingness, love, respect, and self-esteem. These needs are like empty spots in our existence that need to be filled. In contrast, growth motivation helps us to *become*, to bring forth the person we were really meant to be.

If growth motivation is frustrated by external circumstances, it will adversely affect the psychological and emotional development of the person. Such frustration may be a contributing factor to behavior pathology.

See also *Maslow, Abraham Harold*; *self-actualization*.

guilt feelings: Self-punitive feelings suggesting that the individual has done, or is about to do, something in violation of his or her moral code. Guilt feelings are often a contributing factor to depression. The individual may give expression to such feelings by saying, "I'm a sinner," or "I cheated my own brother," or "I lied to my wife."

According to Freud, guilt feelings arise from the critical judgments of the superego. In Freudian theory, the superego is the internalization by the individual of the parents' values. The parents' values are themselves a reflection of the parents' own religious and cultural ties. Thus, in Freudian theory, the superego is *acquired*, not inborn.

However, it is possible to argue that some guilt feelings arise from a deeper source within the individual. It is possible to speak of *existential guilt*, the remorse that arises when one feels that one has not used one's time on Earth wisely. The individual may give expression to existential guilt by saying, "I wasted my life," or "I never amounted to anything because I was too lazy," or "I've ruined everything I've ever touched." Existential guilt is often felt by middle-aged and elderly people when they reflect on their younger days and are convinced they wasted their talents and opportunities.

Guilt feelings are, within limits, normal. However, it is obvious that some people are too hard on themselves. They whip themselves with guilt feelings for real or imagined offenses that would seem trivial to most of us.

See also *existential neurosis*; *Freud, Sigmund*; *superego*.

H

habit: A learned behavior pattern that can be performed on an automatic basis with very little conscious attention. It is possible to have cognitive, emotional, or motor habits. A cognitive habit is a routine, predictable way of thinking. Some people have what the psychiatrist Aaron Beck calls *automatic thoughts*. Emotional habits are routine, predictable ways of feeling. We have "pet peeves." Some people become depressed every time they hear a certain song. Motor habits are routine, predictable ways of acting. We use motor habits to drive a car, operate a typewriter, and speak.

Habits can be adaptive or maladaptive. Adaptive habits help us to cope and adjust. Thus some people have "good" habits of sleep, eating, work, and so forth. Maladaptive habits interfere with our ability to cope and adjust. Thus some people have "bad" habits. They think irrational thoughts, situations easily make them anxious or angry, and they may smoke, drink, or eat too much.

Behavior therapy is designed to help individuals with maladaptive habits.

See also *automatic thoughts*; *behavior therapy*; *classical conditioning*; *habit disorders*.

habit disorders: In general, any behavioral disorder in which maladaptive habits play a dominant role. However, in practice, the term is usually reserved for children. Thus habit disorders are usually thought of as such problems as eating disorders, encopresis, enuresis, sleepwalking, stuttering, and tics.

See also *eating disorders*; *encopresis*; *enuresis*; *sleepwalking disorder (somnambulism)*; *stuttering (stammering)*; *tic disorder*.

halfway house: An alternative facility to a mental hospital. A halfway house is a midpoint (i.e., "halfway") between the community and an institution. A typical halfway house is governed to a large extent by the residents themselves; a clinical psychologist or psychiatrist is on call. As first conceived, a halfway house provided aftercare to help a newly released mental patient make a smooth transition back to the community. Studies have shown that the support provided by the halfway house lowers the likelihood of being rehospitalized.

Going beyond its first conception, halfway houses are now often used to provide an option for troubled persons who are candidates for hospitalization. It often helps them to stay out of a mental hospital.

Halfway houses are usually funded by governmental agencies and philanthropic foundations.

See also *community mental health center*.

Hall, Granville Stanley (1844–1924): One of the principal founders of American psychology. Hall is credited with earning the first Ph.D. in psychology in the United States, obtaining the degree in 1878 under the sponsorship of the eminent William James. In 1887, he was responsible for the publication of the first journal of academic psychology in the United States, the *American Journal of Psychology*. Hall helped to organize the American Psychological Association and became its first president in 1892.

Hall invited Sigmund Freud and Carl Jung to lecture in the United States on psychoanalysis at Clark University in 1909. These presentations did much to establish psychoanalysis as an important force in American psychology.

Hall's research was primarily in the areas of developmental and educational psychology. One of his methods was to explore the thinking processes of children by asking them sets of questions. Two of Hall's principal works are *The Contents of Children's Minds* (1883) and *Adolescence* (1904).

See also *Freud, Sigmund*; *James, William*; *Jung, Carl Gustav*; *psychoanalysis*.

hallucination: A false perceptual experience that carries the force of reality. The external stimulus needed to produce the experience is absent but, nonetheless, seems to be there to the person producing the hallucination. Thus, in a *visual hallucination*, the individual sees something that is not present to other observers. For example, a patient suffering from a schizophrenic disorder saw his dead grandfather walking across the room and tried to touch him. Hallucinations can occur in any sensory modality. Therefore, in addition to visual hallucinations, there are *auditory, olfactory, tactile*, and *gustatory hallucinations*.

The presence of hallucinations is a strong sign that an individual is suffering from a disturbed mental state. They often are associated with either organic deterioration or functional disturbances.

A combination of visual and auditory hallucinations may be so vivid that a patient will hold a conversation with an invisible presence.

See also *delusion*; *dementia*; *hallucinogens*; *hallucinosis*; *illusion*.

hallucinogens: Drugs capable of producing hallucinations. (Hallucinogens are also known as *psychedelic drugs*.) Hallucinations experienced under these conditions are, of course, not a symptom of a mental disorder. Instead, they represent, in most cases, a temporary alteration in the perceptual processes.

Hallucinogens have been used in a variety of ways. First, they have been used for recreational purposes. When used in this manner, they have a substantial potential for abuse. Second, they have been used for religious purposes, as a way of opening doors to mystical experiences and "other realities." Third, they have been used in psychotherapy (primarily research projects) to help patients gain access to different viewpoints on life. At present, there is little or no use of hallucinogens in psychotherapy.

See also *lysergic acid diethylamide-25 (LSD)*; *marijuana*; *mescaline*; *phencyclidine (PCP)*; *psilocybin*.

hallucinosis: A biological state in which the nervous system is somewhat more likely to produce hallucinations. For example, a stroke victim might complain that he or she smells onions frying. A person with a brain tumor might complain that music is always playing. The toxic effects of drugs can produce hallucinosis. Delirium tremens, associated with alcohol withdrawal, is an example. Also, hallucinogens produce a state of hallucinosis through their biochemical action.

See also *delirium tremens*; *hallucination*; *hallucinogens*.

haloperidol: See *major tranquilizers (antipsychotic drugs)*.

hashish: A narcotic drug with intoxicating effects obtained from the sprouts of the hemp plant. The plant that produces hashish is a first cousin to the plant used to obtain marijuana. The word *assassin* is derived from "hashish." During the time of the Crusades, the drug was used by opponents of the Christians.

See also *marijuana*.

hebephrenic schizophrenia: An older term for what today is called *schizophrenia, disorganized type*. The word *hebephrenic* is derived from Hebe, the goddess of youth in Greek mythology. The person who is hebephrenic is very infantile in his or her behavior. In other words, the individual has regressed to "youth."

See also *schizophrenia*.

hemophobia: An irrational fear of blood. Most commonly, the person suffering from hemophobia is made faint or emotionally upset by the sight of blood. Another name for hemophobia is *hematophobia*.

See also *phobia*.

heroin: A narcotic derived from opium. It is related to morphine and codeine. Heroin is capable of providing some relief from pain, fostering relaxation, and inducing euphoria. Frequent users of heroin require larger and larger doses because of habituation to the action of the drug. It is frequently abused and has a tendency to produce an addiction at both a physiological and psychological level.

At one time, heroin was used as an analgesic by physicians. However, it is not currently used in this way in the United States.

It is estimated that there are about one-quarter million people in the United States addicted to heroin. *Methadone*, a synthetic narcotic, is sometimes used in therapy programs designed to help addicted persons break free from heroin.

See also *drug addiction*; *methadone*; *narcotic drugs*.

heterosexuality: An orientation in which the individual desires sexual relations with members of the opposite sex. The person with heterosexual interests finds individuals of different gender to be sources of erotic experience. Freud believed that heterosexuality was normal, not homosexuality. He associated heterosexuality with the last stage of psychosexual development, the *genital stage*.

See also *genital stage*; *homosexuality*; *psychosexual development*.

histrionic personality disorder: A kind of personality disorder characterized by melodramatic behavior. (This disorder has also been called *hysterical personality disorder*.) Talking loudly, making grand gestures with the hands as in a silent movie, expressing emotions with great force, and so forth are some of the specific kinds of actions associated with this disorder. Persons with the disorder tend to always want to be the center of attention.

Behaviors such as those described here reach the level of an actual disorder only if they greatly interfere with personal relations or make it highly difficult for the person to meet everyday responsibilities. For example, a married person who suffers from this disorder makes a sort of living hell out of home life.

The disorder is common, but no exact statistics are available. Also, women are somewhat more likely to be identified as suffering from the disorder than men. However, this may be due to a certain amount of cultural bias. (Almost everyone has heard the pejorative term *hysterical woman*.) Individuals with a histrionic disorder are somewhat more likely than others to simultaneously suffer from a substance use disorder.

The causes of histrionic personality disorder are obscure. One can only speculate in a general way that the individual's developmental history has produced a state of low self-esteem. The theatrical behavior can be thought of as (1) a defense system designed to repress feelings of helplessness and inadequacy and (2) a way of manipulating and controlling others.

The basic treatment for this disorder is psychotherapy aimed at helping the individual understand the psychological and emotional roots of the maladaptive behavior.

See also *hysteria*; *personality disorders*; *psychoactive substance use disorders (substance use disorders)*.

holistic viewpoint: The viewpoint that the "mind" and the "body" are two aspects of a unified whole, the living organism. Applied to behavior pathology, adjustment problems are viewed in a large framework encompassing biological, psychological, and socio-cultural factors. All of these factors interact with each other when maladaptive behavior is manifest.

The holistic viewpoint should be contrasted with *dualism*, the point of view that (1) the "mind" arises from a supernatural world associated with the soul and (2) the "body" arises from the natural world of cause and effect. Dualism in effect places a wedge between mind and body, making it difficult to deal with many problems.

The holistic viewpoint has gained a good deal of ground in medicine, psychiatry, and clinical psychology in the past two or three decades. For example, the American Psychiatric Association's *Diagnostic and Statistical Manual of Mental Disorders* gives explicit weight to a combination of the factors identified here when a diagnosis is made.

The holistic viewpoint is also of particular importance when an attempt is made to understand psychosomatic (i.e., psychophysiological) disorders.

See also Diagnostic and Statistical Manual of Mental Disorders; *psychosomatic disorders*.

homosexuality: A distinct erotic attraction to, or a preference for sexual relations with, persons of one's own gender (i.e., male-male or female-female). There have been many sexual surveys, and the general incidence of homosexuality is fairly well-known. The following percentages are conservative ones. Among males, it is estimated that about 4% have an exclusively homosexual orientation; about 10% have had a homosexual experience. Among females, it is estimated that about 2 or 3% have an exclusively homosexual orientation; about 6 or 7% have had a homosexual experience. When a female has homosexual desires, she is more likely to maintain bisexual behavior than is a male with homosexual desires.

The American Psychiatric Association's *Diagnostic and Statistical Manual of Mental Disorders* does not identify homosexuality as a mental disorder. Therefore, it would not seem to require explanation. However, persons with a heterosexual orientation are often puzzled by homosexuality, finding it very difficult to understand. Therefore, psychiatry and psychology do make some attempt to explain homosexuality. A number of explanations have been offered. Some of the principal ones follow. First, it is possible that there is an inherited tendency toward homosexuality. Correlational studies of identical twins give some credibility to this idea. Second, it is possible that abnormal changes in a mother's hormone levels during pregnancy may in some way affect the sexual development of a fetus; this may affect adult sexual orientation in a way that is not yet clear. Third, psychoanalysis hypothesizes that fixations of libido, caused by emotional traumata, during the phallic stage of development may be a principal cause of homosexuality. Fourth, learning theory suggests that copying the behavior of a parent of the opposite sex (e.g., a boy copying the behavior of his mother) may play a role in subsequent homosexuality.

Although homosexuality is not a mental disorder, it is of some interest to note that, up until fairly recently, a formal distinction was made between ego-dystonic and ego-syntonic homosexuality. *Ego-dystonic homosexuality* was defined as a kind of homosexuality in which the homosexual individual was greatly distressed by his or her sexual orientation. *Ego-syntonic homosexuality* was defined as a kind of homosexuality in which the homosexual individual was content with his or her sexual orientation.

Although the distinction between ego-dystonic and ego-syntonic homosexuality no longer has any formal status, the ego-dystonic diagnosis can still be made if a clinician deems it useful or proper. This is accomplished by reference to a general category in the *Diagnostic and Statistical Manual of Mental Disorders* used to classify sexual disorders not otherwise identified. However, the diagnosis appears to be rarely made.

See also *bisexual behavior*; Diagnostic and Statistical Manual of Mental Disorders; *gay*; *lesbian*.

Horney, Karen (1885–1952): One of the principal founders of psychoanalysis in the United States. Horney received her academic training in Germany; she earned an M.D. degree and obtained her psychoanalytic training at the Berlin Institute of Psychoanalysis under the guidance of the eminent psychoanalyst Karl Abraham. In 1932, Horney became a resident of the United States.

Although Horney is known as a psychoanalyst, she felt no great loyalty to Freud's specific theories. She accepted the broad concepts that mental life has unconscious roots, that ego defense mechanisms are important, and that anxiety plays an important part in neurotic conflict. However, she believed that Freud placed too much emphasis on biological factors in development and not enough emphasis on the role of interpersonal relationships and the influence of society in general. She is considered to be a neo-Freudian and a major revisionist of Freud's theories.

Horney was a principal founder in 1942 of the American Institute for Psychoanalysis. The Karen Horney Clinic was founded in 1955 in New York, and it became an important center for psychotherapy and the training of analysts. Horney wrote highly readable books for the general public, and through these books exerted a wide influence. Two of her books are *The Neurotic Personality of Our Time* (1937) and *Self-Analysis* (1942).

See also *Freud, Sigmund*; *neurosis*; *psychoanalysis*.

hostility: A negative emotional state characterized by an antagonistic and unfriendly attitude. Hostility is often directed toward another person; this is particularly true if the other person is perceived as a source of frustration. Thus a husband may feel hostile toward his wife because he is convinced that she is keeping him from fulfilling a long-standing ambition. A child may feel hostile toward a parent because the child believes that the parent is restricting his or her freedom.

Hostility can be manifest or latent. When hostility is manifest, it often is expressed in the form of cutting remarks or aggressive behavior. Its presence is obvious. When hostility is latent, it may be masked with smiles or kind deeds; the "sugar" covers the poison. Sometimes the individual himself or herself represses the hostility to an unconscious mental level; then there is self-denial of the hostility. This kind of hostility, when present in human relations, is harder to deal with than manifest hostility.

A fairly high level of hostility is often present in persons who suffer from mental disorders. In psychotherapy, latent hostility is often ferreted out and expressed.

See also *emotion*.

humanistic therapy: A general term denoting any kind of psychotherapy that tends to focus on the theme of self-actualization.

Humanistic therapy aims to help the person grow and to become the individual he or she was meant to be. Although in one sense, all psychotherapy would seem to have these general aims, in fact only certain specific kinds of psychotherapies, emphasize the goals identified. The kinds of psychotherapies usually mentioned as fitting in the humanistic category are client-centered therapy, Gestalt therapy, and individual psychology.

Humanistic therapy is a broadly conceived approach to psychotherapy, not a specific kind of therapy. It is very similar in nature to another broadly conceived approach, *existential therapy*. Humanistic therapy tends to emphasize the importance of growth, the positive side of life. Existential therapy tends to emphasize the importance of overcoming alienation and loss of meaning in existence, coping with the negative side of life. Thus the difference between the two is more one of emphasis than anything else.

See also *client-centered therapy*; *existential therapy*; *Gestalt therapy*; *individual psychology*; *self-actualization*.

Huntington's chorea: An inherited disease of the central nervous system involving a degenerative process of neurons located in the frontal portion of the brain. (Huntington's chorea is also known as *Huntington's disease* and *hereditary chorea*. Informally, it is sometimes referred to as *Woody Guthrie's disease*.) George Huntington, a neurologist, identified the disease in 1872. Symptoms include jerky random movements of the entire body and mental deterioration. The word *chorea* is from a Greek word meaning "dance." (Note the similarity to the familiar word *choreography*.) The idea is that the person with the disease makes involuntary dancelike motions. Huntington's chorea is a progressive disease and usually leads to death in 10 to 20 years. At present, there is no known cure for the disease. Treatment consists of drugs and sometimes surgery to alleviate symptoms.

The disease is caused by a dominant gene and can be carried by either a male or female. Assume that a father is carrier and that a mother is not. Because the gene is dominant, the statistical odds are that one-half of this couple's children will have the disease. The father, the carrier, will develop the disease himself.

However, he is likely to pass it on to his children before he experiences symptoms. This is because in most cases the disease is latent until the individual is 30, 40, or even more years of age. It is estimated that there are presently about 50,000 latent cases in the United States.

Potential parents who suspect that they are carriers of Huntington's chorea should consider obtaining genetic counseling prior to having offspring. Such counseling can play a role in preventing the spread of the disease.

See also *genetic counseling*.

hydrocephalus: An abnormally large head caused by excessive amounts of cerebrospinal fluid trapped within ventricles (i.e., openings) in the brain. (In terms of its Greek roots, hydrocephalus means "a head filled with water.") The condition may be present at birth or may develop later as a result of an infection. If untreated from infancy, the victim often develops a very large head and is mentally retarded. The mental retardation is due to brain damage caused by excessive pressure on the brain. In the case of an adult, trapped cerebrospinal fluid will not lead to an enlarged head because the skull has lost its plasticity. However, mental retardation can still result.

Treatment consists of surgery designed to drain off excessive cerebrospinal fluid. If this is done in the early years, the head will grow normally, and the child will be saved from mental retardation. Adults can be treated with a similar procedure.

See also *mental retardation*; *microcephaly*.

hydrotherapy: In general, any use of water to treat a disease. In the instance of psychiatric treatment, this usually consists of having an agitated mental patient relax in a tub of warm water. The use of water in this way often has a tranquilizing effect. The patient reclines on a canvas hammock in the water and is restrained by a second canvas cover over the tub. The duration of treatment is usually 1 hour, and vital signs (i.e., pulse, temperature, respiration) are carefully monitored by an attendant.

Another kind of hydrotherapy used to control agitation is to wrap a patient in cool wet sheets. This usually produces an initial shock and a subsequent tranquilizing effect as the body warms the water in the sheets.

Hydrotherapy of the type described here is fast becoming a thing of the past as drugs are used more and more to tranquilize patients. However, it should be noted that hydrotherapy has the advantage of having fewer toxic side effects than many prescription drugs.

See also *drug therapy*; *somatic therapy*.

hyperkinetic (hyperactive) disorder: One of the two basic kinds of attention deficit disorders.

See also *attention deficit disorder*.

hyperobesity: Great obesity. One criterion that is often used is this one: ideal weight plus 100 pounds. Thus if one's ideal weight is 120 pounds, one is hyperobese if the total weight is 220 pounds.

See also *compulsive eating*; *eating disorders*; *obesity*.

hypertension: High blood pressure. Usually there are no symptoms of high blood pressure, and this is why it has been called the "silent killer." In most cases, the cause of hypertension is obscure. However, in some cases, it is clearly organic (e.g., a tumor on the adrenal gland or hardening of the arteries). In the obscure cases, it is hypothesized that psychological factors may play a role. Emotional conflicts or psychosocial stressors may induce or aggravate hypertension.

Treatment consists of a set of recommendations depending on the particular case. Some of these are reducing salt intake, reducing if overweight, exercise, and the taking of antihypertensive medication. Counseling and psychotherapy can be helpful in some cases, helping the individual change thoughts and attitudes that produce chronic anger. Behavior therapy may be useful in assisting the person to make life-style changes.

See also *psychosomatic disorders*; *Type A behavior*.

hyperventilation: Very rapid breathing. In the framework of mental health, hyperventilation is a symptom of anxiety and is often associated with panic disorder. Hyperventilation may lead to fainting.

An immediate self-treatment that is often recommended is to cover the nose and mouth with a paper bag, rebreathing the air in the bag a total of 8 to 12 times. This is effective in inhibiting the hyperventilation because it is caused by rapidly lowered levels of carbon dioxide in the blood. The air exhaled into the bag has a higher level of carbon dioxide than the surrounding air. Thus, the rebreathing procedure helps to restore carbon dioxide levels in the blood to normal levels.

Long-range treatment consists of psychotherapy for anxiety and/or panic disorder.

See also *anxiety*; *panic disorder*.

hypnosis: An altered state of consciousness characterized by selective attention and increased suggestibility. The word *hypnosis* is derived from a Greek word meaning "sleep." However, hypnosis only superficially resembles sleep. It mimics sleep because the hypnotic subject who is concentrating on one stimulus is often unaware of other stimuli (i.e., lights and sounds in the room). Thus he or she may appear to be "unconscious."

There has been much debate among researchers as to whether or not hypnosis really is an altered state of consciousness or a kind of subconscious role playing. The weight of evidence tends to support the hypothesis that it is quite definitely a unique mental state as indicated before.

One of the principal personalities in the history of hypnosis was Franz Anton Mesmer (1733–1815). Working in France, he produced many "cures" of nervous ailments through the use of what he called "animal magnetism." A team of scientists, including Benjamin Franklin, decided that his claims were excessive and that he was a charlatan. For many years after Mesmer's death, hypnotism had a bad name. Even today many persons think of it as vaguely evil in nature.

The English surgeon James Braid (1795–1860) restored some of hypnotism's credibility. He demonstrated that it could be used to alleviate pain in operations. Also, he is responsible for giving it its present name.

There are five traditional categories of hypnosis: (1) insusceptible, (2) hypnoidal, (3) light trance, (4) medium trance, and (5) deep trance. As indicated by their names, each category suggests a step "down" into the hypnotic state. In a deep trance, it is possible to give posthypnotic suggestions and induce hallucinations. A *posthypnotic* suggestion is one that takes effect *after* the trance is over. For example, it is possible to suggest during the trance that a person will feel very thirsty one-half hour after coming out of the trance. Let's assume the individual came out of the trance at 8:00 P.M. At 8:30, the individual goes to the sink, takes a glass of water, and announces loudly, "Boy, it's hot in here. A cool drink sure feels good!" It is obvious to observers that the cause of the behavior is beneath the level of the subject's awareness.

See also *hypnotherapy*; *mesmerism*.

hypnotherapy: The use of hypnosis to treat disorders. In the framework of mental health, hypnosis is used in several ways. First, hypnosis can be used in psychotherapy to facilitate insights into the unconscious aspects of mental life. It can be used, for example, to bring repressed memories to consciousness. Freud used it this way at one time but rejected this approach in favor of free association. One of the problems is that unconscious material may be brought forth too quickly without adequate safeguards. Some therapists fear that this approach can precipitate a psychotic process in some patients. Others argue that if the patient has sufficient ego strength, the risk is minimal.

Second, hypnosis can be used to remove symptoms. Through the use of posthypnotic suggestions, a person can be helped to manage problems such as nail biting, smoking, compulsive eating, and so forth. Although this approach can be useful, its effects are often temporary. Direct symptom removal is usually combined with psychotherapy in general and is seen as an adjunct to it.

Third, hypnosis can be used to induce relaxation. It can be helpful in the treatment of individuals who suffer from tension and anxiety. Also, the induction of relaxation can be useful when combined with the behavior therapy technique known as systematic desensitization.

Naturally, all of the uses described here should be conducted only under the auspices of a licensed therapist. Unfortunately, a number of persons with minimal qualifications are more than willing to take on trusting persons for a fee.

Under the proper conditions, hypnotherapy is a credible treatment modality. In 1958, The Council of Mental Health of the American Medical Association reported favorably on the therapeutic uses of hypnosis.

See also *desensitization therapy*; *hypnosis*; *mesmerism*.

hypoactive sexual desire disorder (inhibited sexual excitement): A sexual disorder characterized by problems revolving around the first and second stages of the sexual response cycle. In males, this manifests itself primarily in the form of erectile problems. In females, there may be an inadequate lubrication swelling response. In either case, the individual is not prepared for sexual intercourse.

Assuming that organic factors have been ruled out, the disorder can be in part explained in psychological terms. Several possibilities exist. First, there may have been an emotional trauma associated with sex in early development. Perhaps the individual was molested or sexually abused. Second, there may be an unresolved Oedipus complex. Third, the patient may have latent hostility toward the partner. Fourth, the patient may no longer find the partner attractive. And, of course, other explanations can be offered.

Treatment consists of psychotherapy aimed at helping the patient understand the psychological causes of the disorder. Specifically, sexual therapy is often recommended.

See also *erectile disorder (erectile insufficiency)*; *frigidity*; *Oedipus complex*; *sexual response cycle*; *sexual therapy*.

hypochondriasis: In its extreme form, a mental disorder characterized by chronic and irrational worry about one's health. (This condition is also known as *hypochondriacal neurosis*.) A person with the disorder is often labeled a *hypochondriac*. For example, the person may have a few headaches and insist that he or she has a brain tumor. Another individual may not have bowel movement for 3 days and become convinced that there is an intestinal obstruction requiring surgery. The excessive anxiety can attach itself to almost any physical function such as eyesight, heart action, digestion, and so forth.

Persons suffering from this disorder often go from physician to physician, seeking to convince one of them that their problems are very serious, that their symptoms should not be taken lightly. If the physician decides that "there is nothing wrong," the troubled individual is seldom reassured.

The disorder is very common, and it seems to affect the sexes in about equal numbers.

Hypochondriasis can be explained to some extent by referring it to an underlying state of chronic anxiety. It is quite possible that the person with the disorder has had a set of experiences in life that make him or her feel threatened and insecure. The resultant anxiety is projected onto the state of one's health.

Treatment for hypochrondriasis is similar to treatment for anxiety disorders. Antianxiety drugs may be prescribed in some cases. Psychotherapy aimed at helping the individual gain insight into the nature of his or her problems is usually recommended.

Hypochondriasis is not to be confused with a psychosomatic disorder. In this case of psychosomatic disorders, there is an actual illness. Also, it is not to be confused with conversion disorder in which anxiety is transformed into a physical symptom.

See also *anxiety disorders*; *conversion disorder*; *psychosomatic disorders*.

hypoglycemia: Low blood sugar. There are two kinds of hypoglycemia, functional and diabetic. *Functional hypoglycemia* is due to obscure causal factors. However, some that can be identified are excessive intake of food at one time, overeating foods with refined sugar (e.g., ice cream, candy bars, and soft drinks), and the drinking of too much coffee. *Diabetic hypoglycemia* is caused by an overly strong response to an antidiabetic drug (e.g., insulin).

Hypoglycemia is of interest in the framework of mental health because it may produce symptoms such as depression and anxiety. If such symptoms are in fact due to hypoglycemia, it is important to know it. Otherwise, the individual might be treated with anti-anxiety agents, antidepressants, and psychotherapy to no avail.

If an individual suffers from functional hypoglycemia, it is recommended that he or she eat more frequently but less heavily at a given time. Also, it is prudent to reduce intakes of caffeine, tobacco, and alcohol. The person should be under a physician's care.

See also *anxiety*; *depression*.

hypomania: A mild form of mania.
See also *bipolar disorder*; *mania*.

hysteria: The original term for what today is called a conversion disorder. The earliest book published on psychoanalysis was *Studies on Hysteria* (1895) by Josef Breuer and Sigmund Freud, and it included the first case in psychoanalysis—the case of Anna O. It was widely believed at that time that hysteria was caused by problems associated with the uterus. (Note that *hyster* is a Greek root meaning "uterus.") Thus it was believed that hysteria was a woman's disorder. Freud went against the conventional thinking of his time by proposing that men can also suffer from hysteria. Today we know this to be correct. The neutral term *conversion disorder* disconnects "hysteria" from its exclusive associations with females.

See also *Breuer, Josef*; *conversion disorder*; *Freud, Sigmund*.

I

id: In Freudian theory, the foundation of the personality. The id consists of the basic biological drives such as hunger, thirst, pain, and sex. The relief of tension created by these drives is perceived by the individual as pleasure. Thus it is said that the id is pleasure-oriented. Also, Freud stressed the importance of aggression, which he thought of as one more inborn drive. There has been substantial debate about this point in psychology. Not all thinkers agree with Freud's point about aggression.

It was Freud's contention that the excessive repression of the drives of sex and aggression are responsible for neurotic reactions. The family and society want the individual to inhibit the sexual drive until marriage, to be faithful to one partner, and to engage in a limited range of sexual behaviors. Also, the family and society want the person to be polite, have good manners, and control outbursts of anger. Naturally, these constraints are necessary if there is to be any kind of culture or progress. However, Freud contended that neurosis is, to some extent, the price paid for civilization.

The id is impersonal and common to all of us. This, indeed, is why it is called the id. The Latin word *id* simply means "it." Thus the id is, in a sense, the "it" of the personality. In Freud's writings in German, he simply refers to the id as the *it*. However, when the psychoanalyst A. A. Brill translated Freud's works into English, he introduced the term *id*.

The other two principal agents of the personality are the ego and the superego.

See also *ego*; *Freud, Sigmund*; *frustration–aggression hypothesis*; *superego*.

identification: A kind of ego defense mechanism characterized by one individual's unconscious association with the attributes of a second individual. The unconscious thought seems to be something such as, "I am you." For example, a boy might want to be "just like daddy." He might try to shave or engage in some other behavior he associates with his father. The identification of children with their parents in early childhood is seen as healthful and one of the ways in which children acquire the values of their culture.

Identification can take place in adulthood. One might admire another person and strive to imitate that person's dress and behavior. The basic psychological process involves the gathering of psychological strength from the real or imagined powers of the second individual. That is why people with low self-esteem are somewhat more likely to overuse identification than are people in general. If one has very low self-esteem, one may identify intensely with another person. Blind following of the more dominant person may be the result.

It is possible to identify with fictional characters and people that one has never met. Thus some people might identify strongly with a hero in a book. Others might identify with sports figures, movie stars, or other celebrities.

See also *ego defense mechanisms*.

identity crisis: According to the psychoanalyst Erik Erikson, a common developmental problem associated with the fifth stage of psychosocial development, the stage of identity versus role confusion. This stage is usually associated with the ages between 12 and 18 (adolescence) but may easily extend into young adulthood.

When one has a well-defined identity, one can say in essence, "I know who I am and I know where I'm going." There is a sense that life has meaning and purpose. On the other hand, an identity crisis exists when there is role confusion, when the individual thinks, "I don't know what to do with my life. I don't know what vocation to pursue." There is the sense that the direction one should follow in life is muddled and obscure. Confusion concerning one's identity can be a contributing factor to chronic anxiety or depression.

See also *Erikson, Erik Homburger*; *psychosexual development*.

idiosyncratic behavior: Behavior that is unique to the individual. We speak of people having quirks, individual peculiarities, personal mannerisms, and oddities of character. These are all ways in which we attempt to describe idiosyncratic behavior in general terms. Many specific examples of idiosyncratic behavior can be given. Joanna never eats the yolks of eggs. Anatole always carries an umbrella. Hanley has not worn a tie in 20 years. Kristina always wears too much lipstick.

Idiosyncratic behavior, or simply idiosyncracies, is considered normal within limits. However, if behavior becomes too odd, or deviant, it becomes a symptom of a mental disorder.

See also *abnormal behavior*; *deviant behavior*.

idiot: A mentally deficient person. The word *idiot* is a very general term lacking precise meaning, and it is also has insulting connotations. For these reasons, it has fallen out of favor as an accurate clinical term. It is better to speak of mental retardation. This opens the possibility of specifying the level of mental retardation.

See also *idiot savant*; *mental deficiency*; *mental retardation*.

idiot savant: A mentally retarded person with some unusual ability or skill. A *savant* is a person of exceptional knowledge. Thus idiot savants would seem to present a contradiction in terms, and to some extent this is so. That is what makes their behavior intrinsically fascinating to many people. Examples of the kinds of behaviors displayed by idiot savants are the ability to perform amazing arithmetical calculations without pencil or paper, unusual musical talent, and the memorization of thousands of facts about a certain subject (e.g., history, geography, or astronomy). Idiot savants astound and amaze because their talents seem so incongruous when compared to their levels of retardation. Many mental hospitals have one or two patients who are idiot savants.

Although the term *idiot savant* has been used for many years, it is somewhat pejorative. It would be kinder, and more accurate, to speak of a "mentally retarded person who is also a savant."

See also *idiot*; *mental deficiency*; *mental retardation*.

illusion: A perception that is at odds with objective sensory information. There are many well-known optical illusions. For example, in one illusion, two lines of equal length appear to be unequal. In a second, parallel lines appear to be warped. In a third, a figure seems to change its spatial orientation even though it in fact remains fixed.

Illusions are not limited to optical ones and can take place in any sensory modality. It is important to realize that these odd perceptions are normal and caused by special arrangements of the sensory elements. Most people will experience them given a specified set of conditions. Illusions should not be confused with delusions and hallucinations. These are pathological and may be signs of a mental disorder.

See also *delusion*; *hallucination*.

imipramine: An antidepressant drug belonging to the class tricyclics. Sometimes it is also prescribed for enuresis (i.e., bed-wetting).

See also *antidepressant drugs*; *enuresis*.

implosive therapy: A kind of behavior therapy characterized by a rapid flooding of the patient with anxiety. The method was pioneered by Thomas G. Stampfl. The purpose of the therapy is to bring about a rapid desensitization to anxiety-arousing stimuli. In this sense, it is similar to systematic desensitization. It differs in that implosive therapy proceeds rapidly, and systematic desensitization proceeds slowly. The word *implosive* suggests a sort of sudden inward explosion of feeling.

Let us say that a patient has a spider phobia. In implosive therapy, the patient might be taken on a guided fantasy by the therapist in which hundreds of spiders were crawling over one's body. The anxiety level would rise to a very high level. However, if the patient is able to tolerate the anxiety without leaving the fantasy, a sort of psychological and emotional numbing to the images will take place. Eventually imagination will produce no anxiety. And neither will actual situations involving harmless spiders.

Implosive therapy is of principal value in treating phobic disorders. It is recommended only for persons who are emotionally stable.

See also *behavior therapy*; *desensitization therapy*; *flooding*; *phobia*.

impotence: An older, and more popular, term for what is more accurately referred to as *erectile disorder*. The word *impotent* means "lack of power." In the case of sexual behavior, it means lack of power on the part of the male to perform the sexual act.

See also *erectile disorder (erectile insufficiency)*.

impulsive behavior: Behavior that takes place spontaneously without prior planning. We say, "I bought it on the spur of the moment" or "I surprised myself by going to a movie last night." Sudden action and lack of forethought are key attributes of impulsive behavior. Although it is obviously normal to act on impulse sometimes, it is also a characteristic of emotionally immature persons. Such behavior is often irresponsible and has adverse consequences. People who steal, cheat, and engage in promiscuous sexual relations on impulse often regret their actions later.

Impulsive behavior is often displayed by children suffering from attention deficit disorder.

Compulsive behavior should be discriminated from impulsive behavior. A compulsion is an urge to act in opposition to one's conscious will or moral standards. Sometimes the behavior that results in response to a compulsion takes place after a lengthy internal struggle. So this kind of behavior is in some ways the logical opposite of impulsive behavior.

See also *attention deficit disorder*; *compulsion*.

incest: Sexual relations with a close relative. The clearest examples of close relatives are (1) parents and their children and (2) siblings. There are borderline cases. If marriage between two persons is forbidden by law or custom, then sexual relations are considered incestuous. Thus some groups might consider sexual relations between first cousins incest. Other groups would not. If a stepfather and a stepdaughter have sexual relations, is this incest? Again, this is a borderline case. They are related by marriage but not by blood. Some groups would consider their sexual relations incest. Again, others would not.

The actual incidence of incest is unknown because it is probably underreported to authorities. Various studies place their estimates between 2% of families and ½ of 1% of families. But these estimates are not considered to be highly reliable. Sexual relations between brother and sister are believed to be about five times as common as between father and daughter. And sexual relations between mother and son are believed to take place very infrequently.

Although estimates suggest that the actual incidence of incest is low, Freud believed that an incest wish is fairly common, particularly in children. This hypothesis forms the basis of what is called in psychoanalysis the *Oedipus complex*.

The *incest taboo*, society's prohibition against incest, arises from good cause. If incest was practiced on a wide and regular scale, there would be a substantial increase in birth defects and recessive genetic disorders.

See also *Electra complex*; *Oedipus complex*.

incoherent speech: Speech that lacks logic and meaning. The term as used in clinical work does not refer to mumbling, stuttering, or the incorrect use of grammar. Instead, it is a sign of a thought distortion. For example, a clinical psychologist asked a patient, "Did you enjoy watching the baseball game on television last night?" The patient answered, "My television is going to the car on the baseball card. If you knew Babe Ruth, why didn't I tell you?"

Persons suffering from schizophrenic disorders and organic mental disorders often display incoherent speech.

See also *confabulation*; *flight of ideas*.

individual psychology: The name given by Alfred Adler to his system of psychology and therapy. Adler, after a period of association with Freud, broke away from psychoanalysis and started his own movement. Although individual psychology has never been as influential as psychoanalysis, it has had an impact of substantial importance on the practice of psychotherapy. Adler is considered one of the founders of contemporary psychotherapy, and the ideas contained in his approach live on.

Here are some important distinctions between Adler's individual psychology and Freud's psychoanalysis:

1. Freud asserted that all neurotic disorders have their origins in sexual conflicts. Adler argued that neurotic disorders are caused primarily by frustrations of the *will to power*, an inborn tendency as important as sex. Adler derived the concept of the will to power from the writings of the German philosopher Friedrich Nietzsche (1844–1900), giving full credit to Neitzsche for the original formulation. Adler said that the will to power provides an impetus toward *superiority striving*, a struggle on the individual's part in the direction of personal growth and self-confidence. (This idea anticipated Maslow's concept of self-actualization and is very similar to it.)

2. Freud made much of the Oedipus complex, a complex revolving around the frustration of incest wishes. Adler paid more attention to a different complex, the *inferiority complex*. The

inferiority complex arises when the will to power is blocked in a particular domain of behavior. For example, if a child strives to understand arithmetic and has significant learning problems, an inferiority complex may arise. The complex is a set of related ideas such as "I'm no good at long division" and "I can't understand fractions" and "I always make mistakes when I add." The child can be said to have a mathematics inferiority complex. It is possible to have an inferiority complex concerning almost any important aspect of life: sex, appearance, athletic ability, speaking ability, and so forth.

3. Freud's preferred mode of therapy was to have a patient recline on a couch and free-associate. Adler asked the patient to sit up in a comfortable chair and have a face-to-face discussion. The emphasis was on two intelligent people attempting to solve a problem together in contrast to the image of the all-powerful therapist and the weak patient. The discussion dealt with the nature of the person's inferiority complex (or complexes). Adler and the patient explored why the complex had formed and what could be done to disassemble it or cope with it.

4. Freud tended to focus on recovering repressed material from the unconscious mental level. Adler tended to focus on what was easily available to the patient in consciousness and accessible memory. As a consequence, Freud was likely to dwell on the past. And Adler was likely to pay more attention to the present and the future.

Individual psychology may be thought of as an important forerunner of today's humanistic therapy.

See also *Adler, Alfred*; *humanistic therapy*; *self-actualization*.

infantile autism: See *autistic disorder (infantile autism)*.

inferiority complex: See *individual psychology*.

informed consent: A legal term indicating that a mental patient has been advised of the benefits, risks, and alternatives to a given treatment. Also, informed consent implies that the mental patient is cooperating and willing to undergo the particular treatment. A psychiatrist needs to obtain informed consent from the patient before administering any treatment, particularly drugs and electroshock therapy. The general principle today is that the mental patient has civil rights and that these should not be violated. It is best that an informed consent be a signed document.

See also *legal aspects of mental health*.

inhibited female orgasm (orgasmic dysfunction): Inability on the part of the female to achieve an orgasm through sexual stimulation of any variety. (The parallel condition in males is called *inhibited male orgasm*.) A woman suffering from *primary* orgasmic dysfunction has never had an orgasm. On the other hand, a woman suffering from *situational* orgasmic dysfunction has had at least one orgasm in her life.

It should be understood that a woman suffering from either kind of orgasmic dysfunction is usually capable of becoming sexually excited and often enjoys sexual intercourse. Thus the label *frigid woman* is inappropriate.

Inhibited female orgasm can be explained in a number of ways. A given explanation may be the correct one for one female and not another. It is possible that the female's clitoris is covered by a heavy foreskin and does not receive enough stimulation during coitus. Or some women have partners who do not provide additional stimulation to the clitoris during sexual relations. Many women require more than simple sexual intercourse to reach an orgasm. Or maybe the female has ambivalent feelings about sexual relations; guilt mixed with desire may block the orgasm. Or the female may have an Oedipus complex (also called an Electra complex in the case of females). Unconsciously, she may perceive her partner as her father; again, guilt may block the orgasm.

Commonsense approaches to dealing with orgasmic dysfunction are often effective. These often include masturbation of the female's clitoris or clitoral area. However, if such pragmatic approaches are ineffective, then a clinical diagnosis should be made, and treatment should be sought. Sexual therapy is often quite effective in helping a female overcome inhibited orgasm.

See also *erectile disorder (erectile insufficiency)*; *frigidity*; *hypoactive sexual desire disorder (inhibited sexual excitement)*; *orgasm*; *sexual therapy*.

inhibited male orgasm (ejaculatory incompetence or retarded ejaculation): A sexual dysfunction affecting males in which there is experienced either great difficulty or total inability to ejaculate when engaged in sexual intercourse. The problem does not appear to be organic in nature, but psychological, because the male suffering from inhibited male orgasm can often ejaculate easily as a consequence of masturbation.

Possible causal factors in inhibited male orgasm are emotional conflicts in which a partner is unconsciously perceived as one's mother, guilt feelings, feelings of shame and disgust, hostility toward the partner, and so forth.

Inhibited male orgasm is not a commonly reported problem. Nonetheless, it does exist. It is perhaps underreported by males because of embarrassment.

Sex therapy may be of value to the male with this problem.

See also *erectile disorder (erectile insufficiency)*; *Oedipus complex*; *premature ejaculation*; *sexual therapy*.

inhibited sexual excitement: See *hypoactive sexual desire disorder (inhibited sexual excitement)*.

inpatient: A mental patient who is a resident in a mental hospital. Mental patients tend to be hospitalized when (1) their problems are very severe, (2) they are unable to care for themselves in a responsible manner, and (3) they are in the acute phase of their illness. Whenever practical, patients are released as soon as possible to a halfway house, a family, or to the community. Then they are treated as outpatients.

See also *halfway house*; *outpatient*.

insanity: Informally, another word for madness or a psychotic disorder. Formally, a legal term indicating that an individual is not completely responsible for his or her actions. Sometimes the term *diminished capacity* is used to suggest that the person has some sense of responsibility but that it is not adequate.

Psychiatrists and clinical psychologists do not use the word *insanity* as a term for a mental disorder. Its technical usage should be confined to its legal meaning.

See also *insanity defense*; *legal aspects of mental health*.

insanity defense: A defense used in criminal cases based on the assumption that an insane person should not be found guilty even if he or she actually committed a criminal act. The logic is fundamentally quite simple: The individual is not responsible and did not consciously intend to violate the law or do harm. A substantial body of jurisprudence upholds the general reasoning behind the insanity defense. For example, the Durham rule and the M'Naghten rule provide legal precedent.

See also *Durham rule*; *M'Naghten rule*.

insight: Seeing into the nature of a problem. The word *insight* is most commonly used in two contexts in psychology: Gestalt psychology and psychoanalysis. In Gestalt psychology, a classical school of psychology stressing the importance of conscious thought processes, insight refers to the ability of a person to perceive how parts relate to a whole. Informally we say, "The pieces went together" or "the light has dawned." Insight is often used by people to solve riddles and mathematical problems, put together jigsaw puzzles, and understand jokes.

In psychoanalysis, insight refers to the patient's capacity to understand the relationship of formerly repressed mental and emotional content to one's conscious mental life. The patient grows in the direction of better self-understanding. One's own personality becomes increasingly perceived in a lucid manner. The individual is less of a mystery to himself or herself.

See also *psychoanalysis*; *repression*.

insight therapy: Any of the therapies that stress the importance of looking inward with the aim of improving one's general understanding of the self and life. A given insight therapy may help a person to connect repressed mental or emotional content to conscious thought processes. Another may focus on thinking more clearly. Another may stress the importance of human relations. Another may attempt to nurture self-esteem. Another may encourage the individual to make the most of his or her talents or potentialities. Another may explore the meaning of life. But all of them give emphasis to the idea that we are conscious beings, that we can think, and that our capacity to understand can help to free us from unnecessary suffering.

See also *client-centered therapy*; *cognitive therapy*; *humanistic therapy*; *logotherapy*; *psychoanalysis*; *transactional analysis*.

insomnia: A disturbed, or abnormal, pattern of sleep. The most common patterns of insomnia are (1) resistance to falling asleep at all, (2) difficulty in staying asleep, and (3) waking up too early in the morning.

There is no one cause of insomnia. Instead, a host of causes have been identified. Any one, or several working together, may explain a given person's insomnia. Examples of possible causes of insomnia include unusual working hours, chronic anxiety, chronic depression, allergic reactions, drinking too much coffee or tea, alcohol abuse, poor physical condition, and abnormal thyroid functioning.

The proper treatment of a given case of insomnia depends on the cause or causes. In some cases, psychotherapy is called for to help the person cope with anxiety or depression. Behavior modification can sometimes help the individual get rid of mal-adaptive sleep habits. In other cases, an underlying medical problem needs to be treated. Often barbiturates are prescribed for insomnia. These drugs help an individual feel less tense and facilitate relaxation. However, barbiturates are not a cure for insomnia and have some drawbacks.

Commonsense self-management approaches to insomnia include (1) not trying to "force" oneself to go to sleep, (2) getting out of bed for 10 or 20 minutes instead of tossing and turning for hours, and (3) drinking a glass of warm milk before retiring.

See also *barbiturates*.

insulin coma therapy: A kind of somatic therapy characterized by the injection of insulin. The excess insulin introduced into the bloodstream creates a condition of hypoglycemia (i.e., low blood sugar), and the body goes into a state of coma. After a period of time in the coma, usually 1 hour, the patient is brought out by an injection of glucose. During the coma, the patient's vital signs must be carefully monitored. The treatment carries with it a certain amount of danger.

Introduced in the 1930s by Manfred Sakel, an Austrian researcher, the shock to the system was believed to have a beneficial effect on schizophrenic disorders. However, the present viewpoint is that, on the whole, the long-range benefits of insulin coma therapy are slight. The potential risk is not offset by the potential gain. Therefore, it is seldom prescribed by today's psychiatrists.

See also *electroconvulsive therapy (ECT)*; *hypoglycemia*; *somatic therapy*.

intellectualization: An ego defense mechanism in which abstract thinking is used as a way to cope with a threatening feeling. The emotional content of an experience is repressed and replaced with a cold analysis. For example, Lathrop is going through a divorce. He obsessively dwells on the reasons for the failure of his marriage.

He has a "theory" based on his reading of several psychology books. And he tries to convince his best friend of the correctness of his theory. All of this mental investment is obviously non-functional. It will not mend his marriage or bring his wife back. But *thinking* is, to some extent, antagonistic to *feeling*. Thus his pain is in part diminished, at least at the conscious level.

See also *ego defense mechanisms*.

intelligence: A very general concept implying the ability of an individual to think logically, solve problems, comprehend relationships, employ mathematical symbols, and grasp concepts. David Wechsler, a leading researcher and test author, defines intelligence as "the global capacity of the individual to act purposefully, to think rationally, and to deal effectively with the environment."

See also *intelligence quotient (IQ)*; *intelligence tests*; *Wechsler intelligence scales*.

intelligence quotient (IQ): The ratio of mental age (MA) to chronological age (CA). The German psychologist William Stern (1871–1938) introduced the concept of the intelligence quotient as a device for obtaining stable measurements of intelligence over a period of years. The basic formula he proposed is:

$$IQ = MA/CA \times 100$$

For example, Katherine's MA is 10. Her CA is 8. $10/8 = 1.25$. $1.25 \times 100 = 125$. Thus her IQ = 125. For a second example, Todd's MA is 12. His CA is 13. $12/13 = .92$. $.92 \times 100 = 92$. Thus his IQ = 92. Note that if MA is higher than CA, the IQ is above average. If the MA is lower than CA, the IQ is below average. Also note that if MA and CA are identical, the IQ will automatically be 100, or average. For example, Melba's MA is 9. Her CA is 9. $9/9 = 1$. $1 \times 100 = 100$. Thus Melba's

IQ is 100. (The 100 is in the formula merely as a device used to move a decimal two places to the right. This makes it easier to read and report IQs.)

The formula proposed by Stern is the original one. However, it should be noted that IQs on contemporary tests are also often arrived at by a statistical method. The statistical method utilizes a measure of variability known as the *standard deviation*. Ranges of scores under a *normal distribution curve*, a bell-shaped distribution, are used to define the IQ when this approach is taken. The statistical method does not alter the basic meaning of the IQ.

A widely used classification scheme used for IQ scores is the one proposed by the research psychologist David Wechsler:

IQ	Classification	Percentage
130 and above	Very superior	2.2
120–129	Superior	6.7
110–119	Bright normal	16.1
90–109	Average	50.0
80–89	Dull normal	16.1
70–79	Borderline	6.7
69 and below	Mental defective	2.2

Thus in the earlier example, Katherine with an IQ score of 125 belongs to the IQ classification Superior, a group comprising 6.7% of a standardized population. Todd with an IQ score of 92 belongs to the IQ classification Average, a group comprising 50.0% of a standardized population.

It is important to realize that IQ is not intelligence itself. It is a *measure* of intelligence. Therefore it is subject to any of the problems involved in measurement. Sometimes it is unreliable. If, for example, a subject is anxious while taking the test, the IQ score may be suppressed. And the individual may in fact be more intelligent than he or she appears to be in terms of the IQ obtained.

In the field of mental health, the IQ has a practical purpose. Its purpose is to assess the amount of intellectual impairment associated with a mental disorder, mental retardation, or organic brain damage. This can be useful information in arriving at an adequate treatment program for the patient.

See also *intelligence*; *intelligence tests*; *mental age (MA)*; *psychological test*.

intelligence tests: Standardized tests of intellectual performance designed to measure intelligence. These tests yield an IQ score. They also provide a profile of an individual's highs and lows in different areas of intelligence such as comprehension, mathematical ability, attention span, or spatial reasoning. Such a profile can be useful if the individual needs counseling. Also the profile can be of diagnostic value if an individual has suffered a cerebrovascular accident (CVA).

The most well-known, and widely used, tests are the Stanford-Binet Intelligence Scale, the Wechsler Intelligence Scale for Children (WISC), and the Wechsler Adult Intelligence Scale (WAIS).

See also *cerebrovascular accident (CVA)*; *Stanford–Binet Intelligence Scale*; *Wechsler intelligence scales*.

intermittent explosive disorder (explosive disorder): An impulse control disorder characterized by a sudden outburst of aggressive behavior. During the outburst, the individual may do substantial bodily injury, often to strangers, and property damage.

Although intermittent explosive disorder is quite rare, it has serious consequences and cannot be dismissed lightly. It is a very serious pathological condition.

It has been argued that in some cases of intermittent explosive disorder, but not most, there is a biological explanation. Brain tumors, epilepsy, and minimal brain dysfunction are possibilities. More commonly, a psychological explanation is used. An individual with a superficially passive personality combined with a large store of repressed rage might reach a sort of critical threshold and manifest explosive behavior. This phenomenon has sometimes been called *snapping*, a sudden loss of self-control.

Anticonvulsant medication is sometimes prescribed for intermittent explosive disorder if it is suspected that there is an underlying brain pathology. Psychotherapy aimed at helping a person cope with frustration and release hostility in a harmless way is the usual treatment of choice.

See also *brain pathology*; *epilepsy*; *impulsive behavior*; *minimal brain dysfunction (MBD)*.

International Classification of Diseases (ICD): A statistical classification system for diseases, morbid conditions, and mental disorders developed and published by the World Health Organization (WHO). The ICD has gone through a number of revisions, and at the time of this writing is in its ninth edition.

The principal system used in the United States for classifying and naming mental disorders is the American Psychiatric Association's *Diagnostic and Statistical Manual of Mental Disorders*, not the *International Classification of Diseases*. The two systems are similar but not identical. One very important difference is that the ICD retains neurotic disorders as a category, and DSM does not.

See also Diagnostic and Statistical Manual of Mental Disorders; *neurosis*.

interpretation: As originally used in psychoanalysis, the effort on the part of the analyst to provide a meaningful link between unconscious thought processes and conscious ones. Thus, in Freud's approach to the interpretation of dreams, the patient is shown how the remembered fragment (i.e., manifest content) of a given dream is a symbolic expression of an unconscious wish (i.e., latent content). Slips of the tongue are also subject to interpretation. A patient says, "I killed my wife last night. Uh—that is, I mean I *kissed* my wife last night." This might be interpreted as a sign of repressed hostility toward the wife. Behavior in general can be interpreted. A patient is frequently very late for appointments. This might be interpreted as a sign of unconscious resistance to therapy. The basic idea of interpretations is to give the patient a clearer understanding of thought and behavior in terms of their unconscious roots.

The concept of an interpretation has been broadened quite a bit beyond its original meaning in classical psychoanalysis. It is possible to say that, in psychotherapy in general, an interpretation refers to any effort on the part of the therapist to help a patient understand the full range and significance of his or her thoughts, feelings, and actions.

See also *dream analysis*; *psychoanalysis*.

intoxication: Broadly speaking, any poisoning of the body. A *toxin* is a poison. As intoxication is used in the mental health field, it usually refers to the excessive intake of a drug such as alcohol, an amphetamine, a barbiturate, a narcotic, or marijuana. It is even possible to speak of caffeine intoxication when a person has had perhaps 12 or more cups of coffee in a short time period. For alcohol intoxication, the words *drunk* or *inebriated* are commonly used.

See also *alcoholism*; *drug addiction*.

intrapsychic conflict: A conflict taking place within one's personality. In classical psychoanalysis, the principal intrapsychic conflict is between the id and the superego. The id gives rise in consciousness to a wish (e.g., "I would like to punch John in the nose"). The superego resists the wish in terms of the individual's value system (e.g., "Nice people don't hit others"). If the ego is strong, it can resolve the intrapsychic conflict and find some realistic working compromise between the crude impulses of the id and the moral restrictions of the superego (e.g., "I'll stop allowing John to take advantage of me").

The intrapsychic conflict described is a fairly mild one. However, intrapsychic conflicts surrounding intense sexual and aggressive feelings can be quite intense. If they are chronic, they can be a contributing factor to mental and behavioral pathologies.

The contemporary concept of an intrapsychic conflict is somewhat more general than the psychoanalytic one. Any internal psychological struggle between opposing tendencies can be thought of as intrapsychic. For example, two opposing values can be in conflict. Noah feels he should spend more time with his aging mother. He also feels he should spend more time with his growing children. If he lives up to one value, he feels he must fail the other one to some extent. He feels caught in the middle and is constantly engaged making a choice between his responsibilities.

An intrapsychic conflict should be contrasted with an *interpsychic conflict*, one taking place between two or more people. Interpsychic conflicts can also be quite intense and may induce maladaptive behavior. Transactional analysis is an approach that gives substantial attention to this kind of conflict.

See also *ego*; *id*; *superego*; *transactional analysis*.

intropunitive: The tendency to punish oneself. Most commonly, this expresses itself as a tendency toward self-blame. The individual may think, "It's all my fault" or "I've let my children down." Intense intropunitive tendencies are associated with self-destructive behavior, masochism, and suicide. In psychoanalytic theory, such intense intropunitive tendencies come from an overly strict super-ego.

See also *masochism*; *suicide*; *superego*.

introversion: A tendency to be preoccupied with the inner world of thoughts and feelings in contrast to the outer world of seeing, hearing, and doing. As originally conceived by Carl Jung, introversion is a psychological attitude characterized by a flowing inward of libido, or psychological energy, toward the psyche (i.e., personality). Thus a person with strong introverted tendencies might prefer a life of contemplation and reflection to a life of business activity or adventure. The opposite attitude to introversion is *extraversion*.

Both introversion and extraversion coexist in most people. However, there is a tendency for one attitude to be dominant. If introversion is dominant, the individual is sometimes called an *introvert*.

Pathology of the personality exists when (1) introversion almost completely eclipses extraversion and (2) the individual is unstable. Thus a person who is highly introverted and simultaneously unstable could be described with words such as *unsociable, pessimistic, rigid,* and *moody.* The approach being described here was developed by the research psychologist Hans J. Eysenck.

See also *extraversion; Eysenck, Hans Jurgen; Jung, Carl Gustav; libido.*

in vivo: Latin for "in life." The term finds its principal use in psychology in the context of systematic desensitization. Often, in systematic desensitization, a patient is presented with guided fantasies designed to induce anxiety. However, it is possible to desensitize the person *in vivo* or "in life." Thus the person who is afraid of spiders may be encouraged to watch the activity of harmless ones or, in time, allow them to crawl on the hand. The person who is afraid to travel in a car may be gently encouraged to go for a ride around the block with the therapist as a first step. *In vivo* desensitization can be quite threatening and must be used judiciously by a therapist, or it can be counterproductive.

See also *behavior therapy; desensitization therapy.*

involutional melancholia: A traditional term for depression associated with middle and old age. The later portion of one's life is sometimes termed an *involutional period,* suggesting both a decline in sexual energy and physical vigor. Early clinicians believed the organic decline played a causal role in the melancholy state when depression occurred in older persons.

Present clinical thought rejects the preceding interpretation. Therefore, involutional melancholia has become essentially an obsolete term. If an older person suffers from severe and chronic depression, it is diagnosed as *major depression.* The individual's age is not a relevant diagnostic criterion.

See also *major depression (unipolar disorder).*

isolation: An ego defense mechanism in which the emotion and the cognitive content of an experience or a memory are divided from each other. The aim of the mechanism is to reduce the individual's level of psychological pain. For example, Jordan, an adult, remembers quite distinctly that his father was physically abusive when Jordan was a child. He can now talk about, and remember vividly, the ways in which he was punished. But no feeling is attached to the memory.

See also *ego defense mechanisms*.

J

Jacksonian epilepsy: See *epilepsy*.

James, William (1842–1910): Highly influential psychologist and
philosopher associated for many years with Harvard University.
James is often referred to as the "dean of American psychologists."
He is considered to be the first American psychologist, established
a psychological laboratory at Harvard, and sponsored the first
Ph.D. degree granted in psychology in the United States. (The
recipient of this degree was Granville Stanley Hall, himself an
influential psychologist.) James helped Clifford W. Beers, a former
mental patient, establish the mental hygiene movement.

James was the father of *functionalism*, a major school of psychology. Functionalism asserts that a principal aim of psychology
is to study the mental life of human beings. It further asserts that
mental life is highly conscious, that consciousness is always flowing
and moving, and that this dynamic aspect of consciousness must
be understood. Functionalism faded into insignificance in academic
psychology in the 1930s and the 1940s due to the rise of behaviorism. However, in recent times there as been a reassertion of
the importance of understanding the conscious aspects of mental
life. This attitude underlies the present great influence exerted by
cognitive-behavior therapy. James can be seen as the principal
forerunner of this contemporary trend.

Two of James's important works are *Principles of Psychology* (1890) and *Varieties of Religious Experience* (1902).

See also *Beers, Clifford Whittingham; behaviorism; cognitive-behavior therapy; Hall, Granville Stanley.*

Janet, Pierre Marie Felix (1859–1947): A pioneer investigator into unconscious mental processes. Janet was the director of the Psychological Clinic of the Salpêtrière and studied under the eminent neurologist Jean Martin Charcot. Charcot was an influence on both Janet and Freud, and many of the observations of Janet and Freud overlap.

Janet did much original work on ego states with the aid of hypnosis. He found he was able to produce dissociative reactions similar to those experienced by multiple personalities, and this line of research produced a deeper understanding of the role of the ego in the personality.

Janet explored how "fixed ideas" can be contributing factors to neurotic problems, and he believed that they did their pathological work from an unconscious level.

As is evident, Janet and Freud had much in common as theoreticians. Although Janet retains a considerable status in the history of psychiatry and psychology, it is also true that Freud has greatly eclipsed him in general reputation.

Two of Janet's books are *The Mental State of Hystericals* (1901) and *The Major Symptoms of Hysteria* (1920).

See also *Charcot, Jean Martin; Freud, Sigmund; multiple personality disorder; neurosis; unconscious mental life.*

Jones, Ernest (1879–1958): A British psychoanalyst and a principal biographer of Freud. Jones was one of Freud's most loyal followers and was influential in introducing psychoanalysis to both the United Kingdom and the United States. In 1911, Jones helped found the American Psychoanalytic Association. Jones made significant contributions to the understanding of neurotic processes and to improvements in psychoanalytic technique.

Jones's approach to therapy is described in his book *Treatment of the Neuroses* (1920). His three-volume biography of Freud, *The Life and Work of Sigmund Freud* (1955), is considered a classic work.

See also *Freud, Sigmund*; *neurosis*; *psychoanalysis*.

Jung, Carl Gustav (1875–1961): A Swiss psychiatrist, early follower of Freud, and major personality theorist. Jung was working as a young psychiatrist in Switzerland with the eminent Eugen Bleuler when Jung became aware of Sigmund Freud and psychoanalysis. Jung visited Freud in Austria and the two men became fast friends. For a number of years, they worked together and cooperated in the formation of psychoanalysis as an influential movement.

In 1909, Jung and Freud traveled together to Clark University in the United States to deliver introductory lectures in psychoanalysis. Due to Freud's instigation, Jung, not Freud, became in 1910 the first president of the International Psychoanalytic Association. Freud was concerned that psychoanalysis might be rejected by a larger community of scientists because of his Jewish origins. Jung was a Christian, and his father was a clergyman.

It eventually became clear to both Jung and Freud that they differed on too many theoretical points to continue their collaboration. Jung established his own approach to therapy and personality theory, calling it *analytic psychology*.

Jung was a prolific writer and published many books in his lifetime. Among his important works are *Modern Man in Search of a Soul* (1933), *Psychological Types* (1933), and *The Archetypes and the Collective Unconscious* (1936).

See also *analytic psychology (analytical psychology)*; *archetypes*; *Bleuler, Eugen*; *collective unconscious*; *extraversion*; *Freud, Sigmund*; *introversion*.

juvenile delinquency: Loosely, the violation of a social norm by a child or adolescent. Formally, juvenile delinquency is the breaking of the law by a minor. A minor is a person who does not yet have the civil and personal rights of an adult. The age of adulthood for certain purposes may be set as young as 16. And, in almost every instance, an individual over the age of 18 is treated as an adult. Exact ages vary from state to state.

Minors basically commit the same kinds of crimes as adults. These may include theft, prostitution, rape, drug selling, drug use, assault, murder, property damage, and so forth. It is conservatively estimated that juveniles are responsible for about 10% to 15% of the crime in the United States.

From the mental health viewpoint, it is important to understand that a personality disorder often underlies juvenile delinquency. Children and adolescents with a history of conduct disorders are often the same ones who transgress against society. In many cases, but certainly not all, the child's problems are a reaction to emotionally cold, authoritarian parents. And such parents may be found at all levels of society.

There are also social and cultural causes of juvenile delinquency. Poverty, lack of opportunity, delinquent peers, and living in a slum all contribute to delinquent behavior. Nonetheless, it is important to note that socially advantaged juveniles are frequently offenders.

Aside from the punishment administered by law, the response to juvenile delinquency is usually a program of rehabilitation and counseling. The aim of such programs revolves around helping the minor develop a better sense of self-esteem and a greater sense of social responsibility. Reality therapy, an approach pioneered by the psychiatrist William Glasser, helps the socially immature individual perceive that there is little or no future in the violation of society's norms and laws.

Juvenile delinquency is a complex problem in our society, presenting problems in both the legal and mental health fields.

See also *conduct disorder*; *reality therapy*.

K

kleptomania: A disorder characterized by an impulse to steal. A key feature of this disorder is that the individual does not steal with any objective aim. The stolen item is not sold for profit, and the individual is not in financial need. Instead, it appears that the act of theft is exciting and intrinsically gratifying. Sometimes the stolen items are given away, secretly returned, or hoarded.

People with this disorder *do* fear arrest and usually make some effort to avoid being caught.

Shoplifting and kleptomania are similar but not identical. It is true that most kleptomaniacs are shoplifters. However, the reverse statement is *not* true. Most shoplifters are not kleptomaniacs. Most shoplifters take items because of their value. They may steal cold-bloodedly and not on impulse at all. The kleptomaniac, on the other hand, seldom thinks ahead about the act of theft.

There is no glib explanation that can be given for kleptomania. However, it is possible to speculate on the meaning of the behavior. It is certainly a way of obtaining a thrill. Risk-taking behaviors such as sky diving and hot-air ballooning provide excitement for some people. The kleptomaniac finds theft exciting. Also, it is a way of feeling powerful. The individual who suffers from low self-esteem may temporarily feel more adequate because theft signifies, "I've outsmarted another person." An individual with a great deal of hostility may unconsciously feel that he or she is punishing other people by depriving them of something of value.

Treatment for kleptomania consists of insight-oriented therapy aimed at helping the troubled individual understand the roots of the irrational impulse. Then the individual is encouraged to find more constructive ways to express conflicting emotional needs.

See also *impulsive behavior*; *insight therapies*.

Klinefelter's syndrome: A set of symptoms characterized primarily by mental retardation and underdeveloped testes. The disorder affects only males. Frequently there is inadequate appearance of secondary sexual characteristics such as facial and pubic hair. There may be little or no sperm production. Often the body tends toward fat and the formation of large breasts. The syndrome was first identified in 1942 by H. F. Klinefelter, an American researcher.

The cause of the syndrome is a chromosomal anomaly. The individual with Klinefelter's syndrome has one male chromosome and two female chromosomes in each cell of his body. *X* is the symbol used to indicate a female chromosome. *Y* is the symbol used to indicate a male chromosome. The normal male has a chromosome structure that may be identified as *XY*. The person with Klinefelter's syndrome has a chromosome structure that may be identified as *XXY*.

Treatment for Klinefelter's syndrome includes shots of the male hormone testosterone, and these often help the individual have a more normal appearance. A sex drive, formerly absent, sometimes emerges as a result of these shots.

See also *androgens*; *chromosomal anomalies*; *mental retardation*.

Korsakoff's psychosis: See *alcohol amnestic disorder*.

Kraepelin, Emil (1856–1926): A German physician, a professor of psychiatry, and director of an important clinic in Munich during the height of his career. Kraepelin was a pioneer in the classification of mental disorders. It was he who introduced the term *dementia praecox* into the psychiatric literature, thus providing a label for madness associated with adolescence and young adulthood. The term *schizophrenia*, suggested subsequently by Eugen Bleuler, has replaced Kraepelin's term.

Kraepelin suggested that psychotic disorders can be divided into two principal categories: (1) disturbances of thought and (2) disturbances of mood. This distinction remains of importance today. Kraepelin had a pessimistic view of severe mental disorders. He believed that they had a biological basis, that their roots resided in genetic, endocrine, or other organic factors. As a consequence, he took the position that they were by and large untreatable.

Contemporary research gives credibility to Kraepelin's emphasis on the importance of biological factors in mental disorders. However, both somatic therapy and psychotherapy suggest that mental disorders are treatable.

Kraepelin's work is regarded as the principal antecedent of the classification system used in contemporary psychiatry, the system reflected in the American Psychiatric Association's *Diagnostic and Statistical Manual of Mental Disorders*.

One of Kraepelin's principal works is *Lectures on Clinical Psychiatry* (1904).

See also *Bleuler, Eugen*; *dementia praecox*; Diagnostic and Statistical Manual of Mental Disorders; *schizophrenia*.

Krafft-Ebing, Richard von (1840–1902): A pioneer in the study of sexual disorders. Krafft-Ebing was a German psychiatrist, a university professor, and for about 15 years the director of the National Insane Asylum in Graz. He made a contribution to the understanding of general paresis and was among a group of researchers who recognized that it was caused by syphilis.

Krafft-Ebing's research helped to make the study of sexual pathology a respectable subject of scientific investigation. His most well-known work is *Psychopathia Sexualis* (1892).

See also *general paresis*; *sexual disorders (psychosexual disorders)*.

L

labile: Unstable. This term is used in psychiatry and clinical psychology to suggest an unstable emotional state. Thus when an individual is described as being *labile*, it suggests that he or she is subject to unpredictable or sudden emotional shifts. This is a characteristic associated in particular with bipolar disorder and cyclothymic disorder.

See also *bipolar disorder*; *cyclothymic disorder*; *emotion*.

Laing, Ronald David (1927–): Scottish psychiatrist and pioneer in the use of existential therapy to treat schizophrenic patients. Laing takes the position that an important causal factor in schizophrenic disorders is alienation from other people. This state is itself traceable to adverse childhood experiences and the pathology of the general society. In brief, the patient is the confused victim of a difficult world he or she did not make.

According to Laing, the standard treatment of schizophrenic disorders with drugs and other kinds of somatic therapies does not address itself to the real problems of the patient. The patient does not need to be administered to according to a prescription or a formula but as an individual with a unique personality. Laing's approach, accordingly, is exceedingly humane. The troubled person is assisted in self-expression, in exploring ways to understand his or her life situation. The patient finds mental health through a gradual process of growth and self-understanding.

Although Laing's work is often understood in the context of schizophrenic disorders, it has general implications for the understanding of troubled persons in general. Two of Laing's books are *The Divided Self* (1965) and *The Politics of Experience* (1967).

See also *alienation*; *antipsychiatry*; *double-bind communication*; *existential therapy*.

language disorder, developmental: See *developmental disorders*.

latency stage: According to Freud, the fourth stage of psychosexual development lasting from about 6 to 12 years of age. During this stage, libido (i.e., psychosexual energy) is dormant.

See also *libido*; *psychosexual development*.

latent dream content: According to Freud, the underlying meaning of a dream. In psychoanalytic theory, a dream is said to have two levels: a manifest level and a latent one. The manifest level consists of the remembered fragments of the dream and its symbols. The latent content is what the symbols point to. The latent content exists at an unconscious level and usually contains a forbidden wish. This forbidden wish tends to be of a sexual or aggressive nature, representing an impulse that is prohibited by the superego (i.e., the moral agent of one's personality). For example, Morton, a man 24 years of age, dreams that he has a boxing match with a masked champion. It is obvious that the masked champion is quite a bit older than he is. Morton soundly defeats the older boxer. In psychoanalytic therapy, Morton discovers that the masked champion stands for his father, and the latent content of the dream is repressed hostility toward his parent.

See also *dream analysis*; *manifest dream content*.

learned helplessness: A tendency to generalize actual helplessness experienced in a first situation to a second situation where the individual is not helpless. For example, Nancy's father was an overcontrolling parent who was insensitive to her feelings when she was a child. She felt that she could "never win" with him. Now she is an adult and married. Her husband is a sensitive and reasonably understanding person. However, if he sometimes behaves in an authoritarian manner, she gets the same helpless feeling that she had as a child. Something in her says, "I can't win." And she does not assert herself but passively succumbs to her husband's wishes. She accepts defeat without a struggle.

Learned helplessness is a phenomenon that his been extensively studied in both animals and people. The researcher Martin E. P. Seligman is responsible for much of the work on the concept. Evidence suggests that learned helplessness is an important factor in depression. Assertiveness training and other forms of psychotherapy can help an individual to overcome learned helplessness.

See also *assertiveness training*; *depression*.

legal aspects of mental health: A substantial body of jurisprudence has arisen surrounding the related topics of mental health and mental disorders. The rights and responsibilities of mental patients have undergone a close scrutiny for many years, and numerous important practices have been established. Traditionally, the legal aspects of mental health have included such domains of concern as (1) the rights of mental patients, (2) the extent of a patient's criminal responsibility when an offense is complicated by the presence of a mental disorder, (3) the use of expert witnesses (e.g., clinical psychologists and psychiatrists) in trials, (4) the importance of obtaining informed consent from families and patients before administering treatment, (5) the determination of competency and incompetency, (6) the establishment of conservatorships to protect incompetent individuals from their own irresponsible or irrational behavior, and (7) the extension of civil rights and due process to juvenile court proceedings.

It is important to realize that a broad legal principle now exists that can be stated as follows: *Mental patients have legal rights.* They cannot be deprived of liberty or subjected to psychiatric treatments without regard to their civil rights. Gone are the days when persons with mental disorders were treated like brainless things. Today the informed consent of the patient and his or her family is essential. Professionals who ignore the legal rights of mental patients are subject to lawsuits.

The term *conservatorship* used in Item 6 refers to the creation of a legal entity similar to a trust. The purpose of this legal entity is to assure that a mentally incompetent person will not deplete a fund of money or property. In order to create a conservatorship, it is essential to establish in a court of law that a given individual is incompetent, meaning he or she is unable to handle matters of finance in a rational and reasonable way. If found to be incompetent, a *conservator*, an individual charged with protecting the property, is appointed.

See also *Durham rule*; *forensic psychiatry and psychology*; *informed consent*; *insanity*; *insanity defense*; *juvenile delinquency*; *M'Naghten rule*.

lesbian: A female homosexual. The word *lesbian* is derived from the Greek island of Lesbos. Legend states that the Greek lyric poetess Sappho and her followers, living in the sixth century B.C. on the island, practiced homosexual behavior.

See also *gay*; *homosexuality*; *sexual disorders (psychosexual disorders)*.

lethality scale: A scale developed by the Los Angeles Suicide Prevention Center with the purpose of assessing the likelihood that a given individual will commit suicide. In other words, the question is, how "lethal" is the person's present situation and state of mind? In order to make an evaluation, a number of scoring categories are used. Some of these include (1) mental symptoms, (2) availability of resources in terms of a family, (3) the existence of psychosocial stressors, (4) the history of suicide attempts, (5) age, (6) sex, and (7) medical health.

The lethality scale is an attempt to develop a way to help mental health workers increase their ability to predict a troubled person's self-destructive behavior.

See also *suicide*; *suicidology*.

libido: As introduced by Freud in the language of classical psychoanalysis, psychosexual energy. The term *libido* is derived from a Latin root meaning "lust." As Freud used the term, he wanted it to indicate that the personality is to some extent shaped by the individual's sex drive. That is why, as Freud meant the word, it is not sufficient to refer to libido as simply the equivalent of sex drive. Freud believed that mental life and sexual life were intertwined. Libido, to Freud, is the energy that makes mental activity possible.

Jung argued that it is not essential to tie the concept of libido to sex drive. Therefore, in Jung's analytic psychology, libido is simply psychological energy. Freud, of course, objected strongly to this usage. However, it has somewhat complicated the meaning of libido. When one sees or hears the word used, the question should be asked: Is Freud's or Jung's meaning intended?

See also *analytic psychology (analytical psychology)*; *Freud, Sigmund*; *Jung, Carl Gustav*; *psychoanalysis*; *psychosexual development*.

Librium: A well-known trade name for a tranquilizer with the generic name *chlordiazepoxide*. Some of the other trade names for this drug are C-Tran, Corax, Libritabs, and Relaxil. Librium is often prescribed to combat anxiety. It is also prescribed to control muscle spasms and symptoms associated with convulsive disorders. Like all drugs, Librium sometimes has adverse side effects. Therefore, it is to be used only by prescription and with medical supervision.

See also *antianxiety drugs*; *drug therapy*.

life change units (LCUs): A concept associated with an inventory entitled the *Social Readjustment Rating Scale* (SRRS). The SRRS was developed in 1967 by the researchers T. H. Holmes and R. H. Rahe, and it is used to evaluate the level of psychosocial stress in a person's life. Life changes that require social readjustment are given a number designed to indicate the change's level of impact. The number is the LCU for that life change. Thus death of a spouse was assigned an LCU value of 100, and this is the maximum value. In descending order, here are some other LCU values: divorce = 73, marital separation = 65, death of a family member = 63, marriage = 50, retirement = 45, change vocations = 36, home foreclosure = 30, trouble with boss = 23, receiving a traffic ticket = 11.

Take note of the fact that even a happy event such as marriage can be stressful. Rahe and Holmes found that LCUs are related to physical illness. If LCUs for a given individual sum to more than 150 over a time interval of 2 years, there is an increased likelihood that the individual will experience an important adverse change in health.

The basic wisdom to be derived from the scale is not that a person should avoid all life changes but that we should make an effort to keep the *frequency* of our life changes at a moderate level. If life changes come at too fast and furious a pace, we have a difficult time adapting to them. If they can be spaced, then social readjustments are more readily made.

See also *psychosocial stressors*; *psychosomatic disorders*; *stress*.

lithium carbonate: The principal tranquilizing drug used to treat bipolar disorder. (An older term for bipolar disorder is *manic-depressive psychosis*.) Lithium carbonate is marketed under several trade names such as Eskalith, Lithane, Lithonate, and Lithotabs. It is hypothesized that lithium carbonate is effective in modulating both mania and depression by (1) regulating the action of neurotransmitters in the central nervous system and (2) producing beneficial cellular changes in neurons.

Although lithium carbonate is not a habit-forming drug, a prescription is required for its use. It has potentially adverse side effects, and the amount taken must be carefully regulated. In very large doses, the drug can be quite toxic.

See also *bipolar disorder*; *drug therapy*; *neuron*; *neurotransmitters*.

lobotomy: A form of psychosurgery in which the frontal lobes of the brain are severed from the rest of the brain. The operation was introduced in 1935 by Egas Moniz, a Portuguese psychiatrist and surgeon. Walter Freeman and James Watts working together pioneered lobotomies in the United States. The origin of the operation starts with Moniz's observation that a lobotomy was capable of tranquilizing a violent chimpanzee. This observation led him to perform the operation on aggressive mental patients, and he reported beneficial results. It is hypothesized that cutting the frontal lobes makes it difficult for a psychotic patient to have delusions and other disordered thoughts.

There are a number of adverse side effects associated with lobotomies. Common ones are (1) development of an apathetic attitude toward life, (2) overeating, (3) decline in social sensitivity, (4) problems controlling urine, and (5) seizures. So it is apparent that the procedure is very serious and should not be undertaken lightly.

Much controversy has surrounded the use of lobotomies in connection with the care of mental patients. Many, perhaps most, mental health professionals seriously question the ethics of irreversible psychosurgery. As a consequence, the use of the lobotomy has declined greatly, and today it is seldom a treatment of choice for psychotic disorders. The use of major tranquilizing drugs has become the principal form of biological therapy for psychotic disorders.

See also *major tranquilizers (antipsychotic drugs)*; *psychosurgery*; *psychotic disorders*.

locomotor ataxia: Lack of ability to coordinate movements. For example, people with locomotor ataxia often have trouble walking. They may also have trouble using their arms in a task requiring their simultaneous activity such as drying dishes. The most well-known cause of locomotor ataxia is infection of the spinal cord caused by the syphilis spirochete.

See also *general paresis*.

locus of control: The perception that one's own behavior has either an external or internal origin. For example, Person A says, "I'm getting divorced. And it's because my parents interfered with my marriage." This statement reflects an *external locus of control*.

Person B says, "I'm getting divorced. I've grown to realize that my marriage is a loveless one, and I made a mistake." This statement reflects an *internal locus of control*. On the whole, an external locus of control tends to suggest that the person feels like a victim, a pawn of fate. An internal locus of control tends to suggest that the person feels a sense of self-control, of choice, of autonomy. A habit of perceiving behavior in terms of an external locus of control may be a contributing factor to depression. A habit of perceiving behavior in terms of an internal locus of control is associated with mental health.

The research psychologist Julian Rotter developed a psychological test used to assess one's tendency to define behavior in external or internal terms, the *Rotter Internal-External Scale*. The subject is asked to answer *agree* or *disagree* with a set of statements designed to reflect internal or external locus of control. For example, an item might say, "I think most people who make a lot of money just happen to know the right people." An *agree* answer with this item suggests an external locus of control. Of course, answers to a single item mean very little. It is a person's overall score on the entire scale that must be used. The test results can be of diagnostic value to psychotherapists.

See also *autonomy*; *personality test*; *psychological test*.

logic-tight compartments: An involuntary cognitive strategy adopted by the individual as a way of avoiding the obvious conflict between incompatible ideas. The person creates two mental "compartments," one for each idea. Then the ideas never meet in consciousness. (Another name for logic-tight compartments is *compartmentalization*.)

Montgomery tells his wife, "I love you, darling, only you." He also has a mistress. When she asks him, "Am I your only love?" he answers, "Yes. You are the only woman I love." When he is with his wife he believes what he says, and when he is with his mistress he believes what he says. He never directly faces the absurd contradiction in his two basically identical statements because he keeps the idea of love for his wife in one "compartment" and the idea of love for his mistress in another "compartment."

By doing this, he is able to reduce the level of his mental and emotional conflicts.

A common example of logic-tight compartments is the businessman who on Sunday thinks, "I love my fellow human beings. Do unto others as you would have them do unto you." And on weekdays he thinks, "It's a dog-eat-dog world. You've got to watch out for Number One or you'll go bankrupt." Sunday thinking is in one "compartment," and weekday thinking is in another "compartment."

Essentially, logic-tight compartments function to reduce anxiety and maintain self-esteem. The strategy is basically an ego defense mechanism.

See also *ego defense mechanisms*.

logotherapy: A kind of psychotherapy pioneered by the European psychiatrist Viktor Frankl. Logotherapy is based on the assumption that human beings have an inborn *will to meaning*, a desire for life to make some sort of sense. The will to meaning is satisfied when one can attain important values, something the individual perceives as worth doing. For some people, this could be raising a child or children. For others, it might be inventing something of use for humankind. For still others, it might be working as a physician or a nurse. Values will vary from individual to individual and from culture to culture. Nonetheless, there is a theme. And that theme is living a useful life in terms of one's society.

Frankl observes that when one is frustrated in attaining important values in life, the result is a kind of emptiness in existence. Frankl calls this state the *existential vacuum* and notes that it frequently plays a role in depression. Many people, particularly in developed countries (i.e., industrialized nations), suffer to some degree from the existential vacuum.

Frankl takes the philosophical position that values are real, that they actually exist. They do not need to be invented by human beings but discovered. Therefore a person who suffers from an existential vacuum might be compared to a person who finds himself or herself in a room with the lights out. There is furniture (i.e., "values") in the room, but they cannot be seen. Someone turns the lights on, and the furniture is immediately observable. The aim of logotherapy is to "turn the lights on" in a person's life in order to illuminate the values a patient has been unable to see.

There is no one way to help an individual see values. It can be done by discussion, examples, and questions. Therapy proceeds in the form of a face-to-face interview between two persons (the therapist and the patient) working toward answers to the most profound questions of life. Sometimes, however, the therapist can facilitate a rapid insight. For example, Natasha, a married woman with three young children, is suffering from depression. She feels overburdened by the pressure of being a young mother. Her husband seems to her to be to be somewhat insensitive to her plight, and he is not helpful around the house or with the children. Also, she wants to go back to college and become a registered nurse, but at present she is able to take only one night class toward her goal. She has a strong tendency to whine and feel sorry for herself. At one point, the therapist asks, "How would you feel if someone kidnapped your children? Then you would be free to pursue your vocational goals. What would you do?"

Natasha reveals her hidden strength of character and answers with passion, "I would go through hell and high water to get my children back! I would never rest until I found them again! No one could do this to me and succeed!"

"There!", exclaims the therapist. "You have just revealed to yourself that raising your children is a value of the greatest importance. Your life is filled with meaning, and you have not been aware of it."

"You're right!" declares Natasha with a sob.

It must be observed that the pursuit of her vocational goals is also a value for Natasha, and it is a value she should realistically find a way to fulfill. However, her timetable might change. Perhaps she decides that she can take more college courses when all of the children are in grammar school for full day sessions.

Frankl was once asked, "What is the difference between psychoanalysis and logotherapy?" He answered with a quip. "In psychoanalysis the patient reclines on a couch and says things that are difficult to say. In logotherapy the patient sits up and hears things that are difficult to hear." Although the quip over-simplifies, it captures in a few words an essential truth about logotherapy.

See also *existential neurosis*; *existential therapy*; *Frankl, Viktor*; *humanistic therapy*.

lunacy: Madness, psychotic behavior. *Lunacy* is an informal word without precise meaning. Therefore, it has no place in a scientific vocabulary describing abnormal behavior. The word is an ancient one derived from the Latin word for moon, *luna*. It is a very old bit of folklore that the full moon brings out the worst in people, that there is an increase in irrational behavior during the waxing of the moon.

A number of researchers have sought correlations between the full moon and crime statistics. Some declare that such a correlation exists. However, the majority of behavioral scientists remain skeptical. They question the methodology of such studies and believe that the evidence in favor of folklore is very weak.

See also *madness*; *psychotic disorders*.

lycanthropy: Two related meanings are associated with lycanthropy. First, lycanthropy is the idea in folklore that some people can turn themselves into wolves. The legend of the *lycanthrope*, or werewolf, is derived from this idea.

Second, lycanthropy is the delusion held by some mental patients that they are wolves or other animals of the wilderness.

See also *delusion*.

lysergic acid diethylamide-25 (LSD): A powerful drug belonging to the class hallucinogens. LSD is an alkaloid substance derived from ergot (a kind of fungus). Very tiny amounts of LSD can produce large alterations in thinking, perception, mood, and actions. Delusions and hallucinations associated with the use of LSD are common. Neurophysiological research indicates the possibility that the drug produces its effect by interfering with the action of *serotonin*, a neurotransmitter. Some people experience flashbacks (i.e., a repetition of a hallucinogenic experience) after they cease using the drug.

Regular use of LSD produces tolerance, a tendency for the drug to induce only modest alterations in consciousness. The drug does not cause physiological dependence. Thus the cessation of its use does not produce significant withdrawal symptoms. However, some individuals do develop a psychological dependence on LSD.

The quality of an LSD "trip" varies greatly. Psychotherapists using LSD in research have found that some subjects have vivid transpersonal experiences that may change their outlook on life. However, "bad trips" can and do take place. Panic reactions, suspicion, a sense of alienation, disorientation, and despair are examples of the kinds of experiences that have been reported. Therefore, substantial warnings have been issued against the recreational use of LSD.

In the 1960s, there was a certain amount of enthusiasm for the possibility that LSD might facilitate the process of psychotherapy. Some research reports supported this hypothesis. However, the present consensus is that LSD has not lived up to its early promise, and, at present, it has no medical or psychiatric use.

See also *delusion*; *flashback*; *hallucinogens*; *neurotransmitters*.

M

macrocephaly: A condition characterized by an unusually large head. Macrocephaly is a cranial abnormality. It is associated with an unchecked growth of the brain's *glia cells*, the cells making up the supporting tissue of the brain. Macrocephaly is an uncommon disorder and is usually identified as congenital (i.e., present at birth). Its cause is obscure, and it is believed that it probably has a genetic basis. The condition produces complications such as visual problems, seizures, and mental retardation. There is no cure for macrocephaly. Treatment consists of adequate medical and psychological care.

See also *hydrocephalus*; *mental retardation*; *microcephaly*.

madness: An informal term that suggests severe mental disturbance. Although madness has no precise clinical meaning, it is associated most closely with psychotic disorders. Madness has a long history of usage in folklore, legends, and novels. Other informal terms such as *crazy*, *nuts*, *and lunacy* are more or less synonymous with madness.

See also *lunacy*; *psychotic disorders*.

magical thinking: A way of thinking often manifested by children between the approximate ages of 2 and 7. This time period defines a developmental stage termed *preoperational*, and it was studied at length by the research psychologist Jean Piaget (1896–1980). Preoperational children have no problem believing that carpets can fly and that Cinderella's fairy godmother can turn a pumpkin into a coach. They also tend to believe that if they just wish for something, it will come true without any effort.

Magical thinking in the preoperational child is normal. However, it is maladaptive when present in an adult. For example, an obese person may go to a physician and expect a series of shots to cure all of his or her weight problems. Subconsciously, the individual is expecting magic; the doctor's needle is perceived somewhat like a magic wand. The reason that magical thinking is maladaptive is that it takes the person in a direction away from the kind of realistic effort required to solve a problem in living.

One of the aims of cognitive-behavior therapy is to help troubled persons rely less on useless approaches such as magical thinking.

See also *cognitive-behavior therapy*.

magnification: A maladaptive form of thinking. In magnification, the individual tends to mentally inflate events. A flat tire is a "disaster." Being caught in a traffic jam is "going through hell." There is a tendency to enlarge things that happen to the self in a downward direction.

However, there may be a tendency to enlarge things that happen to others in an upward direction. A friend's daughter gets married, and she is "the most beautiful bride I've ever seen." Or a relative has a good business income, and he or she is "rich, a millionaire." The tendency to distort downward for oneself and upward for others can be a contributing factor to depression.

Magnification is one of the thought errors identified by cognitive therapy.

See also *cognitive therapy*.

major depression (unipolar disorder): A very severe mood disorder characterized by a number of related symptoms. Some, but not all, of the following symptoms may be observed in a given patient:

changes in appetite, insomnia, weight fluctuations, low self-esteem, self-criticism, inability to pay attention, preoccupation with the end of life, feelings of hopelessness, the idea that life has no meaning, finding very little pleasure in anything, loss of interest in friends, thoughts of suicide, complaints, and lack of energy.

Major depression is sometimes called *unipolar* because moods do *not* alternate between mania and depression as they do in bipolar disorder. In major depression, they remain on the "down" side.

Major depression is not different from mild or moderate depression in a qualitative sense. The difference is primarily one of degree, of intensity. For a more complete discussion, see the entry for depression.

See also *depression*; *mood disorders (affective disorders)*.

major tranquilizers (antipsychotic drugs): Tranquilizers that have a beneficial effect on psychotic disorders, disorders characterized by severe thought distortions. These drugs help ameliorate delusions, hallucinations, and agitation in mental patients. The first major tranquilizer used in the United States was *reserpine*, a drug introduced in the 1950s by the psychiatrist Nathan Kline. Reserpine was made from a chemical taken from the roots of the East Indian snakeroot plant.

The next important step in what has been called the "drug revolution" in the care and treatment of mental patients came with the introduction of *chlorpromazine*, marketed under such trade names as Thorazine, Chloramead, and Promapar. It is estimated that about 4,000,000 prescriptions a year are written for chlorpromazine.

Recently new classes of major tranquilizers have been developed to treat persons who do not respond well to chlorpromazine and drugs with a similar chemical structure. An example is *haloperidol*, marketed under the name Haldol.

In some patients, the major tranquilizers can produce adverse side effects. Common ones are dryness of mouth and nasal passages, fidgety feelings, and tardive dyskinesia (a condition involving involuntary muscle contractions).

It is important to understand that the major tranquilizers do not cure psychotic disorders. They are, however, effective in the treatment of these severe conditions. They help to control symptoms and, in many cases, make patients amenable to psychotherapy.

See also *chlorpromazine*; *drug therapy*; *psychotic disorders*; *tardive dyskinesia*.

maladaptive behavior: Behavior that works against adjustment and personal growth. Maladaptive behavior tends to be self-destructive, self-defeating, and of little long-range value to the individual or the culture. Sometimes the word *pathological* is used in connection with maladaptive behavior to suggest that it is "sick."

Many of the symptoms of the various mental disorders identified in this encyclopedia can be thought of as kinds of maladaptive behaviors. Delusions, hallucinations, agitation, inability to concentrate, irrational fears, chronic anxiety, chronic anger, suicidal impulses, compulsive eating, drug abuse, and more all fit in this general category.

Drug therapy and psychotherapy alike aim to modify maladaptive behavior, seeking to replace it with *adaptive behavior*, behavior that meets the real needs of the individual, the family, and society.

See also *abnormal behavior*; *symptom*.

maladjustment: Lack of harmony with oneself and the external world. The focus in some maladjusted individuals may be on lack of inner adjustment. Such individuals are the ones who suffer from anxiety disorders and other disturbances of emotion. They are troubled *within*. They seem to be at war with themselves. The early researchers in psychoanalysis used the word *neurosis* to describe such a state of affairs. Although "neurosis" is no longer a formal clinical category, it still is used to describe in a loose way the condition of the person who has an inner conflict.

The focus in other maladjusted individuals may be on lack of outer adjustment. Such individuals are the ones who inflict suffering on others. An example of this kind of person is provided by an individual who has an antisocial personality disorder. A person can be maladjusted in terms of the family or the culture but may have little sense of anxiety or guilt.

Maladjustment can be thought of as a component of every mental disorder. Therefore, there are as many causes of maladjustment as there are causes of mental disorders. Examples of general causes are (1) an inadequate developmental history, (2) learned maladaptive habits, (3) frustration of important desires, (4) association with peers who provide maladaptive role models, and (5) lack of opportunity. A general cause that has been debated at length is genetic predisposition. It is too easy to say that a person has "bad blood" or "it's all in the genes." On the other hand, there is evidence from genetic research that certain traits of temperament and behavior may have an inborn basis. The general trend of contemporary professional thought is to agree that genetic factors can *contribute* to maladaptive behavior. However, there is no simple one-to-one link between genes and behavior. Therefore, it is inaccurate to say that a person was "born bad" or "doomed to be neurotic."

See also *antisocial personality disorder (psychopathic personality; sociopathic personality)*; *genetic predisposition*; *maladaptive behavior*; *neurosis*.

male erectile disorder: See *erectile disorder (erectile insufficiency)*.

malingering: Acting sick as a device to avoid one's work or duty. A commonly expressed attitude is that mental patients are not sick at all. They are just pretending to be sick to escape responsibilities. A more sophisticated version of this is to say that a particular mental patient acts sick as a way to control others, to manipulate them toward his or her own ends. The symptoms of a mental disorder are seen as power tactics, not symptoms of an underlying illness at all.

Although it is true that, in a certain paradoxical sense, sickness does give the afflicted person a sort of power, it seems doubtful that this is the explanation of either most physical illness or most mental illness. Possibly one should seek ways to *not* reinforce symptoms; and this *is* done in behavior modification approaches to the treatment of mental disorders. However, it is much too simplistic a position to dismiss mental disorders by labeling all of them forms of malingering.

On the contrary, people with mental disorders, in most cases, *suffer*. They need emotional support and treatment in the same way that persons with physical illnesses do.

There is a class of mental disorders characterized by false symptoms. These are the *factitious disorders*. However, even these disorders are not explained in terms of malingering.

See also *behavior modification*; *factitious disorders*.

Malleus Maleficarum: The Latin name of a book written by the monks Johann Sprenger and Heinrich Kraemer. The English title of the book is *The Witches' Hammer*, and it was published in the fifteenth century. The work is based on the assumption that witches are possessed by the devil and must be destroyed. Methods of finding witches and verifying that they practice witchcraft are described in detail. This book had a long and influential history in Europe.

From the present point of view, it seems likely that most "possessed" people of past centuries suffered from mental disorders. Therefore, it appears probable in retrospect that many individuals persecuted as witches were simply poor unfortunates who were ill.

See also *demonology*.

mania: A state of agitation and excitement so intense that behavior becomes irrational. Some of the signs of mania include (1) unwarranted euphoria, (2) excessive activity, (3) talking rapidly, (4) flight of ideas, (5) excessive self-confidence, (6) a tendency to become highly irritable if contradicted, (7) lack of interest in sleeping, and (8) inability to sustain attention.

For example, Archibald, an unemployed screenwriter, is in a manic state. He is hospitalized and rushes up to the nurse on the ward. Archibald's eyes are bright, and there is a spittle on his lips. He begins to shout at the nurse, "I want to tell you about the greatest idea for a movie that anyone has had in a century. This will be a blockbuster if there ever was one! Bigger than *Star Trek*! I'm writing a screenplay combining an invasion of aliens from outer space with an earthquake in Los Angeles that's a 10 on the Richter scale! Oh God, oh God, oh God, I've got to get out of this place and get to a phone! I've got to tell somebody at the studio about this *right now*!"

See also *bipolar disorder*; *depression*.

manic-depressive psychosis: The original term for what today is called a bipolar disorder.

See also *bipolar disorder*.

manifest dream content: According to Freud, the surface of a dream. The manifest content consists of the dream symbols. In psychoanalytic theory, these stand not for themselves but for something else, something hidden at an unconscious level (i.e., the latent content). The idea is that one dare not dream in a knowing way about a particular subject because it is too threatening to the ego, the conscious self. Thus, depending on the circumstances, a queen might stand for one's mother. A gun might stand for a penis. Pins scattered on a chair might stand for a group of sperm. A dying plant might stand for a dying person.

It is critical to realize that Freud rejected the notion of universal symbols. Therefore the previously mentioned meanings could be quite different for different dreamers. One cannot tell from the symbol alone the nature of the latent content of the dream.

Freud believed that the interpretation of dreams was a "royal road to the unconscious." The manifest content of the dream provides the point of entry to that road.

See also *dream analysis*; *latent dream content*.

marijuana: A hallucinogen obtained from the hemp plant. Marijuana is related to hashish. The chemical name for marijuana is *cannabis*. Street names include "grass," "pot," and Acapulco gold. Marijuana cigarettes are referred to as "joints" or "reefers." Sometimes marijuana is called Mary Jane (i.e., "mari" + "juana").

Although it is true that marijuana *is* an hallucinogen, it is usually classified as a mild one. It does not usually produce alterations of consciousness as vivid as those produced by lysergic acid diethylamide-25 (LSD), phencyclidine (PCP), mescaline, and psilocybin. Some of the adjectives used by users to describe the effects of marijuana are "euphoria," "self-confidence," "less shy," "exhilaration," "relaxed," and "floating." The use of marijuana tends to make the user less inhibited. Therefore there may be impulsive acting out of sexual or aggressive feelings. However, it is important to quickly add that a 1972 report of the National Commission on Marijuana and Drug Abuse found no particular link between the use of the drug and violent criminal behavior.

Although the use of marijuana is illegal, this has not stopped its widespread use. It is estimated that about 50% to 60% of people between the ages of 21 and 29 have tried marijuana at least once. It should be realized that there is quite a bit of distance between trying a drug once, frequent use, and abuse. Many persons who have tried marijuana do not repeat the experience with any great frequency. Although it *is* possible for some people to develop a psychological dependence on marijuana, there is little or no tendency to acquire a physisological dependence. Withdrawal from the drug's use does not present a medical crisis.

There has been much discussion about marijuana's effects on health. Smoking marijuana with regularity does present clear-cut health hazards. Medical problems associated with respiration (e.g., bronchitis and emphysema) are common. People with heart disease may put an undue strain on their hearts by using marijuana. There have been studies that suggest regular marijuana use may have (1) an adverse effect on the immune system, (2) lower testosterone levels in males, and (3) do chromosome damage. However, a general medical consensus does not exist on the results of these studies. At present, the situation is inconclusive. However, the safest approach would obviously be to avoid use of the drug.

On the psychological side, it has been suggested that the regular use of marijuana produces a general reduction in ambition. This is termed the *amotivational syndrome*. The pros and cons of the reality of the amotivational syndrome are discussed elsewhere in the encyclopedia.

See also *amotivational syndrome*; *hashish*; *lysergic acid diethylamide-25 (LSD)*; *mescaline*; *phencyclidine (PCP)*; *psilocybin*.

marital schism: A "split" between the partners in a marriage. A marital schism exists when husband and wife do not agree at all on important values or standards of behavior. They may have very different ideas of right and wrong, what is moral and immoral, and how to spend leisure time. Research suggests that a marital schism has an adverse effect on the development of a child's personality. Specifically, it has even been suggested that marital schism is a contributing factor in schizophrenic disorders.

See also *double-bind communication*; *schizophrenia*.

marital therapy: Therapy with the principal goals of (1) improving communication and (2) reducing conflict between a couple. There is no single theory of therapy that applies uniquely to marriages. Therefore, a given therapist might take a psychoanalytic, behavioral, or humanistic approach, depending on his or her convictions and training. However, it should be noted that transactional analysis is particularly well-suited to helping individuals understand self-defeating patterns of communication.

The word *conjointly* is used when members of the couple are seen together. Although this is the most common mode used in marital therapy, sometimes the husband or the wife is seen individually.

Some therapists and counselors prefer terms such as *couple therapy* or *couple counseling* to marital therapy. They note that many couples who need counseling are unmarried.

Although the focus in marital therapy is on enhancing a relationship, sometimes it is recognized that a given marriage is, in fact, ending. One, or both, partners may be unable to forgive real or imagined transgressions. There may be irreconcilable differences in attitudes and moral standards. In such cases, marital therapy can at least help the partners understand clearly *why* their marriage is coming to a close. Their feelings can be explored, and animosity can be reduced to a minimum. Clear thinking can in part replace emotional confusion.

See also *couple counseling*; *family therapy*; *transactional analysis*.

Maslow, Abraham Harold (1908–1970): A research psychologist and a principal founder of American humanistic psychology. In 1934, he received a Ph.D. degree from the University of Wisconsin. For a number of years, he was associated with Brooklyn College and subsequently with Brandeis University. He served as president of the American Psychological Association in 1967.

In his early professional years, Maslow was favorably impressed by behaviorism. However, as his thinking matured, he decided that the inner world of people was too rich a territory to exclude from psychological theory. He decided to study human beings in their fullness—with their hopes, ambitions, and dreams.

His researches led him to the conclusion that human motivation follows a sort of ladder of needs from lower to higher. Low on the ladder's rungs are physiological needs and the need for safety. These are primary and important. However, they are not unique to human beings; they are shared with animals.

The uppermost rung of the ladder of needs is *self-actualization*, an inborn tendency to maximize one's talents and potentialities. It is the frustration of this need that causes many people to become anxious, depressed, and otherwise troubled. Maslow explored ways to help people become more self-actualizing, to bring forth by their own actions the person they were meant to be.

Humanistic psychology, as advocated by Maslow, is sometimes referred to as a *third force* in psychology. This terminology is used because traditionally the two dominant forces in American psychology have been behaviorism and psychoanalysis.

Maslow's most influential book is *Toward a Psychology of Being* (1968). Another important work is *Motivation and Personality* (1970).

See also *behaviorism*; *peak experience*; *self-actualization*; *therapy*.

masochism: The tendency to obtain pleasure from pain or suffering. In *sexual masochism*, the individual derives pleasure from punishment or humiliation during sexual activity. When someone has *masochistic personality traits*, he or she invites insults and abuse in a personal relationship. An Austrian novelist named Leopold V. Sacher-Masoch (1835–1895) described characters who "enjoyed" pain during sexual activity, and this is the basis of the word *masochism*.

Sexual masochism is classified as a sexual disorder. Individuals with this disorder find that their principal way of becoming sexually excited is to be tied down, insulted, hit, or otherwise abused. Some persons with the disorder engage in self-mutilation as a way of obtaining sexual excitement.

The term *masochistic sabotage* is used in psychoanalysis to describe self-destructive behavior. The idea is that one undermines one's own accomplishments. For example, a person unconsciously seeks to ruin a business he or she has built with great personal effort. Another person unconsciously finds ways to undermine a seemingly happy marriage.

A fairly convincing explanation of masochism is offered by psychoanalysis. Psychoanalysis defines masochism in terms of an overly punitive superego. The individual feels guilt for sexual desire or other desires in life. He or she does not feel free to simply enjoy pleasurable actions. The superego says, "This is wrong. You are bad for wanting or doing this." Therefore the superego must be appeased. Punishment is the price paid for an opportunity to engage, temporarily, in guilt-free forbidden pleasure.

Masochistic tendencies often start in childhood. Once established, they tend to be quite persistent. Psychotherapy may help an individual reduce the intensity of masochism.

See also *sadism*; *sexual disorders (psychosexual disorders)*; *superego*.

masturbation: Manual stimulation of the genital organs. The usual implications of masturbation are that both self-stimulation and orgasm are associated with the act. An antiquated name for masturbation is *onanism*. In Genesis, there is the concept of the sin of Onan. God commanded Onan to marry the wife of his dead brother, Er. Onan was further commanded to procreate, and he defied God's wishes. He had sexual intercourse with his wife, but he withdrew prior to ejaculation, thus "spilling his seed on the ground." This is the sin of Onan, the wasting of "seed" or sperm.

Masturbation has also been called *self-abuse* because of the implication that it is somehow harmful to the body and the mind. There is no evidence whatsoever that this is so. Masturbation does not cause blindness, heart disease, or psychotic disorders (i.e., "insanity" or madness). It *is*, of course, possible that if one worries about masturbation because of the belief that it is sinful, then it can have negative effects on mental health. But if, on the other hand, one holds the belief that masturbation is a normal sexual outlet under conditions where a sexual partner is not available, then sexologists agree that it in fact *is* a normal sexual outlet.

Masturbation is a very common behavior. Numerous studies of sexual behavior agree on this statement. A consensus of studies suggests that about 95% of men and 70% of women have masturbated at least once.

The all-too-common belief that masturbation causes psychotic disorders is probably based on the observation that mental patients masturbate. Lacking privacy, they are often "caught in the act" by a nurse or attendant. However, in the case of hospitalized individuals, cause and effect are mixed up. Patients are not mentally ill because they masturbate. Instead, they masturbate because they are human beings with sexual drives, and they do not have sex partners during confinement.

See also *orgasm*; *sexual deviations*; *sexual disorders (psychosexual disorders)*.

medical viewpoint: The viewpoint that a mental disorder is caused by an underlying illness. A distinction is made between the illness itself and its symptoms. For example, delusions are said to be symptoms of schizophrenic disorders. Irrational fears are symptoms of phobic disorders.

The illness can be organic (i.e., have a biological basis). This is known as the *medical viewpoint, organic version*. It is also known as the *biomedical viewpoint*.

It is also asserted that the illness can be functional. The disease entity might be identified in general terms as a "neurosis." Or it might have a very specific identification such as an Oedipus complex. This is known as the *medical viewpoint, functional version*. It was the general orientation used by Sigmund Freud. (There is nothing physically "wrong" with the mind in this case. It is more a question of the mind's *working wrongly*. That is what is meant by "functional.")

The medical viewpoint, both versions, is frequently used to help us explain mental disorders. The value of the medical viewpoint has been challenged (see *mental illness*).

See also *biomedical viewpoint*; *Freud, Sigmund*; *Oedipus complex*.

megalomania: A highly exaggerated sense of self-worth or self-importance. Persons suffering from megalomania may think that they are rich, famous, geniuses, dictators, religious prophets, and so forth. If the ideas supporting the megalomania are sufficiently fantastic, they are said to be delusions of grandeur.

Although megalomania is not associated with any particular mental disorder, it tends to be found most frequently in narcissistic personality disorder, the manic phase of bipolar disorder, and delusional (paranoid) disorders.

See also *bipolar disorder*; *delusional (paranoid) disorder*; *narcissistic personality disorder*.

megavitamin therapy: Prescribing very large doses of vitamins as a treatment for mental disorders. This approach is also known as *orthomolecular psychiatry*, obtaining the "right molecules" for mental health. (The Greek root *orthos* means "right.")

The biochemist and Nobel laureate Linus Pauling has had much to do with stimulating the interest in megavitamin therapy. Pauling, with David Hawkins, a physician, published the encouraging book *Orthomolecular Psychiatry* in 1973.

The megavitamin approach to mental health is based on the assumption that vitamins play a crucial role in the synthesis of neurotransmitters. If one does not have optimal nutrition, then the biochemistry will be defective. It is assumed that too many people have inadequate nutrition, and it is possible that they need vitamin replacement therapy. For example, there is ample evidence to link depression to deficiencies in the supply of the neurotransmitter norepinephrine. If the body lacks the substances it needs to produce norepinephrine, it stands to reason the individual will suffer from depression.

In practice, the emphasis in megavitamin therapy has been on the B-complex vitamins. They appear to play a critical part in the chemistry of neurotransmitters.

Although the logic behind megavitamin therapy has much to recommend it, there is no consensus concerning its effectiveness. Advocates give glowing reports. Skeptics say the methodology of studies on megavitamin therapy leave much to be desired.

See also *biomedical viewpoint*; *neurotransmitters*; *norepinephrine (noradrenalin)*.

melancholia: Great depression, deep sadness. In the American Psychiatric Association's *Diagnostic and Statistical Manual of Mental Disorders*, a major depressive episode with melancholia is characterized by a loss of joy in existence. Activities that are usually pleasurable cease to be so.

The word *melancholia* has an ancient meaning. It can be traced back to the teachings of Hippocrates (c. 460–377 B.C.). Hippocrates said that extreme sadness was caused by excessive quantities of black bile. (The Greek root *melas* means black, and *chole* means bile.) Although Hippocrates's idea seems quaint today, it is worth noting that it is a forerunner of biochemical theories of depression.

See also *depression*; *major depression (unipolar disorder)*.

meningitis: Inflammation of the *meninges*, the membranes covering the brain and the spinal cord. There is a spectrum of causes of the inflammation, and these include viral infections, bacterial infections, fungi, and autoimmune responses. Medical symptoms include fever, vomiting, and headache. The principal psychological symptom is delirium (i.e., mental confusion). Convulsions, violence, agitation, and illogical talk are common behaviors associated with the delirium.

With proper medical treatment (e.g., antibiotics in the case of bacterial infections), victims of meningitis usually make a full recovery. However, in a small percentage of cases, there is some permanent residual brain damage.

See also *delirium*; *organic mental syndromes (organic brain syndromes)*.

mental age (MA): A measure of intellectual development obtained by comparing a child's performance on an intelligence test with his or her peers of the same chronological age (i.e., actual age in years). For example, let us say that the average child 8 years of age can answer 40 questions correctly on a given intelligence test. Donald's chronological age is 10. However, he answers only 40 questions correctly on the test. His mental age is 8 because he performs no better than the average child of 8. On the other hand, Leanne's chronological age is 7. She is not expected to answer 40 questions correctly on the test but does. Therefore, she has a mental age of 8. Obviously, mental age can be above, or below, chronological age.

Because mental age is, on the whole, correlated with chronological age, it is not a constant measure of intelligence. It tends to keep growing from year to year. Therefore, a preferred measure is the intelligence quotient (IQ), which compares mental age to chronological age.

See also *intelligence quotient (IQ)*.

mental deficiency: An early term for what today is called mental retardation.

See also *mental retardation*.

mental disorder: A disorder characterized by a pathology of thought, feeling, or action. Such terms as *mental illness, abnormal behavior, maladaptive behavior,* and *maladjustment* are used to broadly identify mental disorders. Examples of pathology of thought are illogical thinking, irrational ideas, and delusions. Examples of pathology of feeling are chronic anxiety, anger, and depression. Examples of pathology of action are alcohol abuse, compulsive eating, and extreme agitation.

The list of mental disorders is long, and it includes both organic and functional disorders. The American Psychiatric Association's *Diagnostic and Statistical Manual of Mental Disorders* provides a complete classification scheme. This encyclopedia provides names, explanations, and treatment possibilities for the principal mental disorders.

See also *abnormal behavior*; Diagnostic and Statistical Manual of Mental Disorders; *maladaptive behavior*; *maladjustment*; *mental illness*.

mental health: A state of well-being characterized by rational thinking, emotional maturity, and effective action. Some of the attributes of rational thinking are facing reality squarely, using logic correctly, having realistic levels of aspiration, estimating accurately the likelihood of outcomes, and effectively planning for the future.

Some of the attributes of emotional maturity are mood stability, freedom from chronic anxiety and chronic depression, and self-control over emotional outbursts. Persons with emotional maturity seldom whine or feel excessively sorry for themselves.

Some of the attributes of effective action are working toward important goals, meeting obligations promptly, and breaking or modifying maladpative habits. In general, it can be said that persons who display effective action are responsible to themselves and others.

It is far easier to spot mental illness than it is to see mental health in other persons. This is because mental illness is vivid. It stands out. And mental health does not. For this reason, there is a tendency of define mental health in negative terms, to think of it as the *absence* of pathology (e.g., delusions, chronic anxiety, compulsive eating).

If an effort is made to see mental health in positive terms, then one must look for the *presence* of positive attributes. Existential and humanistic psychologists have pointed to two attributes of particular importance. Abraham Maslow asserts that self-actualizing persons have more *peak experiences*, moments of rapture or joy. Viktor Frankl asserts that persons with mental health have discovered *meaning in life*, the conviction that life has purpose and value.

See also *Frankl, Viktor*; *logotherapy*; *Maslow, Abraham Harold*; *mental disorder*; *mental illness*; *peak experience*; *self-actualization*.

Mental Health Association: A national organization dedicated to promoting mental health and combating mental illness. Four times a year it publishes a journal entitled *Mental Hygiene*. The association has a practical orientation and is a patron for research projects. Also, it is an important resource base for information on mental health and mental hospitals.

The prior name of the association was the National Association for Mental Health. It was established in 1950 and was the result of the uniting of several organizations.

The Mental Health Association is not a government organization. Its work is entirely voluntary.

See also *mental health*; *mental illness*.

mental illness: A term that has almost the same meaning as mental disorder but not quite. The term *mental illness* suggests a division between an underlying *disease* and its *symptoms*. This is known as the *medical viewpoint*. The underlying disease may be either organic or functional in nature, but the important point is that it *is there* and it is causing trouble.

There are those who question the value of the medical model and the whole concept of mental illness. For example, the psychiatrist Thomas Szasz wrote an influential book in 1961 entitled *The Myth of Mental Illness* in which he argued that mental illness is a confused and murky concept. Mental patients have problems in living; they are troubled. But they do not "have" a sickness. Behavior therapists tend to agree. They accept no arbitrary division between an illness and its symptoms. The argument is made that, in the case of mental illness, the maladaptive behavior *is* the "illness."

As a consequence of the preceding considerations, it is today thought to be generally preferable to speak of *mental disorder*, not *mental illness*. A "disorder" does not necessarily imply the two levels of symptom and illness. Nor does it rule them out. It is simply a more neutral term than illness.

Note that the American Psychiatric Association publishes the *Diagnostic and Statistical Manual of Mental Disorders*. The word *disorders* is featured prominently in the title, not *illnesses*.

See also *mental disorder*.

mental retardation: A lack of normal mental ability as measured by a standardized intelligence test. Examples of such standardized tests are the Stanford–Binet Scale and the Wechsler Intelligence Scales.

Subnormal mental ability is defined as an intelligence quotient (IQ) score of about 70 or below. Four categories of mental retardation are identified: (1) mild (IQ = 50–55 to about 70), (2) moderate (IQ = 35–40 to 50–55), severe (IQ = 20–25 to 35–40), and profound (IQ below 20 or 25). It is estimated that roughly 1% of the population scores in the mentally retarded range.

The term *mental retardation* is preferred over the older term *mental deficiency*.

There are a number of biological causes of mental retardation. Genetic disorders such as Down's syndrome, Turner's syndrome, and phenylketonuria (PKU) account for a substantial percentage of mental retardation. Other biological causes include rubella (German measles) during pregnancy and antagonistic blood categories between infant and mother.

Mild mental retardation often has little or no organic basis. This kind of retardation is called *familial mental retardation* (see entry).

There is no cure for mental retardation. However, the condition can be treated with much success, depending on the severity of the retardation. Persons with mild and moderate retardation can often be trained to be quite productive and self-sufficient. Persons with severe and profound retardation often require institutional care. However, even under these circumstances, much can be done through training programs to greatly enhance the quality of life.

See also *Down's syndrome*; *intelligence*; *mental deficiency*; *phenylketonuria (PKU)*; *Stanford–Binet Intelligence Scale*; *Turner's syndrome*; *Wechsler intelligence scales*.

mescaline: A hallucinogenic drug. It is derived from the peyote cactus plant. Street terms for mescalaine include *barf tea, big chief,* and *cactus.* There is a long tradition in Central and South America of using mescaline to alter consciousness and open perceptual doors to religious experiences. Mescaline is somewhat similar in its effects to lysergic acid diethylamide-25 (LSD). And the same reservations associated with the recreational use of LSD apply to the use of mescaline.

See also *hallucinogens*; *lysergic acid diethylamide-25 (LSD)*.

mesmerism: Another term for hypnosis. The word *mesmerism* is derived from Franz Anton Mesmer, a popular hypnotist of the eighteenth century. Mesmer was exposed as a quack by a distinguished committee of scientists that included Benjamin Franklin.

See also *hypnosis*; *hypnotherapy*.

methadone: A synthetic narcotic. Methadone is used in some medical and psychiatric programs to help an individual withdraw from an addiction to heroin. The idea is for methadone to provide a supporting bridge as the individual makes an effort to give up heroin. Methadone can sometimes be helpful because it meets physiological demands of the addicted individual without providing the euphoria of heroin. Therefore the individual can engage in gainful employment. The psychological dependence on heroin is thus broken first; then the individual proceeds to give up the physiological dependence by withdrawing from the methadone.

Methadone treatment has its opponents and advocates. Opponents point out that methadone is, like heroin, an addictive drug and that it, too, is subject to abuse. Advocates say that it provides important support during the critical withdrawal period from heroin. At present, there is no professional consensus.

See also *drug addiction*; *heroin*; *narcotic drugs*.

methylphenidate: A stimulant used to treat attention deficit disorder, drowsiness, fatigue, and narcolepsy. (Two trade names for methylphenidate are Methidate and Ritalin.) The functional action of methylphenidate is to increase alertness and general arousal.

It is interesting to note that it is often prescribed for attention deficit disorder in children. One of the symptoms of this disorder is hyperactivity, a condition in which there seems to be too much arousal. However, methylphenidate appears to have a paradoxical effect. Instead of stimulating the child with attention deficit disorder, the child is frequently calmed. The mechanism by which this takes place is somewhat obscure. However, it is possible to speculate that the relationship between arousal and stimulation is like an inverse U. The child who is suffering from attention deficit disorder may be on the crest of the U. A stimulant moves the child off the crest and thereby has a tranquilizing effect.

Like most drugs, methylphenidate sometimes has adverse side effects. Common ones include changes of mood, sleep disturbances, headaches, and loss of appetite. A prescription is required in order to take the drug.

See also *attention deficit disorder*.

Meyer, Adolf (1866–1950): A psychiatrist and a pioneer in the mental hygiene movement in the United States. Meyer is often called the "dean of American psychiatry." His land of birth was Switzerland, and he received his medical degree from the University of Zurich. He emigrated to the United States as a young adult to work as a pathologist in a mental hospital. In 1910, Meyer became a professor of psychiatry at Johns Hopkins Medical school and remained associated with the school for over 30 years.

Meyer was an early advocate of the holistic viewpoint, the viewpoint that the "mind" and the "body" are two aspects of a unified whole, the living organism. As a consequence, he stressed the importance of understanding mental patients as complete persons. He advocated the taking of a case history in order to gain an understanding of how factors in the patient's life may have contributed to his or her mental disorder.

Meyer tended to look upon mental disorders as primarily problems in adaptation to the challenges of life. The mental patient has learned maladaptive ways of responding. What is learned can be unlearned, and, as a consequence, many very troubled persons are treatable and can improve.

Meyer was not a prolific writer. However, his existing articles and essays were collected and published after his death under the title *Collected Works* (1951).

See also *Beers, Clifford Whittingham*; *holistic viewpoint*.

microcephaly: A condition characterized by an unusually small head. Microcephaly is a cranial abnormality. Persons suffering from this condition have a brain that is below average in size. And the condition is linked to mental retardation. The degree of mental retardation is usually more than moderate.

Biological factors play a major part in microcephaly. Some cases are probably caused by a recessive gene. A common cause is infection of the mother during pregnancy. An example is rubella (German measles). Exposure during pregnancy to extremely high levels of radiation has also been linked to microcephaly.

The condition is not curable. It is, however, treatable to some slight degree. In most cases, an individual with the disorder is cared for in a supportive institutional environment. Training programs aim at helping the individual develop the maximum amount of self-sufficiency.

See also *macrocephaly*; *mental retardation*.

migraine headache: A particularly severe kind of headache associated with dilation of blood vessels in the scalp. Symptoms include blurred vision, pain on one side of the head, upset stomach, vomiting, and bloodshot eyes.

To some extent, it is possible to distinguish a migraine headache from a tension headache. As indicated before, a migraine headache is associated with *dilation* of blood vessels. Pain receptors in the blood vessels respond to their stretched and excessively opened condition. In a tension headache, the pain arises from *constricted* muscles and blood vessels in the scalp. Not all researchers agree that the distinction between a migraine and a tension headache is a sharp one. For example, a tension headache can precede a migraine headache. Thus the two headaches may be different phases of the same problem.

Both biological and psychological factors can cause migraine headaches. Biological causes include responses to the menstrual cycle, the effects of oral contraceptives, and an allergic reaction to some foods. For example, chocolate has been found to induce migraine headaches in some people.

One of the important psychological factors that has been identified in the case of migraine headaches is an overcontrolling personality. Persons with this kind of personality tend to be perfectionists. Everything *must* go their way. They try to run a tight ship and strive with great energy toward their goals. The migraine headache usually hits them during a period of relaxation such as the evening hours or when on vacation. Migraine headaches are, to some extent, properly classified with the psychosomatic disorders.

More than one treatment has been recommended for migraine headaches. Aspirin is sometimes used; however, in some cases aspirin seems to aggravate migraine headaches. Pain-killing drugs are sometimes prescribed. A cold compress applied to the scalp can be of aid. An old treatment is to place the hands in a basin of warm water, and this may be effective in some cases. The warm water dilates the blood vessels in the hands, and this action is antagonistic to dilated blood vessels in the scalp. As the vessels in the hands open, the ones in the scalp become more constricted.

The warm water treatment described here has led to an approach used in biofeedback training. The sufferer is taught to gain voluntary control over blood vessels in the hands. Learning to open these vessels at will is a way of preventing and controlling migraine headaches.

See also *biofeedback training*; *psychosomatic disorders*.

milieu therapy: The *milieu* is the environment, the surroundings. Thus, in the broadest possible sense, milieu therapy refers to any attempt to help a troubled person by prescribing a vacation, a change in jobs, a change in life-style, and so forth.

However, more specifically the term usually refers to the inpatient treatment in a hospital. The idea is that both the staff and patients should generate a *therapeutic community*, a community dedicated to helping patients recover. This can be done in several ways. Patients can be encouraged through behavior therapy to be as responsible for themselves as possible. Social groups formed by patients can provide important recognition and help individuals avoid emotional isolation. There should be ongoing events such as the celebration of birthdays. Occupational therapy and music therapy should be provided. In this way, the total environment, or milieu, is involved in the healing process.

See also *behavior therapy*; *therapy*; *token economy*.

minimal brain dysfunction (MBD): A general term used to suggest a set of related cognitive and behavioral disturbances. The assumption is that these disturbances are caused by a slight amount of damage in the brain stem, the region of the brain that controls arousal. It is hypothesized that, in most cases, the damage was caused during the birthing process. An infant deprived of oxygen, for example, may suffer such damage. Slight damage to the brain stem does not affect intelligence, but it does affect attention span and motor activity. Therefore persons with the problem are somewhat more likely than most persons to have problems in concentration. Also, they tend to be restless and do not like to sit still for very long.

Minimal brain dysfunction is one of the principal explanations of conditions such as attention deficit disorder and developmental reading disorder.

See also *attention deficit disorder*; *developmental reading disorder (dyslexia)*.

minimization: A maladaptive form of thinking. In minimization, the individual tends to mentally deflate events. Winning an important award is "nothing" or "just luck." Compliments are discounted. "Someone else deserved the honor, not me." There is a tendency to perceptually belittle desirable things that happen to the self. One young woman after working many years to attain a college degree said, "Well, big deal. So what do I do for encores?" A tendency toward minimization makes it difficult for the individual to extract gratification from rewarding life events and may be a contributing factor to depression.

Minimization is one of the thought disorders identified by cognitive therapy.

See also *cognitive therapy*; *magnification*.

Minnesota Multiphasic Personality Inventory (MMPI): A standardized paper-and-pencil test of personality. It is more widely used than any other personality test and is considered to have a high degree of reliability. There are 550 items, and they can be answered *true*, *false*, or *can't say*. Each item makes a reference directly or indirectly to the self. The following items are *not* on the test proper but give an indication of the flavor of the test:

T F ? 1. My father was very kind and understanding.
T F ? 2. I have trouble sleeping most nights.
T F ? 3. I hear voices that tell me to do terrible things.
T F ? 4. I hate to meet people for the first time.
T F ? 5. Aliens from outer space live among us in disguise.
T F ? 6. I have to take laxatives frequently.
T F ? 7. It's all right to hurt people if they hurt you.

Developed in the 1940s by psychologists at the University of Minnesota, the test measures more than one dimension (i.e., phase) of personality. The aim of the test is to identify pathology. Therefore, when scored, the test yields a set of *clinical scales*, scales that report the degree of disturbance an individual has in given personality areas.

Here are the 10 principal clinical scales associated with the MMPI:

1. *Hypochondriasis*. Measures a tendency to have irrational health worries.
2. *Depression*. Measures a tendency to be emotionally low, to find little pleasure or joy in everyday events.
3. *Hysteria*. Measures a tendency to convert anxiety into a physical symptom such as imagined blindness, deafness, or paralysis.
4. *Psychopathic deviation*. Measures a tendency to have very little conscience, a poorly developed moral sense.
5. *Masculinity-femininity*. Measures a tendency to be at odds with traditional gender identity roles.
6. *Paranoia*. Measures a tendency to mistrust the motives and actions of others.
7. *Psychasthenia*. Measures a tendency toward "neurotic" problems such as anxiety disorders, phobic disorders, or obsessive-compulsive disorder.
8. *Schizophrenia*. Measures a tendency toward disordered thinking (e.g., delusions) and perceptual distortions (e.g., hallucinations).
9. *Hypomania*. Measures a tendency to become agitated and overly excited.
10. *Social introversion*. Measures a tendency to withdraw from contact with other people.

See also *personality test*; *Rorschach Test*; *Thematic Apperception Test (TAT)*.

minor tranquilizers: See *antianxiety drugs*.

M'Naghten rule: A landmark legal decision in the history of the insanity defense. In 1843, the House of Lords in England ruled that an individual is not responsible for a crime if the person in question "was laboring under such a defect of reason from disease of the mind as not to know the nature and quality of the act; or, if he did know it, that he did not know that what he was doing was wrong." The spirit of the M'Naghten rule lives on and is still applied in many criminal cases.

See also *Durham rule*; *insanity defense*; *legal aspects of mental health*.

mongolism: An outmoded term for Down's syndrome. See *Down's syndrome*.

monoamine oxidase (MAO) inhibitors: A class of antidepressant drugs. MAO inhibitors are marketed under several trade names including Marplan, Nardil, and Parnate. Research data suggests that a common biochemical cause of chronic depression is low levels of neurotransmitters such as serotonin and norepinephrine. These neurotransmitters are destroyed by the enzyme monoamine oxidase. The MAO inhibitors act by blocking the action of mono-amine oxidase, thus having the effect of increasing the net levels of serotonin and norepinephrine in the central nervous system.

The tricyclic derivatives are more frequently prescribed than the MAO inhibitors. This is because it is believed that tricyclic agents may be somewhat more effective, although this is open to question. Also, the tricyclic agents do not carry the food restrictions associated with MAO inhibitors. These agents interact in an adverse way with *tyramine*, a substance with the function of regulating blood pressure. The adverse reaction itself is a dangerous increase in blood pressure. Tyramine is contained in various foods and drinks including some red wines, some breads, some fruits, and some meats. A patient taking an MAO inhibitor is given a list of foods to avoid.

See also *antidepressant drugs*; *drug therapy*.

mood disorders (affective disorders): Types of mental disorders characterized primarily by disturbances in mood. A *mood* is an emotional state. Thus, if a person manifests inappropriate elation or depression, it is possible that a mood disorder is present. This is particularly true if the mood state is chronic and resists returning to the normal range.

The causes of mood disorders are both biological and psychological. It is believed that severe disturbances of mood in which there is loss of reality contact have a biological basis. A genetic predisposition or a biochemical imbalance may be primary causes. Severe mood disorders are usually treated with either drug therapy or electroconvulsive therapy.

More moderate disturbances of mood are believed to be caused primarily by psychological factors such as repressed anger, learned helplessness, or psychosocial stressors. Moderate disturbances are usually treated with psychotherapy.

See also *bipolar disorder*; *cyclothymic disorder*; *dysthymic disorder (unipolar disorder)*; *major depression (depressive neurosis)*.

moral therapy: A nonspecific kind of therapy that helps mental patients recover by treating them with kindness and understanding. The basic idea is to treat a human being like a human being, not like a disturbed animal. Moral therapy was an influential approach in the early nineteenth century and was an outgrowth of the decent treatment of mental patients encouraged by such pioneers as Philippe Pinel in France and William Tuke in England.

As a distinctive movement, moral therapy no longer exists. However, its effects remain evident in the contemporary attitude in psychiatry and clinical psychology that mental patients need help, guidance, and understanding.

See also *antipsychiatry*; *milieu therapy*.

moron: An individual with an IQ score between 50 and 70, indicating mild mental retardation. Moron is from a Greek root meaning "stupid." Unfortunately, popular usage has given the word *moron* a belittling meaning. Therefore it has become a somewhat obsolete term in clinical usage. Today it is recommended that we restrict ourselves to "mild mental retardation" in place of "moron."

See also *mental retardation*.

morphine: A narcotic drug with analgesic properties. Street names for morphine include *dope*, *morpho*, and *white stuff*. The word *morphine* is derived from the Greek legend of Morpheus, the god of dreams. Morphine is an alkaloid compound derived from opium. It has a place in medical practice and can be used to control pain. However, the body gets used to it quickly, and its effectiveness is limited. Because morphine induces pleasant states ranging from relaxation to euphoria, it is a frequently abused drug. It is addictive and both a physiological and psychological need for the drug tend to develop in the regular user.

Treatment for a person addicted to morphine requires both medical management and supportive counseling. There will be unpleasant physical reactions such as excessive sweating, stomach cramps, nausea, and shakiness during the physiological withdrawal period. Once physiological withdrawal is accomplished, it is important to treat psychological dependence. The wish to take the drug remains even after the body no longer needs it.

See also *drug addiction*; *heroin*; *methadone*; *narcotic drugs*.

multiple personality disorder: A type of dissociative disorder characterized by the presence in a single person of two or even several personalities. The disorder is classified as dissociative because the ego loses some of its integrity; the self is "disconnected" to some extent.

Let us say that a patient named Alice manifests two personalities. Alice is the original personality, and she is serious, responsible, and somewhat humorless. She has two children, is sexually faithful to her husband, and is a full-time homemaker. Her second personality is Joan, a sexually promiscuous hell raiser. When Alice is eclipsed by Joan for 2 or 3 days, Alice has a blackout for the time period that Joan was dominant. Alice has no conscious knowledge of what Joan was doing. Joan, on the other hand, is aware of Alice's behavior. She spies on Alice and criticizes her when talking to a therapist. Note that the inferior personality has a kind of power not held by the superior personality.

As indicated, it is possible for the person suffering from multiple personality to present a number of distinct personalities complete with names and traits. The condition appears to be a real one. Although pretense, role playing, and malingering are possible interpretations in some cases, this is not the correct interpretation in all cases.

Females are somewhat more likely to suffer from the disorder than are males. Although the disorder has received a great deal of publicity, it is in fact quite uncommon.

It is not possible to pinpoint a single set of causes of the disorder; however, it has been found that child abuse is a common factor in the developmental history. In general terms, the psychological meaning of the disorder seems to be fairly clear. The inferior personalities are usually impulsive and emotionally immature. Therefore, it is reasonable to hypothesize that they allow an outlet for emotional expression in persons who are usually responsible and socialized. Forbidden sexual and aggressive wishes can be acted out without guilt because there is no conscious knowledge of the offensive behavior.

The disorder sometimes makes its first appearance in childhood. However, it may not be clearly identified until adolescence or adulthood. It is often a stubborn condition with a long history in a given person.

It is important to realize that multiple personality is *not* a schizophrenic disorder. Multiple personality is, loosely speaking, a neurotic condition. Schizophrenic disorders are psychotic conditions.

The most common treatment for multiple personality is psychotherapy with a psychoanalytic orientation. This approach is designed to encourage insight. Sometimes hypnosis is used to bring forth one of the personalities. The aim of the therapy is to foster the eventual reintegration of the two or several personalities into one.

See also *dissociative disorders*; *schizophrenia*.

mutism: Not speaking over a protracted period of time. The individual who does not speak may behave this way for several reasons. There may be an organic problem. A child who is born deaf and does not receive the proper kind of training will be unable to speak. A person with a neurological impairment may be partially or completely mute.

Mutism caused by psychological problems divide into two related categories. *Elective mutism* is voluntary; the individual refuses to speak. This is often interpreted as a form of hostility, a kind of passive-aggressive behavior. *Involuntary mutism* is outside of the individual's conscious control. This kind of mutism may also be an expression of hostility, but it is not willed or planned. Involuntary mutism is frequently seen in catatonic schizophrenic disorders.

Mutism is also frequently present in autistic disorder. The categories identified above blur somewhat in the instance of this condition. The child is mute for at least two reasons. Children with the condition are not prone to make social contact and therefore do not tend to have the kind of experiences important in the acquisition of speech. This is probably the primary cause of the mutism. And then it is possibly aggravated by hostility on the child's part. Behavior therapy with children suffering from autistic disorder usually includes speech training.

See also *autistic disorder (infantile autism); schizophrenia.*

myxedema: Chronic fatigue caused by a deficiency of *thyroxin*, a hormone produced by the thyroid gland. Myxedema has related physical and psychological symptoms such as obesity, emotional instability, lack of comprehension, mental confusion, impaired memory, and dulled speech. The term *hypothyroidism* can be used to describe the cause of myxedema.

Severe cases of myxedema may induce psychotic symptoms such as delusions and hallucinations. The individual may be mistakenly thought to be suffering from a schizophrenic disorder.

The treatment of myxedema is thyroid replacement therapy. The condition usually responds well to treatment.

See also *endocrine system.*

N

narcissism: A kind of ego defense mechanism characterized by self-absorption. Another term for narcissism, one that sometimes appears in psychoanalytic literature, is *ego erotism*. The Greek myth of Narcissus tells the story of a youth who fell in love with his own image as it was reflected in a pool of water. He was overcome with longing for the beautiful youth in the pool, and he eventually starved to death. The myth contains a warning: Excessive self-love can be destructive. A person with a healthy personality cares not only about himself or herself but about others.

Here are two examples of persons using narcissism. Bianca, an adolescent who has doubts about her attractiveness, spends an inordinate amount of time picking out clothes and worrying about makeup. Orson, a young adult who is short of stature, is a compulsive body builder. Both of the examples reveal that the individuals in question use narcissism to defend the ego against threats to its sense of integrity and worth.

See also *ego defense mechanisms*; *narcissistic personality disorder*.

narcissistic personality disorder: A kind of personality distinguished primarily by an exaggerated tendency to perceive oneself as important. Some of the traits that may be associated with this disorder include dreaming of doing almost impossible things, craving admirers for almost all of life's tasks, having anger when great plans are challenged, and significant problems in personal relationships. The individual with this disorder is using the defense mechanism of narcissism to a pathological degree in order to cover up feelings of inadequacy.

If, from time to time, the defense system breaks down, the individual will become temporarily depressed. Then he or she will express ideas such as, "I'm never going to amount to anything," or, "I've failed at everything I've ever attempted." However, if the person actually suffers from a narcissistic personality disorder, depression will not be the person's dominant emotional state. On the contrary, most of the time the individual will appear to be "up" and rather willful.

The roots of narcissistic personality disorder appear to be in underlying feelings of low self-esteem. At a usually unstated level, the individual has grave doubts about his or her capacity to meet life's challenges.

A narcissistic personality disorder may cause the individual serious problems in living. It is difficult for a person with this disorder to be a loving partner. He or she has very little to give to another. On the other hand, there is great emotional need. And the "normal" partner may feel sucked dry of love.

The primary treatment for the disorder is insight-oriented psychotherapy.

See also *narcissism*; *personality disorders*.

narcolepsy: A tendency to fall suddenly and involuntarily asleep. Usually the period of sleep is brief in duration (e.g., a few minutes). Symptoms often associated with narcolepsy are chronic drowsiness, insomnia, and abrupt loss of muscle control.

Narcolepsy can be biological or psychological in origin. A biological cause of narcolepsy is dysfunction in the *reticular activating system*, an arousal control center in the brain stem. Another biological cause of narcolepsy is encephalitis. A psychological cause of narcolepsy is an unconscious wish to run away from responsibilities. This interpretation places some cases of narcolepsy in a category similar to psychogenic fugue.

If the cause of narcolepsy is thought to be biological, the treatment is usually drug therapy. Amphetamines are often prescribed. They are stimulants and, in some cases, have a beneficial effect. If the cause is psychological, the treatment of choice is insight-oriented psychotherapy.

Narcolepsy is an uncommon condition. The word *narcolepsy* is unfortunately similar to the word *epilepsy*. However, narcolepsy is *not* a form of epilepsy.

See also *encephalitis*; *epilepsy*; *fugue*.

narcotherapy: The use of narcotic agents in medical or psychological therapy. These drugs can be used to reduce pain. Opiates are sometimes prescribed for persons suffering from chronic pain associated with a severe illness. They are also prescribed for either postoperative pain or the pain resulting from an accident.

Narcoanalysis is a specific kind of narcotherapy. It is the use of narcotics to assist in the exploration of a patient's unconscious mental life.

See also *narcotic drugs*.

narcotic drugs: In general, drugs that produce a stupor. More specifically, the term *narcotic drugs* tends to be limited to opium, morphine, codeine, and heroin. Sometimes methadone, a synthetic drug, is also listed as a narcotic. Morphine is derived from opium. Codeine and heroin in turn are derived from morphine.

See also *heroin*; *methadone*; *morphine*; *opium*.

nature–nurture controversy: A running controversy in psychology over the relative importance of nature (i.e., heredity) versus nurture (i.e., environment) in the determination of behavior. Applied to abnormal psychology, the controversy focuses on the relative importance of the two factors in the determination of mental disorders. Advocates of the importance of nature argue that it plays the dominant role in the causation of mental disorders. For example, there is evidence that genetic factors play a significant part in schizophrenic disorders. Advocates of the importance of nurture argue that it plays the dominant role in the causation of mental disorders. For example, there is evidence that the conflicting communication styles in some families tend to foster schizophrenic disorders in children.

In the late nineteenth and early twentieth centuries, advocates of the importance of nature had great prestige. Exciting discoveries in genetics and biology in general seemed to suggest that mental disorders could be explained primarily in physical and organic terms. With the rise of behaviorism in the 1910s and 1920s, there was a great surge of interest in the environmental approach. The individual's learning history seemed to be the key to unlocking the mystery of mental disorders. Freud's emphasis on the importance of the person's developmental history also gave great weight to the environmental viewpoint.

Today the pendulum of opinion has swung to a middle position between an extreme nature viewpoint and an extreme nurture viewpoint. The contemporary approach is to emphasize the importance of the *interaction* between heredity and environment. They affect each other in a complex way, and a certain amount of weight must be given to both nature and nurture if one wants to obtain a complete explanation of a mental disorder. Thus a great deal of wind has gone out of the sails of the traditional nature–nurture controversy.

See also *behaviorism*; *double-bind communication*; *genetic predisposition*.

negativism: An attitude or behavioral trait characterized by a tendency to resist commands or requests. Two basic kinds of negativism are identified: (1) passive and (2) active. In *passive negativism* the individual may resist by "forgetting" to do something, by performing a task slowly, or by completing work inadequately. In *active negativism*, the individual does the opposite of what is requested. For example, a mental patient asked to display his open hand instead clenched it into a fist.

Negativism often appears in early childhood and again during adolescence. It is considered to be normal at these times and is interpreted as an expression of the individual's need for autonomy. In most cases, it is the expression of a developmental stage and usually will pass with maturation. If it does not pass, then negativism can become a personality trait. Sometimes it is a component factor in a personality disorder.

Negativism is often displayed by patients suffering from a schizophrenic disorder of the catatonic type. Examples are refusing to get out of bed, to eat, to speak when spoken to, and so forth. One way to understand this kind of negativism is to look on it as a sign of anger. Unable to safely express anger openly, the patient expresses it indirectly in the form of negativism.

See also *autonomy*; *schizophrenia*.

neo-Freudian: Loosely, any psychoanalytic approach that accepts many of Freud's major assumptions but rejects specific details. The combining form *neo* is from Greek roots meaning "new." Neo-Freudian psychoanalysts feel free to revise Freudian personality theory and psychoanalytic technique in accordance with their own clinical experience and research.

The assumption that human beings have an unconscious mental life is *the* key assumption that is never rejected by a Freudian or a neo-Freudian. There is no way that a viewpoint can be called Freudian in any sense of the word if this assumption is not utilized.

The assumption that gaining insight into the nature of one's unconscious mental life is therapeutic is a second assumption that is characteristic of both classical psychoanalysis and neo-Freudian thought.

The assumption that we use defense mechanisms to protect the ego against the harsher aspects of reality is a third assumption associated with both classical psychoanalysis and neo-Freudian thought.

Some well-known neo-Freudians are Erik H. Erikson, Karen Horney, and Harry S. Sullivan. Some authorities include Carl Jung, Alfred Adler, and Otto Rank as neo-Freudians. This is debatable because they strayed very far from Freud's basic teachings. Anna Freud and Ernest Jones are identified simply as Freudians.

See also *Adler, Alfred; ego defense mechanisms; Erikson, Eric Homburger; Freud, Anna; Horney, Karen; insight; Jones, Ernest; Jung, Carl Gustav; Rank, Otto; Sullivan, Harry Stack; unconscious mental life.*

neologism: Either (1) the coining of a new word or phrase or (2) the use of standard words in new and idiosyncratic ways. The use of neologisms is not necessarily pathological. For example, a creative writer might make use of them for the purpose of artistic effect. On the other hand, they are a common characteristic of the speech of persons suffering from schizophrenic disorders. Under these conditions, neologisms are a communication barrier. One of their psychological purposes is to help the patient retain a certain amount of power. They succeed in keeping the mental health professional at a distance. It is as if the patient is speaking in code and the helping individual is a kind of enemy.

One patient said, "I will jotling make my ketlo." It turned out this meant, "I will not make my bed." She had coined the words *jotling* and *ketlo* for "not" and "bed." Another patient said, "I want to go home thermos." This was decoded to mean, "I want to go home tomorrow." The existing word *thermos* was substituted for "tomorrow."

See also *clang associations; confabulation; echolalia; flight of ideas.*

nervous breakdown: A catchall term without any precise clinical meaning. It is *not* a standard diagnostic category in the American Psychiatric Association's *Diagnostic and Statistical Manual of Mental Disorders*. The term *nervous breakdown* is used by the general public to label almost any serious problem the individual has in coping adequately with the challenges of life, particularly if the problem leads to hospitalization. In general it is best to avoid the term because it communicates only a vague and highly inadequate meaning.

See also Diagnostic and Statistical Manual of Mental Disorders; *mental disorder.*

neurasthenia: An outdated term once used to label a condition characterized by chronic fatigue. The literal meaning of the word *neurasthenia* is "weakness of the nerves." It was once believed that overwork and other demands on the individual actually wore out the nerves at a biological level. This general viewpoint is still reflected in such phrases as "My nerves are all shot" and "My boss gets on my nerves." Thus neurasthenia once was based on the assumption that an organic basis for ongoing weakness and a low energy level was actual wear and tear on the nerves.

Subsequently, it was recognized that chronic fatigue could have a psychological basis. And neurasthenia came to be looked upon as a neurotic condition. The disorder was seen as functional in nature, not organic.

Today neurasthenia has no formal clinical status. It is not a diagnostic category in the American Psychiatric Association's *Diagnostic and Statistical Manual of Mental Disorders*. Presently the concept of neurasthenia has been subsumed under the category *dysthymic disorder*. The term *neurasthenia* is sometimes used in an informal sense to describe symptoms associated with that disorder.

See also *dysthymic disorder (depressive neurosis)*.

neurodermatitis: An irritation or inflammation of the skin believed to have its origins in emotional conflict. Itching and dryness of the skin are two of the common symptoms associated with this disorder. Neurodermatitis is classified as a psychosomatic disorder.

Treatment of the disorder may include both medical care and counseling or psychotherapy.

See also *psychosomatic disorders*.

neurology: A medical specialty concerned with the health and treatment of the nervous system. A *neurologist* is a medical doctor who has made an intense study of neurology. Much of Freud's early training was in neurology, and many of his first patients had complaints such as blindness, deafness, and paralysis. These complaints seemed to have their origins in nervous system pathology. Freud, and others, recognized that some ailments that seem to have a neurological origin are psychological in nature. Emotional conflicts are sometimes converted into physical symptoms. Thus historically there is a close connection between neurology and psychiatry.

See also *conversion disorder*; *hysteria*.

neuron: The basic building block of the nervous system. A neuron consists of a single cell specializing in the transmission of information. The principal parts of a neuron are (1) one or more *dendrites*, structures that receive information either from the outside world or from other neurons, (2) the *cell body*, the bulging central portion of a neuron, (3) the *nucleus* of the cell, containing both ribonucleic acid (RNA) and deoxyribonucleic acid (DNA), (4) the *axon*, a structure that transmits information to other neurons or to muscle cells, and (5) the *end foot*, a structure providing a point of functional contact with other neurons. It is the end foot that releases *neurotransmitters*, chemical messengers.

A neuron transmits information in a wavelike action from the dendrite and cell body to the axon. This wavelike action is known as *depolarization*, a change in electrical potential from a resting negative state to a positive state, then back to a negative state again. Informally, scientists often speak of neurons "firing" instead of depolarizing.

Three basic kinds of neurons are (1) *sensory neurons*, neurons that pick up information from the external world, (2) *association neurons*, neurons that communicate with other neurons, and (3) *motor neurons*, neurons that stimulate muscle fibers to contract.

Neurons are arranged in complex structures, including the autonomic nervous system and the brain. It is the highly sophisticated way in which neurons are arranged that makes thinking and action possible. When there is infection or damage to the nervous system, neurons often suffer or die. The resulting changes in personality and behavior are often dramatic. Cerebrovascular accidents and alcohol amnestic disorder are just two examples of disorders involving the pathology of neurons.

See also *alcohol amnestic disorder*; *autonomic nervous system*; *cerebrovascular accident (CVA)*; *neurology*; *neurotransmitters*.

neuropsychological evaluation: An evaluation of a patient's neurological and psychological health. More than one professional person may be involved in such an evaluation. The joint efforts of a psychiatrist, a neurologist, and a clinical psychologist are often required. Interviews, neurological tests, and psychological tests are the principal tools used to make an overall assessment.

Frequently, the chief aim of such an evaluation is to determine the level of organic involvement residing behind a patient's symptoms. Thus patients who have recently had a cerebrovascular accident, are suspected of suffering from Alzheimer's disease, or are suffering from other organic disorders are often referred for a neuropsychological evaluation.

See also *Alzheimer's disease*; *cerebrovascular accident (CVA)*; *organic mental disorders*.

neuropsychology: A field of psychology that studies the relationship of the brain and nervous system to behavior. Research conducted in neuropsychology is of value in more than one way. For example, knowledge gained in neuropsychology has made possible safer and more effective drug therapy. For a second example, findings from neuropsychology help us reach a better understanding of how to provide treatment for organic mental disorders.

See also *drug therapy*; *organic mental disorders*.

neurosis: A general term loosely suggesting a mental disorder characterized by chronic anxiety or emotional conflict. The term *neurotic disorder* has no formal clinical meaning in the United States and is not be be found as a basic category in the American Psychiatric Association's *Diagnostic and Statistical Manual of Mental Disorders*. However, it is correct to speak of a *neurotic process* to suggest unconscious mental and emotional conflicts capable of producing significant symptoms and problems in adjustment. It should be understood that "neurotic process" is not a diagnosis.

On the whole, it is considered appropriate by American mental health professionals to use the word *neurotic* as an adjective, not a noun. This usage preserves the traditional meaning of the word, recognizes that neurosis is a pathological mental and emotional process, but rejects neurosis as a specific disease or disorder. Thus we can correctly speak of a "neurotic paradox" and a "neurotic style" in a broad descriptive way.

The earliest meaning of the word *neurosis* was an organic pathology of the nerves themselves. Freud and others recognized that the symptoms of neurological problems could be presented by patients with emotional conflicts. Thus Freud made a formal distinction between the *actual neuroses* and *psychoneuroses*. Actual neuroses were organic in nature. Psychoneuroses were due to emotional difficulties. In time, the unadorned word *neurosis* came to refer primarily to the psychoneuroses, and that is its present usage.

Note that, in the first paragraph of this entry, a point is made of stating that the American Psychiatric Association's diagnostic manual avoids identifying neurosis as a specific disorder. However, the overall picture is confused to some extent by the fact that the *International Classification of Diseases* (ICD) does in fact list a set of neurotic disorders. As already indicated, this is not the approach of choice in the United States.

One reason for favoring the U.S. system is that the word *neurosis* is a bit too much of a catchall. It covers a very wide spectrum of symptoms and is somewhat too general. A second reason is that the word *neurosis* implies a specific theoretical approach, primarily a psychoanalytical one. Behavior therapy and cognitive therapy, for example, do not necessarily accept the theories of psychoanalysis.

In sum, there has been much debate about how to use the word *neurosis* correctly. In the United States, the preferred usage is to avoid using it as a diagnostic category. However, the richness and utility of the word is preserved in its usage as an adjective to describe troubled emotional processes.

See also Diagnostic and Statistical Manual of Mental Disorders; *Freud, Sigmund*; International Classification of Diseases (*ICD*); *neurotic paradox*; *neurotic style*.

neurosyphilis: The spread of a syphilitic infection to the nervous system, including the brain and spinal cord. The resulting pathology can lead to dementia and general paresis.

See also *dementia*; *general paresis*.

neurotic paradox: The tendency of some emotionally troubled persons to engage in self-defeating behavior. These individuals often seem to be their own worst enemies. They program themselves for failure. The seemingly useless behavior tends to present a persistent pattern and is quite resistant to change. It sometimes seems almost to be a style of life.

The psychology behind the neurotic paradox is that the self-defeating behavior is a way of reducing anxiety. For example, a person might falter in a business endeavor as a way of avoiding the threat of confining himself or herself to a career chosen by parents. Or another person might avoid earning much money as a method of avoiding the responsibilities of marriage.

See also *neurosis*; *neurotic style*.

neurotic style: A general approach to life colored by an underlying neurotic process. Thus the person who manifests a neurotic style will be emotionally troubled, engage in much self-defeating behavior, be plagued by chronic anxiety, and have an inadequate overall adjustment. A neurotic style of life does *not* imply that the individual in question is irresponsible. On the contrary, such persons are sometimes compulsively responsible. They tend to have a perfectionistic streak. On the other hand, much of what they do is *ineffective*. They do not succeed in reaching their goals.

Alfred Adler was one of the first psychologists to speak of the importance of one's style of life. He noted that some persons live by *neurotic fictions*, meaning they pursue unrealistic and impractical goals. Thus, on the whole, they doom themselves to failure. The pursuit of neurotic fictions is a common aspect of neurotic style.

See also *Adler, Alfred*; *neurosis*; *neurotic paradox*.

neurotransmitters: Chemical messengers released by the end foot of a neuron. Neurotransmitters released by a first neuron have three principal functions: They may (1) excite a second neuron, causing it to depolarize, (2) inhibit a second neuron, keeping it from depolarizing, and (3) stimulate a muscle fiber to contract. From a biochemical point of view, neurotransmitters are complex organic molecules capable of releasing minute amounts of energy.

In recent years, neurotransmitters have received a great deal of attention and study. One reason for this interest in the action of neurotransmitters is because of their important role in mental health. It is now recognized that biochemical imbalances can be causal factors in mental disorders. For example, a low level of the neurotransmitter norephinephrine is a factor in some kinds of depression. And an imbalance of the neurotransmitter dopamine is believed to be a factor in schizophrenic disorders.

See also *dopamine*; *neuron*; *norepinephrine (noradrenalin)*.

nicotine dependence (tobacco dependence): A substance use disorder characterized by an inability to stop using products containing nicotine such as cigarettes, cigars, snuff, and chewing tobacco. A person who uses these products voluntarily, who has no desire to quit, and who has no obvious health problems should not be diagnosed as suffering from nicotine dependence.

However, if one or more of the following behaviors or symptoms is present, then nicotine dependence probably exists. First, the individual has made repeated efforts to stop without success. (The person seems to be a living example of Mark Twain's famous statement, "It's easy to stop smoking. I've done it hundreds of times.") Second, the individual suffers withdrawal symptoms (e.g., headache, stomach distress, anxiety, and general crossness) when abstaining from nicotine. Third, the individual has a medical problem that is complicated by the use of nicotine (e.g., heart disease or bronchitis).

Nicotine dependence is obviously a problem of substantial size in our society. Millions of people smoke, and thousands chew tobacco. Not all of these people are dependent, of course. However, it is estimated that as many as one-half of users eventually want to give up tobacco. Those who reach this point and find themselves unable to successfully carry out their intentions may be thought of as nicotine-dependent.

Many approaches and treatments have been tried with nicotine dependence. Nicotine gum can be chewed in place of smoking. Tranquilizers or sedatives are sometimes prescribed during a period of withdrawal to help the individual cope with nervous tension. However, this approach carries the very real risk of becoming dependent on the drug prescribed. Some hospitals and clinics offer group meetings designed to help persons stop using tobacco. Hypnotherapy is sometimes helpful. Aversion therapy may also be helpful.

Probably the most effective general approach is behavior therapy aimed at helping the individual break the various individual habits that support the nicotine dependence.

See also *aversion therapy*; *behavior therapy*; *hypnotherapy*; *psychoactive substance use disorders (substance use disorders)*.

nihilism: In philosophy, the viewpoint that life is meaningless and existence is absurd. This way of looking at the world is often a feature of depression. The thoughts and ideas of chronically depressed persons often reflect a nihilistic orientation. One patient said, "Life is pointless, and nothing makes any sense." Another patient said, "Shakespeare was right when he wrote that life is a tale full of sound and fury, told by an idiot, signifying nothing."

Approaches such as cognitive therapy and logotherapy are designed to help the depressed person see that nihilism is not a *fact* about the world but a way of *construing* the world.

See also *cognitive therapy*; *depression*; *logotherapy*.

nomadism: An ineffective way of dealing with psychosocial stressors characterized by restlessly moving about the country or frequently changing occupations. The nomadic person in essence runs away from difficult situations. Instead of standing one's ground, the individual takes flight. Nomadism bears some similarity to the condition known as fugue.

See also *fugue*.

nondirective therapy: See *client-centered therapy*.

noradrenalin: See *norepinephrine (noradrenalin)*.

norepinephrine (noradrenalin): One of the neurotransmitters. Norepinephrine plays an important role in emotional adjustment and mental health. Low levels of this substance are a causal factor in endogenous depression. The principal function of drugs such as the monoamine oxidase (MAO) inhibitors and tricyclic antidepressants is to increase the functional level of norepinephrine in the central nervous system.

See also *depression; monoamine oxidase inhibitors; tricyclic antidepressants*.

norm: See *abnormal behavior*.

nuclear magnetic resonance (NMR): A procedure making it possible to generate a surprisingly lucid picture of the brain or other soft tissue. The nuclear magnetic resonance process takes advantage of positive and negative polarities of atoms contained within human tissue. A magnetic field is used to align the atoms into orderly patterns. Then a radio signal makes it possible to translate the patterns into visual images. And these can be preserved in printed form.

Nuclear magnetic resonance imaging is a useful diagnostic tool for psychiatry and neurology. Tumors, damage due to strokes, and atrophy of brain tissue can be evaluated to some degree. The process is of substantial use in the diagnosis and evaluation of organic mental disorder.

See also *computerized axial tomography (CAT); positron emission tomography (PET)*.

O

obesity: Informally, a condition in which the individual is quite fat, or corpulent. Various formal clinical definitions have been suggested. One that seems practical is a condition in which the individual is 20% or more over a normal weight according to standard height–weight charts. Twenty percent suggests slight obesity. Persons who are 40% over a standard weight are *moderately obese*. The term *morbid obesity* is reserved for those individuals who are 50% or more over a standard. *Hyperobesity* is the word used to describe individuals who are 100 pounds over their ideal weight.

Obesity is a major health problem in the United States. Survey data suggest that between 10 to 20% of U.S. citizens range from slightly to moderately obese. And obesity is also a complicating factor in a host of chronic illnesses extending from high blood pressure to diabetes.

Causal factors in obesity include those at both a biological and psychological level. Genetic factors appear to play a role in some cases of obesity. Experiments with rats suggest that fat-making genes exist. And some strains of rats have a definite tendency to become easily obese. The same seems to be roughly true for human beings, although the data are less convincing. It has been suggested that a basic body type termed *endomorphic* has more fat cells than other body types. And this is believed to be an inherited tendency. Obesity of the kind described in this paragraph is termed *genetic obesity*.

Endocrine disturbances can contribute to obesity. Persons with a low production of the hormone thyroxin tend to have a slow metabolic rate and may not burn excess calories easily. The unburned calories are stored as fat. Some individuals with a tendency toward hypoglycemia (i.e., chronic low blood sugar) may suffer from defective carbohydrate metabolism. It is possible that they, too, store unburned calories as fat. Obesity of the kind described in this paragraph is termed *endogenous obesity*.

From a psychological viewpoint, an important factor in much obesity is compulsive eating. For this reason, obesity may be categorized as a psychosomatic disorder. Some obesity seems to result primarily from the excess intake of calories. There may be no obvious genetic factor or metabolic problem, and one is not always thought to be present. Obesity of the kind described in this paragraph is termed *dietary obesity*, and it is probably quite common.

Of course, genetic, biochemical, and psychological factors can all interact and, in the case of a particular obese individual, all may play some role.

Much thought and research have gone into the treatment of obesity. If the problem appears to be primarily of a biological nature (i.e., genetic or endogenous obesity), then medical management is recommended. A prudent diet, hormone therapy, appetite-suppressant drugs, and regular exercise-are all treatment approaches that have been used with mixed success.

If the problem appears to be primarily of a psychological nature (i.e., dietary obesity), then psychotherapy is recommended. Usually the therapy attempts to (1) help the individual understand *why* he or she overeats and (2) offer practical behavior modification strategies designed to curtail the excessive intake of food.

See also *compulsive eating*; *eating disorders*; *hyperobesity*; *Overeaters Anonymous (OA)*.

obsession: An idea or behavioral impulse that intrudes on the individual's consciousness against one's will. Usually obsessions have a stubborn quality; they are tenacious and recurring.

An obsession can be part of a neurotic process or a schizophrenic disorder. If the obsession is part of a neurotic process, the individual recognizes that it is foolish or irrational. However, this recognition does not make the obsession go away. Here are selected examples of neurotic obsessions manifested by some patients: (1) driving a car after 3:00 P.M. is unlucky, (2) even new paper cups have germs, and (3) my hair is too thick.

If the obsession is part of a schizophrenic disorder, the individual may believe the idea is "true" or the behavioral impulse is "right." Under these conditions, the obsession becomes part of a delusion. Here are selected examples of schizophrenic obsessions manifested by some patients: (1) getting wet from the rain causes cancer, (2) avoid people with dead eyes because they carry disease, (3) if you eat olives or peanut butter, you will die young, and (4) I must kill all nurses with blond hair. The distinction between neurotic and schizophrenic obsessions is not a sharp one. However, schizophrenic obsessions seem to have a somewhat more bizarre quality.

See also *neurosis*; *obsessive-compulsive disorder (obsessive-compulsive neurosis)*; *schizophrenia*.

obsessive-compulsive disorder (obsessive-compulsive neurosis): An anxiety disorder characterized by the presence of either obsessions or compulsions (or both). An obsession is experienced in the case of this disorder as both irrational and involuntary. The term *ego dystonic* is used to describe its intrusive quality. The presence of the obsession often induces a substantial anxiety in the individual. Often the obsession suggests that some dreaded event or disaster is about to befall the individual. For example, "If I happen to pass a fire hydrant on the way to work, I will get sick today."

A compulsion is an intense, almost irresistible impulse to carry out a ritual or other fixed pattern of action. For example, a person may have the compulsion to hold on to water faucets one minute before either turning them on or off. Or another person may need to tap a foot seven times on the floor before entering a bedroom.

Quite often, the function of a given compulsion is to reduce the anxiety associated with a given obsession. For example, a person may think, "If I touch doorknobs without gloves, I will get a heart attack before midnight. But if I wash each finger three times, it will undo the damage I did when I touched the doorknob." So the person touches the doorknob, then goes to the bathroom to carry out the compulsion. Note that counting to "magical numbers" is often part of a ritual compulsion.

Adolescents and young adults are the most common sufferers from obsessive-compulsive disorder. Both sexes seem to suffer from the disorder in approximately equal numbers. Although such a disorder complicates life, it seldom creates a major psychological disability. No exact statistics are available on the frequency of the disorder, but it is not thought to be too common.

Not much is known about the causal factors involved in obsessive-compulsive disorder. It is believed, however, that proneness to depression may be associated with the disorder. Psychoanalysis sees obsessive-compulsive behavior as a part of a neurotic process. Early childhood experiences are thought to contribute to a pattern of chronic anxiety. The anxiety can take the concrete form of obsessions, and the anxiety associated with them is reduced by compulsions. The psychoanalytic viewpoint is not, however, accepted by all clinicians.

Left untreated, the disorder tends to resist change. In fact, the compulsions may gain strength because they reduce anxiety, and this is very reinforcing.

One treatment that seems to be of some assistance in alleviating the symptoms of an obsessive-compulsive disorder is the prescription of tricyclic agents. These drugs are usually prescribed for depression, but some data suggest that they may be useful in breaking up the circular thinking involved in an obsession.

Insight-oriented therapy is often used to treat obsessive-compulsive disorder. Behavior therapy has also been used with some success. One of the behavior therapy methods sometimes used is called *response prevention*. The anxiety associated with the obsession is invoked, the therapist is present, and the patient is encouraged to resist the compulsion. This approach can, in some cases, bring about a gradual extinction of the compulsive tendency.

See also *anxiety disorders*; *neurosis*; *obsession*; *obsessive-compulsive personality disorder (compulsive personality disorder)*.

obsessive-compulsive personality disorder (compulsive personality disorder): A kind of personality disorder characterized by perfectionistic tendencies and a lack of flexibility. It is difficult for individuals with this disorder to spontaneously express warmth. Thus it is common for such persons to lack adequate emotional closeness in their important human relationships. Other traits associated with this disorder are a tendency to be dominating, great involvement in one's vocation, and difficulty in making decisions. Although any of these traits can be more or less "normal," in the person with an obsessive-compulsive personality disorder, they are excessively prominent.

Persons with this disorder often find that it interferes with their effectiveness in life. It impairs their ability to adequately play important social roles such as spouse or parent. It also interferes with job performance.

Psychoanalysis hypothesizes that fixations of libido in the anal stage of development are a contributing factor to obsessive-compulsive personality disorder. There is, however, no consensus among mental health professionals concerning the predisposing factors associated with this disorder.

No good estimates exist, but the disorder is believed to be fairly common, particularly among men.

If a person with this disorder is sufficiently distressed by his or her behavioral traits, then psychotherapy may be of some value. There is no easy cure with drug therapy. The individual with an obsessive-compulsive personality disorder needs to participate voluntarily in the process of behavioral change.

See also *anal character traits*; *obsessive-compulsive disorder (obsessive-compulsive neurosis)*; *personality disorders*.

occupational therapy: A kind of therapy that focuses on providing a mental patient with an opportunity to engage in constructive or creative activity. Examples of such activities are drawing or painting pictures, playing a musical instrument, learning to type, woodworking, modeling in clay, writing a story, needlecraft, and so forth. Often one or several large well-lit rooms in a hospital are set aside for these activities. Occupational therapy is not thought of as a primary therapy but is secondary to drug therapy or psychotherapy.

A primary goal of occupational therapy is to encourage a mental patient to be less withdrawn, to make social contacts with other people. Another goal is to raise self-esteem through the visible evidence of a valued accomplishment.

Occupational therapy is a specialty in its own right. A registered occupational therapist is required to have a 4-year college degree in occupational therapy plus supervised training.

See also *psychotherapy*; *therapy*.

Oedipus complex: In psychoanalysis, a set of unconscious motives and ideas characterized by (1) an incest wish toward the parent of the opposite sex, (2) guilt over the wish, and (3) fear of punishment from the parent of the same sex. According to Freud, the conflict surrounding the forbidden incest wish reaches crises proportions toward the end of the phallic stage (around the age of 5 or 6) and is "solved" by the defense mechanism of repression. Repression brings about a period of psychosexual latency lasting from about the ages of 6 to 12.

The term *Oedipus complex* is derived from the Greek tragedy *Oedipus Rex* in which a man inadvertently slays his own father and marries his own mother. Freud believed that the play revealed a universal theme and that all children must cope with their incest wishes. Although the word *Oedipus* suggests a male, the term *Oedipus complex* is appropriately used to refer to either males or females. However, the term *Electra complex* is sometimes used as a synonym for the Oedipus complex when talking about women.

There is no consensus among clinicians concerning the importance of the Oedipus complex. Many believe that Freud exaggerated its importance. Others argue that it is far from universal.

However, it can be noted that, at least in some cases, patients have incest wishes or incest fantasies toward their opposite-sex parents. In these instances, Freud's hypothesis that incomplete repression of an Oedipus complex can be a factor in sexual disorders certainly seems to be of some value.

See also *Electra complex*; *latency stage*; *phallic stage*; *psychosexual development*.

olfactory hallucinations: Hallucinations involving the sense of smell. For example, one patient regularly complained that he smelled frying onions. Another patient complained that others on the ward smelled of lemon juice. Olfactory hallucinations are sometimes a symptom of brain damage but not necessarily. They can also arise in connection with schizophrenic disorders.

See also *delusion*; *dementia*; *hallucination*.

onanism: An antiquated name for masturbation.

See also *masturbation*.

operant conditioning: A kind of conditioning in which an action is followed by a reinforcer. The action is called *operant behavior* if it is functional in some way, if it "pays off." A *reinforcer* is any stimulus that increases the likelihood that the operant behavior will be repeated. Assume that a rat is trained to press a lever in order to obtain pellets of food. Under these conditions, lever pressing is operant behavior, and the pellets are reinforcers.

Various key aspects of operant conditioning were studied extensively by the behavioral psychologist B. F. Skinner and his associates. Skinner has argued convincingly, in a series of books and articles, that operant conditioning is an important way of describing much human behavior. A general conclusion that can be derived from his extensive experiments with both animals and human beings is that *behavior is shaped by its own consequences*. This principle underlies behavior modification, an approach that is quite useful in helping troubled persons deal with maladaptive learned behavior patterns.

See also *behavior modification*; *Skinner, Burrhus Frederic*; *token economy*.

opiates: See *opium*.

opium: A narcotic drug derived from the fluid in the pods of the opium poppy plant. Chemical substances derived from opium are also narcotic drugs and are designated *opiates*. These include morphine, codeine, and heroin. Opiates are capable of relieving pain. As a consequence, they have legitimate medical uses.

Opiates are also capable of inducing pleasurable states of relaxation and euphoria. For this reason, they are subject to substantial abuse. Unfortunately, a physiological tolerance to the opiates builds quite rapidly, and ever-increasing dosages are required to maintain the wanted drug response. As a consequence, an addiction to an opiate tends to cost more and more money. And the body is forced to endure higher toxic levels of the drug. Opium and its derivatives are addictive in both the physiological and psychological senses. The body develops a "need" for the drug. And a craving for the drug may remain even after a physiological dependency is broken.

See also *drug addiction*; *heroin*; *methadone*; *morphine*; *narcotic drugs*.

oppositional defiant disorder: A disorder associated with childhood and adolescence characterized by a negative and hostile attitude toward adults in positions of authority, particularly parents. Examples of specific behaviors that suggest the presence of the disorder are temperamental outbursts, arguing with parents, refusing to do household chores, acting in an annoying manner on purpose, refusing to accept responsibility for mistakes and errors, and using foul language. On the whole, a picture emerges of an extremely troublesome and willful child or adolescent.

The disorder is a problem primarily within the family setting.

It is important to realize that the maladaptive behavior is displayed with an intensity and a frequency that is substantially greater than average for children and adolescents of the same age. This needs to be established before a diagnosis of oppositional defiant disorder is warranted.

In children, the disorder is more common in males. In adolescents, the disorder is equally common in both sexes.

Not much reliable data exists concerning the causal factors involved in this disorder. However, it is reasonable to speculate that the causal factors are similar to those involved in conduct disorder. Three of particular importance appear to be emotionally cold parents, too much punishment, and absence of a stable home environment. Informally, it appears that parents who are not affectionate and who also rely on an authoritarian parental style are somewhat more likely to induce, or aggravate, an oppositional defiant disorder.

Oppositional defiant disorder is very similar to conduct disorder and in some cases progresses into it. A conduct disorder is more severe than an oppositional defiant disorder.

Treatment for oppositional defiant disorder is similar to treatment for conduct disorder. It consists of counseling and psychotherapy. An approach such as reality therapy in which the troubled child or adolescent is helped to see the adverse long-run consequences of defiant behavior may be helpful.

See also *conduct disorder*; *reality therapy*.

oral character traits: According to psychoanalytic theory, character traits caused by fixations of libido (i.e., psychosexual energy) during the oral stage of development. These fixations can be induced either by emotional wounds or overindulgence. Sucking, biting, chewing, spitting, and so forth are examples of oral behaviors common in infancy. These same behaviors have their adult counterparts. When oral behavior becomes a part of one's character, or personality, it is thought to take either an oral-passive or an oral-aggressive form. One person with an *oral-passive* personality may eat soft foods compulsively. Another may take in information uncritically. He or she does not "chew" information but is gullible. One person with an *oral-aggressive* personality may be sarcastic (i.e., make "biting" remarks). Another may eat in wolflike fashion, taking big ripping bites out of chicken legs and hamburgers.

Excessive eating, talking, smoking, and drinking are all examples of oral character traits.

See also *libido*; *oral stage*; *psychosexual development*.

oral stage: According to Freud, the first stage of psychosexual development. The oral stage is associated with infancy and lasts from birth to about 18 months of age. Freud hypothesized that libido (i.e., psychosexual energy) was concentrated in the oral zone during this time period. Thus this zone is the first erogenous zone (i.e., zone of sexual pleasure).

See also *erogenous zones*; *libido*; *psychosexual development*.

organic brain syndromes: See *organic mental syndromes (organic brain syndromes)*.

organic mental disorders: Mental disorders that are assumed to have a basis in organic (e.g., neurological or biochemical) pathology. These disorders are divided into three general groups: (1) disorders associated with aging, (2) disorders associated with the abuse of substances (e.g., alcohol, amphetamines, and cocaine), and (3) disorders associated with either a physical condition or of obscure origin.

See also *alcoholism*; *Alzheimer's disease*; *amnesia*; *amphetamines*; *barbiturates*; *caffeine intoxication*; *cocaine*; *delirium tremens*; *dementia*; *hallucinogens*; *hallucinosis*; *marijuana*; *opium*; *phencyclidine (PCP)*; *stimulants*.

organic mental syndromes (organic brain syndromes): Syndromes (i.e., sets of symptoms) that appear in general to have a biological basis but of indefinite or questionable origin. Ten principal specific organic syndromes are identified. These are:

1. *Delirium*, characterized by a clouding of consciousness. Clear thinking is impaired.
2. *Dementia*, characterized by a deterioration in functional intelligence.

3. *Amnestic syndrome*, characterized by memory difficulties.
4. *Organic hallucinosis*, characterized by hallucinations (i.e., false perceptions).
5. *Organic anxiety syndrome*, characterized by irrational worry and concern.
6. *Organic delusional syndrome*, characterized by delusions (i.e., irrational or false beliefs).
7. *Organic mood syndrome*, characterized by mood and emotional difficulties.
8. *Organic personality syndrome*, characterized by such problems as emotional outbursts, lack of social wisdom, impulsive behavior, and petty theft.
9. *Intoxication*, characterized by irrational actions associated with the abuse of alcohol or other drugs.
10. *Withdrawal*, characterized by irrational actions associated with the recent cessation of the use of alcohol or other drugs.

See also *amnesia*; *anxiety*; *delirium tremens*; *delusion*; *dementia*; *hallucinosis*; *intoxication*; *mood disorders (affective disorders)*; *personality disorders*.

organic viewpoint: See *biomedical viewpoint*.

organ susceptibility hypothesis: The psychoanalytic hypothesis that, in a given individual, a "weak" or susceptible organ will be the target of a psychophysiological (i.e., psychosomatic) disorder. Thus one individual with underlying emotional conflict will develop heart problems, another will develop lung problems, and still another will develop stomach problems. The personality unconsciously "chooses" the path of least resistance, and this path takes it to the weak organ.
    See also *psychosomatic disorders*.

orgasm: The third stage of the sexual response cycle. An orgasm is experienced as the peak of sexual pleasure for both males and females. The pleasure is sustained briefly over a time span of about 3 to 10 seconds.

In males, an orgasm and the ejaculation of semen occur simultaneously. The ejaculation of semen is associated with the contraction of bladder muscles and the relaxation of compressor muscles in the penis surrounding the urethra. A sex flush, a reddening and roughening of the skin, is often associated with sexual excitement and the orgasm in both males and females. This sex flush quickly fades after orgasm. In both sexes, there is increased general muscle tension prior to an orgasm.

In females, the primary physical basis of an orgasm is involuntary wavelike contractions of the *pubococcygeus (PC) muscle* surrounding the vaginal channel. The rate of the contractions is slightly under 1 per second. The uterus also undergoes systematic contractions. There are frequently associated contractions of the sphincter muscles of the rectum.

The appearance of an orgasm in sexual relations is not a completely stable behavioral phenomenon. It is involuntary and does not appear at will. Also, it is inhibited or modified by a spectrum of factors including general health, level of sexual excitement, attitudes toward sexuality, resentments toward the partner, chronic anxiety, and depression. Sexual difficulties are relatively common. Fortunately, they often respond well to therapy.

See also *erectile disorder (erectile insufficiency)*; *frigidity*; *hypoactive sexual desire disorder (inhibited sexual excitement)*; *sexual disorders (psychosexual disorders)*; *sexual therapy*.

orthomolecular psychiatry: See *megavitamin therapy*.

outpatient: A patient who is not hospitalized. Such a patient usually makes regular visits to a clinic, hospital, or mental health professional in private practice. Drugs, psychotherapy, or a combination of both are usually prescribed. Today's approach to therapy tends to favor outpatient treatment over hospitalization whenever possible. It is, of course, less expensive to treat the patient. More important, avoiding institutionalization often helps foster a positive self-concept and may be therapeutic in itself.

However, there are times when a mental disorder is so severe or psychosocial stressors are so overwhelming that hospitalization is essential. Even then, the impetus of modern therapy is to think in terms of eventual release, not prolonged confinement.

See also *community mental health center*; *halfway house*.

outreach programs: Programs designed by governmental agencies and hospitals to bring into communities outpatient clinics and counseling offices. Professional staffing includes psychiatrists, clinical psychologists, and social workers. These are "storefront" clinics and provide easy access for local residents. The basic idea is to take services directly to the public as opposed to keeping the same services at a distance.

See also *community mental health center*; *outpatient*.

overanxious disorder: A disorder associated with either childhood or adolescence characterized primarily by persistent anxiety. The young person's mental and emotional life is clouded by irrational apprehension, consternation over real or imagined mistakes, misgivings concerning ability, and dread of coming events. Related symptoms include tension, headaches, and upset stomach. If the disorder continues past the age of 18, it often develops into one of the anxiety disorders.

The disorder occurs with a relatively high rate of frequency. Males are more often afflicted than females. The oldest child in the family is more likely to have the disorder than other siblings. Children in large families tend not to display the disorder. It is speculated that a small family in which the child carries a large burden of emotional responsibility, in which the parents are over-controlling and set very rigid high standards, contributes to the formation of the disorder. It is also reasonable to hypothesize that inborn traits of temperament may make some contribution to the disorder.

Psychiatric treatment for the disorder includes the prescription of tranquilizing drugs. However, this approach is recommended only if the disorder disables the patient. Often counseling and therapy designed to help the child or adolescent express feelings more openly and to become more assertive are helpful.

See also *anxiety disorders*.

Overeaters Anonymous (OA): A self-help organization patterned after Alcoholics Anonymous (AA). If there is an OA group nearby, it can be located through a local telephone directory. No charge is made for attendance. People who are either obese or abuse food are the principal participants.

Overeaters Anonymous assumes that compulsive eating is a disease and that personal recovery from the disease is difficult, if not in some cases impossible, without the help and support of other people. It also assumes that a Higher Power, greater than the sufferer, can restore some semblance of order to a confused existence. These assumptions form the basis of a 12-step recovery program.

See also *Alcoholics Anonymous (AA)*; *bulimia nervosa*; *compulsive eating*; *eating disorders*.

overprotection: As formulated in psychoanalysis, the concept of overprotection refers to an attribute of the parent–child relationship. An overprotective parent will attempt to shield the child from the natural risks and hazards of life. One can speak of overprotection only if the parental behavior is excessive and rather obviously pathological. For example, an overprotective parent might not allow a child to learn to roller skate because it is possible to sprain an ankle or break a leg while roller skating. Another overprotective parent might insist that a child wear a sweater if there is the slightest breeze. The concerned parent is, of course, protective in a rational way.

Psychoanalysis interprets overprotection in terms of a reaction formation, an ego defense mechanism. The basic idea is that the parent in question has repressed hostility toward the child. At an unconscious level, it is possible that the child is wished harm. In order for the parent to protect his or her ego, to maintain a positive self-concept, this hostility is converted to conscious affection. The artificial quality of the affection is betrayed by the compulsive watchdog attitude toward the child's welfare.

The psychoanalytic interpretation certainly seems appropriate in some cases. However, it is possible to interpret overprotective behavior in other ways. A car owner is often overprotective toward a new car. This is hardly unconscious hostility toward the car. The excessive care and caution manifested toward the car almost certainly arises from the fact that the car may, for the moment, be overvalued in the owner's eyes. It is also possible for a parent to feel the same way. Parents who have only one or two children, who waited a long time for children, or who had to go through fertility counseling in order to conceive a child may all have a tendency to be overprotective.

It has been suggested that overprotection can have an adverse affect on a child's development. Psychoanalysis hypothesizes that it may be a contributing factor to a neurotic process.

See also *ego defense mechanisms*; *neurosis*; *reaction formation*.

P

panic disorder: One of several anxiety disorders. Panic disorder is characterized by a series of abrupt and intense episodes of irrational anxiety. Related symptoms include labored breathing, heart palpitations, chest pain, faintness, and the sensation that one is about to die. The attacks usually take place over several days or weeks. The source of the anxiety is obscure and is not based on real danger. For example, the individual may be walking to work or shopping.

Panic disorder seems to occur with a relatively high rate of frequency and is seen more often in females than in males. The disorder tends to be associated with young adulthood. Sometimes the disorder is aggravated by the simultaneous presence of agoraphobia.

It is difficult to specify a set of specific causal factors in a person's life history that lead to a diagnosis of panic disorder. However, there are children who manifest a disorder termed *separation anxiety disorder*, characterized by unreasonable apprehension surrounding temporary partings from parents or the home. Young adults with a history of this disorder appear to be more likely to develop panic disorder. A factor that may precipitate a panic disorder is the recent loss of someone or something of great personal value (e.g., a loved one, an important relationship, or a large sum of money). It is possible to speculate that a neurotic process is responsible in a general way for the pathology underlying the disorder.

The treatment for panic disorder includes antianxiety medication and psychotherapy. It is important that the individual be given emotional support and reassurance. Although, in some cases, the disorder tends to be persistent, quite often it ebbs quickly.

See also *agoraphobia*; *anxiety disorders*.

paradoxical intention: A psychotherapeutic technique developed by the psychiatrist Viktor Frankl in the framework of logotherapy. A patient is told to either (1) try to make happen that which is feared or (2) attempt to inhibit that which is wished for. For example, a patient who is afraid of a heart attack is told to try to make one take place by an effort of will. Or a patient who is afraid of fainting in public is told, "Go ahead. Make yourself faint right now. Let me see what a good fainter you are." Or a female patient who seldom has an orgasm is told, "Next time when you are engaged in sex do your best to try to *not* have an orgasm."

The paradoxical attempt to make a feared event happen often demonstrates to the patient that many fears are groundless. They do not happen even if they are willed to happen. The attempt to inhibit a wished for response, on the other hand, often has a relaxing and freeing effect. The individual stops fighting himself or herself.

Although paradoxical intention is presented in the larger context of logotherapy, a therapy that deals with the deep issue of finding meaning in life, it is essentially a behavioral technique. And it can sometimes be quite an effective tool.

See also *behavior therapy*; *Frankl, Viktor*; *logotherapy*.

paranoid disorder: See *delusional (paranoid) disorder*.

paranoid personality disorder: A kind of personality disorder distinguished primarily by suspicion and mistrust. Related symptoms include being overly secretive, taking great offense when criticized, having difficulty relaxing, finding it difficult to laugh easily, and maintaining a distant cool attitude toward others, even loved ones. It is important to realize that these are *not* psychotic symptoms.

Paranoid personality disorder appears more frequently in males than in females, and it often interferes with marital adjustment as well as other human relations. A paranoid personality disorder is a handicap but often a relatively moderate one. Because the individual's reality contact is intact, he or she can often compensate for the maladaptive personality trends to some degree.

Persons with this disorder tend to avoid treatment. Because they lack a sense of trust, they doubt that a therapist can help them. Also, they do not perceive themselves as the source of their problems. It is situations and other people that cause problems. As a consequence of this tendency to avoid treatment, it is difficult to evaluate the overall frequency of occurrence of this disorder.

If treatment does take place, it is usually psychotherapy with a focus on practical ways of changing attitudes and behavior in the direction of a more trusting and optimistic outlook.

See also *delusional (paranoid) disorder*.

paranoid schizophrenia: See *schizophrenia*.

paraphasia: A tendency to speak in a mixed-up or garbled way. For example, the individual may say, "Went to I store loaf more" instead of "I went to the store for a loaf of bread." Paraphasia is often a sign of brain damage or neurological problems. However, it can also be displayed by persons with schizophrenic disorders or other serious mental disorders. It is not associated with a specific kind of mental pathology.

Paraphasia can be thought of as a milder form of aphasia.

See also *aphasia*; *confabulation*.

paraphilias: Sexual behaviors that are at odds with the conventional sexual behavior of a given culture. (The word *paraphilia* is from Greek roots suggesting "love" of "peripheral things.") Paraphilias used to be called "sexual perversions." However, this usage is no longer recommended because it connotes pathology. A paraphilia may or may not be pathological in terms of the individual's overall adjustment. The term *sexual variance* is suggested as a practical synonym for paraphilia.

See also *bestiality*; *exhibitionism*; *homosexuality*; *incest*; *lesbian*; *masochism*; *pederasty*; *pedophilia*; *sadism*; *sodomy*; *transsexualism*; *transvestic fetishism (transvestism)*; *voyeurism*.

paraprofessionals: Persons who assist professionals in the offering of services. Usually a professional in the mental health field is thought of as an individual with a higher degree or one with a long history of specialized training. Psychiatrists, clinical psychologists, psychiatric nurses, and psychiatric social workers are usually thought of as occupying professional status. The principal paraprofessional position is that of psychiatric technician.

See also *clinical psychologist*; *psychiatric nurse*; *psychiatric social worker*; *psychiatric technician*; *psychiatrist*.

paresis: See *general paresis*.

paresthesia: An unusual feeling or perception such as a numb sensation in the skin, an itch, a ringing in the ears, and so forth. These are sometimes signs of a neurological problem. However, they can also be symptoms of a conversion disorder. The paresthesia in itself does not reliably indicate the presence of a specific problem.

See also *conversion disorder*; *neurology*.

Parkinson's disease: A neurological disorder characterized by an impairment in voluntary muscle control. Related symptoms include tremors, shakiness, partial paralysis, lack of coordination, and absence of mobile facile expressions.

A principal causal factor in the disease appears to be a deficiency of the neurotransmitter dopamine. An important clinical observation is that Parkinson's disease is almost never associated with a schizophrenic disorder. This finding lends some credibility to the *dopamine hypothesis*, a hypothesis that states that one of the causal factors in schizophrenia is excessive activity of dopamine.

The disease is chronic and is not thought of as curable. However, it can be treated and managed. Various medications exist that reduce the symptoms of the disease.

It is important to realize that Parkinson's disease is *not* a mental disorder. Because of changes in facial expression and the voice, the individual may give the impression of declining mental ability. This is usually not the case.

See also *dopamine*; *neurology*; *neurotransmitters*; *schizophrenia*.

passive-aggressive personality disorder: A personality disorder characterized by masked hostility and its expression in disguised form. Related symptoms include postponement of important tasks, sloppiness, lack of cooperation, and inattention when spoken to. Subjectively, the individual often suffers from low self-esteem and feels helpless in the presence of authoritative persons.

A passive-aggressive personality disorder is a handicap primarily in the area of human relations.

Adults who were stubborn and recalcitrant as children are somewhat more likely to develop a passive-aggressive personality disorder. It is possible to speculate that a causal factor in the individual's developmental history is a parental style consisting of a combination of authoritarianism and lack of emotional closeness.

No reliable data are available concerning the frequency of occurrence of the disorder. Nor is it known if one sex is more affected than the other.

Treatment usually consists of psychotherapy focusing on helping the patient find adequate ways to cope with frustration and constructively express hostility. Assertiveness training can be helpful.

See also *personality disorders*.

pathological gambling: An impulse control disorder characterized by a lack of ability to manage the desire to gamble. Related symptoms may range from brash overconfidence to depression and anxiety. Associated aspects of the disorder include troubled family relationships, inability to make payments on loans, writing worthless checks, obtaining money at an excessively high rate of interest because of poor credit, and taking too much time off from work. Sometimes discouragement becomes so severe that the victim of the disorder contemplates suicide as a release from a seemingly impossible burden of life problems.

Frequency of occurrence of the disorder is higher among males than among females. The course of the disorder tends to be chronic, often lasting for many years of the individual's adult life. Pathological gambling is often first evident during the adolescent years.

Causal factors associated with pathological gambling disorder include loss of a parent in childhood, ineffective parents, early contact with betting behavior, a tendency to overvalue the tokens of success such as expensive clothing, a lack of focus on long-range financial plans, a tendency toward unconventionality, an excessive desire for thrills, a tendency to be superstitious, and an intense need to be admired.

Research by B. F. Skinner and others has demonstrated that when reinforcement is partial, or intermittent, a learned tendency becomes highly resistant to extinction. Gambling behavior is reinforced on an irregular basis and, as a consequence, often tends to become a very strong habit. For this reason, it usually takes a substantial therapeutic effort to treat pathological gambling with any degree of success.

Nonetheless, psychotherapy can be effective in some cases. Insight-oriented therapy may help the individual to understand neurotic processes underlying compulsive gambling. Behavior therapy may be useful in helping the individual to develop practical self-management strategies.

An important option that is available to victims of pathological gambling is the one afforded by Gamblers Anonymous.

See also *Gamblers Anonymous (GA)*; *impulsive behavior*.

Pavlov, Ivan Petrovich (1849–1936): A Russian physiologist and researcher into the process of classical conditioning. Pavlov received his medical degree from the University of St. Petersburg in 1883 and won a Nobel Prize in 1904 for his research on the physiology of the digestive glands. It was subsequent to the winning of this award that he turned to the experimental investigation of conditioned reflexes in dogs.

In one of his sets of experiments, Pavlov was able to demonstrate that it was possible to create behavioral pathology in dogs that had been previously agreeable by forcing the animals to make difficult discriminations. This phenomenon is called *experimental neurosis*, and it has suggested to many students of abnormal psychology that a similar process may operate in human beings.

Pavlov took the point of view that science alone can bring enlightenment to the human race. He asserted that behavior can be explained without recourse to vague or mysterious forces. On the contrary, he believed that behavior is a part of the natural world and can be understood as such. This outlook on Pavlov's part had a great influence on John B. Watson, the father of behaviorism.

Pavlov is looked on as the father of modern learning theory. His work remains an inspiration to behavior therapists.

One of Pavlov's principal works is *Conditioned Reflexes* (1927).

See also *behavior therapy*; *classical conditioning*; *Watson, John Broadus*.

peak experience: A high moment of exceptional personal meaning. Words such as *rapture*, *joy*, and *ecstasy* are often associated with peak experiences. One person may have a peak experience when watching a child take his or her first steps. A second person may have a peak experience at the moment when an important goal is attained. According to Abraham Maslow, peak experiences are associated with the process of *self-actualization*, a tendency to maximize one's talents and potentialities. Persons who use their possibilities wisely, who act on their options in life, are likely to have more peak experiences than persons who are somewhat more passive.

See also *Maslow, Abraham Harold*; *self-actualization*.

pederasty: A paraphilia characterized by homosexual relations between adult males and boys. The usual implication is that the adult male practices anal intercourse on the boy.

See also *homosexuality*; *paraphilias*; *pedophilia*; *sodomy*.

pedophilia: A sexual disorder, also a paraphilia (i.e., sexual variance), characterized by fantasies or actual behaviors on the part of an adult in which a prepubertal child is the sexual partner. A parallel characteristic is a preference on the part of the adult for this kind of activity over conventional adult relations.

The individual suffering from pedophilia is often termed a *pedophile*.

Pedophilia occurs at a fairly high level of frequency. About one-third of sex offenses fall into the category of child molestation. Most of the victims of this disorder are males, and they are most commonly in their middle years. Frequently the individual is low in intelligence, has a schizophrenic disorder, abuses alcohol, or is socially withdrawn.

It is important to note that one-half or more of child molestation occurs with a person familiar to the child such as a relative or a family friend.

Causal factors in pedophilia include a lack of adequate sexual education in childhood, a highly moralistic attitude toward sex, rigid religious training, inability to establish meaningful human relations with adults of the same age, homosexual tendencies, beginning senility, and lack of sexual confidence.

Individuals with pedophilia are often prosecuted and may spend some time in a prison or a mental hospital. Various treatment approaches have been used with pedophilia. A medical treatment is the prescription of drugs designed to inhibit testosterone production and reduce the individual's sexual drive. Insight-oriented psychotherapy is often used aiming to help the individual understand the roots of the disorder. More recently, various kinds of behavior therapies have been used aiming to help the individual modify both sexual focus and actions. In particular, aversion therapy (a type of behavior therapy) has been used to help the individual develop negative associations with the desires and actions of the disorder. All of the treatment approaches have met with limited success. The disorder tends to be highly resistant to therapeutic intervention.

See also *aversion therapy*; *behavior therapy*; *child abuse*; *paraphilias*; *pederasty*; *sexual disorders (psychosexual disorders)*.

pellagra: A disease characterized by such symptoms as dermatitis (skin irritation), soreness of the mouth, upset digestion and diarrhea, and disturbed mental functioning. The disturbed mental functioning may include delusions, hallucinations, and depression. Left untreated, severe pellagra can lead to death. (The term *pellagra* comes from Italian root words meaning "aggravated skin.")

The cause of pellagra is a deficiency of *niacin*, one of the B-complex vitamins. The relationship of a niacin deficiency to disturbed mental function adds a certain amount of credibility to the possible value of megavitamin therapy, at least in some cases. In particular, persons who abuse alcohol or other drugs and some older people are sometimes prone to a niacin deficiency.

See also *megavitamin therapy*.

penis envy: An early psychoanalytic concept hypothesizing that women in general have an unconscious wish to have a penis. Freud proposed that the wish has its origin in the phallic stage of development (i.e., during the preschool years). The girl may see the penis of her father or of a brother and develop the idea that something is missing in her anatomy.

A more mature version of penis envy is to suggest that the female does not literally wish for a penis but envies the status and power that being a male confers on the individual. She wants not the penis itself but what the penis can bring. This describes a revision of classical psychoanalysis and is not what Freud had in mind.

In psychoanalytic theory, the well-adjusted woman has given up the infantile wish for the penis, has made her peace with the facts of life, and accepts the cultural role associated with her gender. Psychoanalysis postulates that highly aggressive and overcontrolling women may be suffering to some degree from penis envy.

The concept of penis envy has been criticized on several counts. First, it suggests that biological normality is perceived as biological abnormality by the young female. Second, it hypothesizes that penis envy is universal among females, which seems highly unlikely. Third, it appears to relegate women to a secondary status. As a consequence of these and similar criticisms, Freud has been accused by some feminists of male chauvinism. Contemporary defenders of Freud argue that he himself was not a male chauvinist but that the concept of penis envy reflects in the psychology of the individual the reality of a sexist culture.

See also *Freud, Sigmund*; *phallic stage*; *psychoanalysis*; *psychosexual development*.

personality disorders: A set of disorders in which enduring traits (i.e., behavioral dispositions) of the individual are maladaptive and impair social functioning. Examples of such traits are mistrust, extreme shyness, dramatic behavior, self-absorption, lack of concern for other people's needs, impulsive behavior, aggressive behavior, overly dependent behavior, and perfectionism. Of course, all of these traits do not usually appear in one individual. In fact, some of them are contradictory. However, if one or two appear in well-defined form, they may provide the basis for a personality disorder.

It is important to realize that a personality disorder does not in any way imply psychosis. People with personality disorders are more often than not free of delusions and hallucinations. Their basic reality contact is unimpaired. Nor does the presence of a personality disorder necessarily suggest the existence of a neurotic process. Frequently persons with these disorders are remarkably free of chronic anxiety. It has been said, with some degree of truth, that they are not so much troubled themselves but troublesome to others.

The subjects of causal factors in, and treatment of, the personality disorders are discussed in the entries in the encyclopedia for the specific disorders.

See also *antisocial personality disorder (psychopathic personality; sociopathic personality); avoidant personality disorder; borderline personality disorder; dependent personality disorder; histrionic personality disorder; multiple personality disorder; narcissistic personality disorder; obsessive-compulsive personality disorder (compulsive personality disorder); paranoid personality disorder; passive-aggressive personality disorder; schizoid personality disorder; schizotypal personality disorder.*

personality test: A type of psychological test used to provide a profile of an individual's outstanding traits (i.e., behavioral dispositions). These traits are conceived of as long-standing or relatively enduring. The aim of a personality test is not to assess a passing mood or transient emotional state. Examples of the kinds of traits evaluated include extraversion/introversion, stability/instability, achievement motivation, need for autonomy, and assertiveness.

The two principal purposes of personality tests are research and clinical diagnosis. Research helps behavioral scientists develop a richer understanding of the human personality. Clinical diagnosis is useful in the development of a treatment program for a patient. Psychotherapists often find the results of a test give them greater insight into the nature of a patient's problems. Test results are also helpful in evaluating a patient's progress.

There is more than one way to conduct a personality test. A person can be observed under controlled conditions through a one-way glass. Or the individual subject can be given a problem to solve, and responses can be evaluated. Or a structured psychological interview can be used. However, in practice, most personality tests are paper-and-pencil tests using a set of standardized materials. These are convenient because they can be administered relatively quickly and evaluated reliably. Published psychological tests usually include test booklets with instructions for administration, scoring, and evaluation.

See also *Minnesota Multiphasic Personality Inventory (MMPI)*; *psychological test*; *Q-sort technique*; *Rorschach test*; *Thematic Apperception Test (TAT)*.

personalization: A kind of cognitive distortion in which one person takes the blame for another person's disappointing behavior. (A *cognitive distortion* is an idea that is the result of a warped or irrational thought process.) Margaret's husband abuses alcohol. She often thinks, "It's all my fault. I'm letting him down. Maybe I don't love him enough, and he's looking for love in a bottle." Michael's two boys are performing poorly in grammar school. He thinks, "I'm not much of a father. I don't spend enough quality time with them. They're goofing off because of my neglect."

Although there may be an element of truth in the individual's self-blaming thoughts, it is often exaggerated. The individual takes *all* of the responsibility for the other person's behavior. This is seldom realistic. It is irrational to think that we have absolute control over another person's actions. That is why personalization is a cognitive distortion.

A tendency to overuse personalization can be a contributing factor to depression. It is actually a form of mental self-abuse.

See also *automatic thoughts*; *cognitive therapy*; *rational-emotive therapy*.

pervasive developmental disorders: See *developmental disorders*.

perversion: Any significant deviation from normal behavior in a pathological or maladaptive direction. The term has been commonly applied to sexual behavior. However, today terms such as *paraphilia* or *sexual variance* are recommended over *sexual perversion*.

See also *paraphilias*.

petit mal epilepsy: See *epilepsy*.

phallic stage: The third stage in Freud's theory of psychosexual development.

See also *psychosexual development*.

phallic symbol: As used in psychoanalysis, a phallic symbol is any object of perception that in imagination can represent the penis. Thus, in a dream, a particular man might see himself shooting a woman in the stomach with a gun. Free association to elements of the dream might reveal that it suggests a rape fantasy. The gun stands for the dreamer's penis. It is his "weapon," and sexual intercourse is seen as an act of aggression. Common phallic symbols are bananas, sausages, cigars, pens, pencils, knives, and so forth.

It is important to realize, of course, that an object that can represent the penis does not always symbolize the penis. It is only when there is a need for the individual to repress awareness of the importance of the penis in a particular context that the symbol comes into play. There is a famous story, possibly apocryphal, told about Freud in this regard. He was once chided because he smoked so many cigars. The critic hinted that possibly Freud's love of cigar smoking represented a repressed wish for homosexual relations. It is reported that Freud smiled and said, "There are times when a cigar is merely a cigar."

See also *dream analysis*; *psychoanalysis*.

pharmacotherapy: The use of drugs to treat pathological conditions, either mental or physical. Note the similarity to the familiar word *pharmacy*, the science and art of compounding and dispensing drugs.

See also *drug therapy*.

phencyclidine (PCP): A hallucinogenic drug popularly known as "angel dust." Although PCP is classified as a hallucinogen, this is somewhat misleading because the taking of the drug seldom causes hallucinations. It is probably more correct to broadly classify

PCP as a *psychoactive drug*. Small doses of PCP produce a reaction in the individual similar to intoxication. The individual becomes somewhat more impulsive and thinking becomes confused. The problem is with high doses. These are capable of producing a delirium. The individual loses the ability to think clearly and becomes very confused.

There are many reports stating that PCP users become violent. The violence seems to be primarily reactive in nature. If left alone, the user will probably sink into a sort of temporary personal oblivion. However, if frustrated, restrained, or arrested by police officers, then aggressive and assaultive behavior can result. It is also reported that PCP users are "hard to stop" when they are fighting off others. This seems to be correct because PCP has anesthetic properties. The person in a PCP delirium "feels no pain."

Because PCP does not induce euphoria, it has been hard for nonusers to see why anyone would abuse the drug or take it on a recreational basis. The key seems to be related to (1) the drug's ability to blot out consciousness and (2) lack of subsequent recall of the PCP state. Thus it can be reasoned that the PCP user is not looking for a "high" or a pleasant experience. He or she is looking for temporary oblivion.

Unfortunately, PCP is an abused drug. It has little practical value for human beings and is not used in the practice of medicine. Frequent use of the drug produces significant adverse effects on intellectual abilities. On the hopeful side, one does not acquire a physiological addiction to PCP. Thus, from the organic point of view, withdrawal is not a great problem. However, it should be noted that psychological addiction can be a problem; the person becomes emotionally dependent on the drug. Therefore counseling and psychotherapy may be required to help the individual stay away from the drug on a permanent basis.

See also *delirium*; *hallucinogens*; *psychoactive drug*.

phenothiazines (phenothiazine derivatives): Drugs that reduce the intensity of the symptoms associated with psychotic disorders. These drugs appear to function principally by blocking the action of *dopamine*, one of the brain's neurotransmitters. Two of the principal agents that fall within the class phenothiazines are chlorpromazine and haloperidol, both discussed in the entry for major tranquilizers.

See also *dopamine*; *major tranquilizers (antipsychotic drugs)*.

phenylketonuria (PKU): A defect of metabolism present in some infants capable of causing mental retardation. (The disease is also known as *phenylpyruvic oligophrenia*.) The neonate with phenylketonuria (PKU) lacks a specific enzyme critical in the digestion of *phenylalanine*, one of the amino acids. If phenylalanine builds up in the blood stream in large amounts, injury to the central nervous system can occur.

Physical symptoms usually become quite evident toward the end of an infant's first year of life. They include an unpleasant smell, digestive upset, and skin problems.

Most states now require that the urine or blood of infants be tested for the presence of *phenylpyruvic acid*, a substance indicating an excess of phenylalanine. If a child has PKU, he or she can be placed on a special diet free of proteins containing phenylalanine. In practical terms, this will be a diet free of meats and animal products such as milk and cheese. Naturally, consultation with a physician and dietician is important to determine the optimal diet for the particular child.

Research suggests that PKU is a recessive inherited disorder. The incidence of PKU in infants is estimated to be between 1 in 10,000 and 1 in 20,000. About 1% of hospitalized patients with mental retardation suffer from PKU.

See also *mental retardation*.

phenytoin: An anticonvulsant drug used primarily to prevent grand mal seizures associated with epilepsy. Trade names for phenytoin include Dilantin, Dantoin, and Di-Phen. The drug is also sometimes prescribed to help control and regulate heart action. Phenytoin acts by reducing the excitability of neurons in the central nervous system.

Common side effects include excessive sleepiness and digestive problems. On the whole, however, the drug is remarkably free of short-term side effects. However, long-term usage for many years may produce pathological changes in bones, lymph glands, and the liver. Therefore, it is a prescription drug and is taken only if necessary.

See also *attention deficit disorder*; *bipolar disorder*; *epilepsy*.

phobia: A kind of anxiety disorder characterized by the presence of an irrational fear. Mild phobias are fairly common, and their presence alone is not enough to justify the diagnosis of an anxiety disorder. The problems associated with the phobia should be either incapacitating or greatly interfere with the course of living before a condition receives a clinical label.

There are three principal kinds of phobia. *Agoraphobia* is characterized by a set of related fears including the fear of being alone, a fear of public places, and fear of traveling any significant distance from home. *Social phobia* is characterized by a fear of placing oneself in situations where others have an opportunity to observe or judge one's behavior. Social phobias are usually specific in nature. For example, the individual may be afraid to speak in public, go to a party and meet new people, use a public rest room, and so forth. *Simple phobia* is characterized by a given irrational fear.

Some well-known simple phobias are (1) *acrophobia*, a fear of high places; (2) *claustrophobia*, a fear of confinement or closed areas; (3) *cynophobia*, a fear of dogs; (4) *demophobia*, a fear of crowds; (5) *haptephobia*, a fear of being touched; (6) *hemophobia*, a fear of blood; (7) *hypnophobia*, a fear of sleep; (8) *necrophobia*, a fear of dead bodies; (9) *nyctophobia*, a fear of darkness or the night; (10) *ophidiophobia*, a fear of reptiles; and (11) *zoophobia*, a fear of animals.

Although both sexes can and do develop phobias, they tend to be more commonly diagnosed in women.

Broadly speaking, there tend to be two general approaches to explaining phobias. First, psychoanalysis tends to see them as symbolical representations. The situation or thing consciously feared is not what is actually feared. The consciously feared stimulus stands for an unconscious wish, one that has been repressed. The actual fear is that one will act on a forbidden impulse, the one contained in the forbidden wish. Thus a fear of heights might be a protective mechanism against the wish to commit suicide by leaping from a tall building. A male who fears snakes might be protecting himself against latent homosexual tendencies. (This assumes the snake can be a phallic symbol.)

Second, behavioral psychology tends to see phobias as having a learned basis. They are generalizations from prior experiences. Thus, a fear of speaking in public might be traced back to prior public-speaking failures. A fear of dogs might be based on the fact that one was once injured badly by a dog.

Although the two general explanations are usually presented as contradictory in nature, they need not be in specific clinical cases. It is certainly reasonable to say that one patient's fear is based on a repressed wish and a second patient's fear is based on generalization from a prior experience.

The treatment for a phobia is usually some kind of psychotherapy. Insight-oriented therapy can be helpful if the phobia has a symbolical basis and unconscious roots. On the other hand, most phobias can be effectively treated with desensitization therapy, a kind of behavior therapy. In fact, the desensitization therapy approach to phobias has been one of the outstanding success stories of the twentieth century. More than one research project has shown the value of treating phobias with desensitization therapy.

See also *agoraphobia*; *anxiety disorders*; *desensitization therapy*; *psychoanalysis*.

physiological addiction: See *drug addiction*.

pica: The eating of substances without nutritional value. Examples of such substances are clay, chalk, ashes, dirt, bits of paper or cardboard, peeling paint, tiny rocks, and dry animal feces. Children, pregnant women, and schizophrenic individuals have all at times exhibited pica. The word *pica* is derived from the Latin word for magpie, an omnivorous bird that eats with little selection.

Pica also has the status of a specific mental disorder associated with infancy or early childhood. Children afflicted with pica usually also enjoy ordinary food. In most cases, children spontaneously outgrow the behavior.

The incidence of pica is low, and it seems to affect both boys and girls in about equal numbers. Pica is rare in older children and adults.

Causal factors in pica include low economic status, mineral deficiencies (particularly iron and zinc), mental retardation, and lack of parental supervision.

Treatment of pica involves a combination of behavior modification for the child and guidance for the parents. In most cases, the behavior can be readily controlled.

See also *eating disorders*.

Pick's disease: A degenerative disease of the brain. The primary symptom is *dementia*, a deterioration in functional intelligence. Related symptoms include memory difficulties, confusion, mood swings, lack of social restraint, becoming tired easily, and lack of interest in living. The onset of Pick's disease is very gradual. It is usually described as a "presenile" disorder because it tends to strike its victims in middle age, not old age.

The disease was first described by the Czechoslovakian psychiatrist Arnold Pick in a publication dated 1892. The disease is rare and is believed to have an inherited basis. Women are somewhat more prone to the disease than are men. There is no known way to prevent Pick's disease. Treatment consists of management and care to relieve the severity of symptoms. However, there is no known cure. A typical victim of the disease will live for 5 or 6 years after the diagnosis in a deteriorating state of health.

It is often quite difficult to tell if a patient has Alzheimer's disease or Pick's disease because their symptoms are very similar. There are, however, subtle differences between the symptoms, and a skilled diagnostician will in most cases be able to make a correct diagnosis. For example, patients with Alzheimer's disease tend to be more anxious and agitated than patients with Pick's disease.

See also *Alzheimer's disease*; *presenile dementias*.

Pinel, Phillipe (1745–1826): A French physician who is famous in the history of psychiatry for freeing mental patients from their chains and shackles. Pinel received his M.D. degree from the University of Toulouse in 1773. During his career, he served as director of the Bicêtre Hospital and subsequently as director of the Salpêtrière Hospital.

It was conventional during the 1700s to look on mental patients as little more than animals. They were objects of scorn and amusement. Pinel took the position that restraining mental patients for prolonged periods of time frustrated them so greatly that they began to act in seemingly inhuman ways.

Instead of punishment and arbitrary confinement, Pinel offered to the patient what has been called "moral therapy." This involved a combination of discussions with the patient, responsible tasks, clean surroundings, and balanced meals. Pinel was gratified by the way patients responded to his ministrations.

See also *Beers, Clifford Whittingham*; *Dix, Dorothea Lynde*; *moral therapy*.

placebo effect: The capacity of a drug or treatment to produce a beneficial effect even though there is no specifiable biological basis for the effect. The word *placebo* standing alone refers to a sham treatment or an inert substance representing an actual drug. (Placebo in Latin means "I will please." Thus a placebo refers to a pleasing substance.)

More than one research project has demonstrated that the placebo effect is quite real. For example, postoperative patients were told in one study that they were receiving shots of morphine for pain. In fact they were being given injections of subcutaneous water. In many cases, a substantial amount of relief from pain was reported. One man took two aspirin in the middle of the night for a headache, went back to bed, and obtained relief. The next morning, he noted that he had inadvertently taken two vitamin C tablets.

The placebo effect is so powerful that research designs on the effects of new drugs must take it into account. In a well-planned experiment, there are at least two groups: the drug group and a placebo group. The two groups are treated alike in all respects. Members of the placebo group receive a sham treatment (e.g., a daily pill). The overall description of the experiment is that it is *double-blind*, meaning that (1) the patients do not know who has been assigned to a particular group and (2) those who summarize the data do not know either. These precautions tend to ensure that little bias enters into the final report. Often the placebo group displays substantial improvement. However, if the new drug is actually effective, then the drug group displays even more improvement. The difference between the improvement of the drug group and the placebo group is a measure of the drug's actual effectiveness.

The reality of the placebo effect can be used to advantage by persons in the healing professions. If a patient is encouraged to have positive expectations for a drug treatment or for psychotherapy, this will *add* to any real effects. However, it is considered unethical to administer only sham treatments.

Recent studies suggest that there may be a physiological basis for the placebo effect, at least in some cases. A placebo may stimulate the body to produce endorphins, and these may bring about a certain amount of relief from pain.

See also *drug therapy*; *endorphins*.

play therapy: A kind of psychotherapy used primarily with children. The child is provided with materials such as clay, blocks, dolls, and toys and encouraged to engage in self-directed activity. The general concept is that children are not as articulate as adults, and they can express themselves more adequately through a set of concrete articles. Also, play therapy is inspired by the psychoanalytic concept of *catharsis*, a process of emotional cleansing. As children play with the toys, they may display both affectionate and hostile feelings. For example, 4-year-old Louise picked up a female doll, hugged it, and said, "This is my mommy. I love her." Then she picked up a male doll and said, "This is my daddy.

He's not nice. I hate him! I hate him!" Then she began banging the doll's head against the floor.

Troubled children who are allowed to express anger through play therapy often develop a certain amount of self-understanding and insight into their relationships with parents and siblings. Thus play therapy helps them make adjustments in the real world. It should also be clear from the preceding description of play therapy that it helps the psychotherapist discover the nature of a child's difficulties. The child in effect states what the family problems are through behavior.

Play therapy should not occur in an emotional vacuum. Parents who bring a child to a therapist with an attitude that says "Fix this problem kid" are misguided. They need to see that, in most cases, the child's emotional problems are a reaction to adverse parental styles such as authoritarianism and emotional coldness. Therefore play therapy should take place in a larger context of family therapy.

See also *catharsis*; *family therapy*; *psychotherapy*.

pleasure principle: In Freudian theory, the basic operating principle of the *id*, the basic foundation of the personality. Pleasure is perceived by the id as reduction of tension. Thus if one is hungry for food, this is a form of tension. Relief from this tension in the form of eating is experienced as pleasure. The same can be said about other drives such as thirst, oxygen hunger, the need for sleep, the need to express aggression, and the desire for sexual release.

Unfortunately, the id is blind. Thus we are not free to act on the pleasure principle without restraint. We need the correction introduced by the *ego*, the conscious agent of the personality. The ego operates in accordance with the reality principle, and it helps us find practical ways to obtain pleasure.

One source of mental health problems is the inability in some persons to find effective channels of expression for the pleasure principle. The ego may be "weak" and somewhat ineffective. In addition, the *superego*, the moral agent of the personality, may impose barriers of its own. The resulting frustration may produce, or complicate, emotional reactions such as anxiety, resentment, and depression.

Psychoanalysis, or psychotherapy with a psychoanalytic orientation, helps the troubled individual find ways to obtain a reasonable amount of pleasure in a practical way.

See also *ego*; *id*; *psychoanalysis*; *reality principle*; *superego*.

positron emission tomography (PET): A diagnostic technique that produces an image of the metabolic activity of the brain. The image itself is usually referred to as a PET scan. Positron emission tomography is accomplished through the injection of weakly radioactive material into the bloodstream. Data from radiation detectors are assembled into the final image.

PET scans are of substantial value. First, they are useful in research on brain processes. Second, they are of diagnostic value in assessing both neurological problems (e.g., epilepsy) and organic damage (e.g., the effects of a stroke). Recent research also suggests that certain kinds of mental disorders may be correlated with metabolic activity in the brain. For example, the blood flow pattern in the brain of a person suffering from a schizophrenic disorder may differ significantly from the blood flow pattern in normal persons.

See also *computerized axial tomography (CAT)*; *nuclear magnetic resonance(NMR)*.

posthypnotic suggestion: See *hypnosis*.

postpartum depression: A depression associated with the period immediately following the birth of an infant. This time period is inexact but is usually identified as about 90 days in length. Although the state of depression is commonly identified with the mother, it can also be correctly applied to some fathers. Mild postpartum depressions are extremely common. Perhaps 40 to 50% of mothers, particularly first mothers, experience them, and they are almost thought of as "normal." However, a significant depressive episode will strike about 5 to 10% of mothers. And in a substantially smaller number of cases, perhaps 1%, there may be psychotic symptoms, including such symptoms as disordered thinking and delusions. When this takes place, the term *postpartum psychosis* is sometimes used. Neither a significant depressive episode nor a postpartum psychosis can be thought of as normal.

Several causal factors may be involved in postpartum reactions. Biochemical changes following delivery may provide a physiological basis for depression. The birth of an infant may be perceived as an anticlimax following the anticipations of pregnancy. Having an infant to take care of is a major life change, a psychosocial stressor, that requires adjusting to. New pressures and demands are associated with the role of parent. And this is particularly true for first-time parents. One or several of these factors interacting can cause postpartum depression.

In most cases, postpartum depression will remiss spontaneously. However, if symptoms persist after the 90-day period, treatment may be indicated. Treatment may include drug therapy for depression and/or psychotherapy aimed at helping the patient cope with the responsibilities of parenthood.

See also *depression*; *psychotic disorders*.

posttraumatic stress disorder (traumatic neurosis): An anxiety disorder in which an unusually traumatic life event causes symptoms that become manifest at some time subsequent to the event itself. Examples of unusually traumatic life events are being confined to a concentration camp, surviving a crash, living through an earthquake, escaping from a fire, going through wartime combat, experiencing a bombing attack, being rescued from a flood, being tortured, and being raped. Posttraumatic symptoms may include nightmares, sleep disturbances, a feeling that the traumatic event is being relived, obsessional memories of the event, lack of zest for life in general, alienation from other people, inability to have deep emotional responses, and loss of joy in life.

Three kinds of posttraumatic stress disorder are sometimes identified. An *acute posttraumatic stress disorder* takes place within a few months of the traumatic event. A *chronic posttraumatic stress disorder* is persistent, tending to be a problem over a span of time. A *delayed posttraumatic stress disorder* surfaces 6 or more months after the traumatic event.

If drug therapy is used to treat a posttraumatic stress disorder, usually an antianxiety drug will be prescribed. If psychotherapy is used to treat the disorder, an issue of particular importance is *survivor guilt*, the feeling that one does not deserve to live when others have died. If survivor guilt can be alleviated, some of the symptoms of the disorder may diminish. A technique that is sometimes used in psychotherapy is to encourage an *abreaction*, in which a patient expresses strongly felt emotions associated with the trauma.

See also *abreaction*; *anxiety disorders*; *stress*.

precipitating cause: A cause that triggers an event. It is the proverbial "straw that breaks the camel's back." In the case of mental disorders, the precipitating cause is usually a traumatic life change, a psychosocial stressor, that makes the symptoms of an underlying problem flare up and become blatant. Thus the death of a spouse, the death of a child, a divorce, the loss of a job, and so forth may shatter a fragile adjustment.

See also *life change units (LCUs)*; *predisposing cause*; *psychosocial stressors*.

predisposing cause: A long-standing, or underlying, cause. Such a cause in the case of mental disorders increases the overall likelihood that the individual in question will eventually display symptoms of the disorder. Examples of predisposing causes are genetic tendencies, biochemical imbalances, neurological problems, and traumatic emotional experiences in childhood. The existence of a predisposing cause does not mean that the individual in question will necessarily fall ill. However, the probability is increased. Actual illness will occur only if there is a precipitating cause.

See also *precipitating cause*.

premature ejaculation: An ejaculation that takes place early during sexual intercourse. The usual implication is that the male reaches his orgasm before the female reaches hers. If the problem is unusually severe or distressing, it can be classified as a sexual disorder.

Premature ejaculation can be explained in more than one way. The correctness of the explanation may depend on the individual involved. Psychoanalysis tends to explain premature ejaculation in terms of unconscious mental conflicts. Perhaps one male harbors latent feelings of hostility toward his partner and involuntarily seeks to deprive her of satisfaction. Perhaps a second male unconsciously perceives his partner as a mother or a sister, feels guilty about sexual relations, and does not allow either himself or his partner full enjoyment. These are distinct possibilities.

However, it is also possible to take a line of reasoning closer to ordinary interpretations. Young men who have a strong sex drive may simply not have gained satisfactory control over the ejaculatory reflex. The Kinsey sexual surveys indicated that about three-quarters of males interviewed reported ejaculating within 2 minutes of penetration. This is not, of course, a "premature" response if both partners are satisfied. However, the data *do* suggest that normal males tend to ejaculate quite quickly if they do not seek ways to inhibit their excitement.

If the problem has unconscious roots, insight-oriented psychotherapy may be helpful. In other cases, a variety of practical approaches may be useful. Some physicians prescribe that a mild anesthetic be applied to the glans penis. This may extend the time to ejaculation by reducing the intensity of stimulation. Or a couple can have sexual intercourse twice within a relatively short time span. The male's second ejaculation is likely to take longer. Or the female can be masturbated to an orgasm, or close to one, prior to male penetration.

Masters and Johnson teach a squeeze technique in which a female partner squeezes the glans penis with her fingers just before a male feels like ejaculating. This trains the capacity to inhibit and extend the ejaculatory reflex.

If problems persist, then sex therapy is recommended.

See also *erectile disorder (erectile insufficiency); inhibited male orgasm (ejaculatory incompetence or retarded ejaculation); sexual therapy.*

premenstrual syndrome (PMS): A cluster of symptoms believed to be caused by the female's physiological state a few days prior to the beginning of her regular menses. Symptoms include cramps, headaches, illogical thinking, depression, and excitability. It is difficult to assess the incidence of PMS. Milder versions of the condition should not be called premenstrual syndrome but *premenstrual tension*. Premenstrual tension is very common, affecting perhaps a majority of women to some degree. However, a diagnosis of premenstrual syndrome is more likely to be reserved for 1% or 2% of the female population.

PMS is *not* a mental disorder. However, it can certainly be a complicating factor in mental disorders. If a woman suffers from PMS *and* chronic depression, cyclothymic disorder, or bipolar disorder, then the mental disorder in question can be substantially aggravated.

Premenstrual syndrome, although it has psychological aspects, is primarily thought of as a biological disorder. Therefore its treatment is essentially medical in nature. Antianxiety drugs, antidepressant drugs, and hormone therapy are some of the treatments that have been prescribed.

The ancient idea that hysteria is due to a wandering uterus may be based on observations that today would be called symptoms of premenstrual syndrome.

See also *bipolar disorder*; *cyclothymic disorder*; *depression*; *hysteria*.

premorbid state: The state of an individual just before the first appearance of significant symptoms of an illness. In the case of mental disorders, these are the "early warning" signs that suggest the eventual appearance of the full-blown disorder. Usually these signs are weaker versions of the eventual symptoms. For example, a schizophrenic patient may have given voice to a few odd ideas that seemed puzzling to friends and family before becoming ill. The premorbid state should be taken seriously. If it can be responded to appropriately, it is possible that early treatment may reduce the impact of the disorder.

See also *diagnosis*.

presenile dementias: Loosely, dementias associated with any time period of a person's life prior to old age. However, in practice, presenile dementias usually refer to dementias appearing in adulthood, usually in middle age (i.e., around ages 40 to 50). Alzheimer's disease is normally classified as a senile dementia because in most cases its onset is in old age. However, in some cases, Alzheimer's disease starts earlier. So it bridges the gap, and it can, in some cases, be thought of as a presenile dementia. The two principal senile dementias are Pick's disease and Huntington's chorea.

See also *Alzheimer's disease*; *dementia*; *Huntington's chorea*; *Pick's disease*.

primary orgasmic dysfunction: See *inhibited female orgasm (orgasmic dysfunction)*.

Prince, Morton (1854–1929): An American psychiatrist who emphasized the importance of understanding the unconscious aspects of mental disorders. In 1879, Prince graduated from Harvard Medical School with an M.D. degree. Like Freud, Prince studied neurology in France in association with Jean Charcot and Pierre Janet. The work of Janet in particular inspired an interest in unconscious mental processes. Prince was one of the key individuals involved in bringing into existence the highly influential *Journal of Abnormal Psychology* in 1906. For more than 25 years, Prince was a leading figure in American psychiatry.

Although there are some similarities between Prince and Freud, primarily their emphasis on the importance of unconscious mental processes, the two men cannot be lumped together as having the same approach. Freud is usually thought of as a systematic thinker; his explanations and treatment of mental disorders all revolved around psychoanalytic theory. Prince, on the other hand, was willing to use ideas from any theory, including behaviorism, in order to provide therapy for patients. For example, Prince believed that maladaptive habits were an important factor in mental disorders. This is the general line of thinking that today underlies behavior therapy.

Prince can be seen as an open-minded thinker who was more interested in helping troubled persons than in the construction of consistent psychological theories. He helped to start American psychiatry down a practical road in which the care and welfare of the mental patient are given first priority.

Two of Prince's books are *The Unconscious* (1913) and *Clinical and Experimental Studies in Personality* (1929).

See also *abnormal psychology*; *behavior therapy*; *Charcot, Jean-Martin*; *Freud, Sigmund*; *Janet, Pierre Marie Felix*.

privileged communication: The information communicated during counseling and psychotherapy sessions. In essence, the concept of privileged communication states that the therapist should not disclose to others what was disclosed in confidence. The patient has a right to privacy. Thus, if a patient reveals that he or she is having sexual relations outside of the marriage, this does not constitute gossip that can be spread by the therapist.

If the information from therapy sessions is to be included in a case history for publication or presentation to a group, the patient should not be identified. Often a false name is used for the patient, and other identifying characteristics such as age and vocation are changed.

However, an ethical problem can arise if the patient discloses that he or she is about to commit a serious crime. Imagine that the patient reveals the plans for a murder. And further assume that the therapist has good reason to believe that the patient is quite serious. What should the therapist do? The principle of privileged communication states that the therapist should remain silent. However, common decency requires that the information be revealed in order to prevent a homicide. In a case such as the one described, both ethical considerations and the therapist's responsibilities under the law suggest that the principle of privileged communication be put aside. However, under most conditions, the principle of privileged communication should be observed.

See also *legal aspects of mental health*; *psychotherapy*.

process schizophrenia: A characteristic of some kinds of schizo-
phrenias in which the onset of the problem is gradual and its
course tends to be chronic. The prognosis of schizophrenia under
these conditions tends to be poor. Treatment is often of minimal
effectiveness.

Process schizophrenia can be compared with *reactive schizophrenia*, in which the onset of the problem is abrupt and its course
tends to be acute. The prognosis for schizophrenia under these
conditions tends to be hopeful. Treatment is often quite effective.

It is hypothesized that process schizophrenia represents an
underlying disease process arising from within the individual.
Reactive schizophrenia, on the other hand, appears to be, to a
large extent, a response to psychosocial stressors, factors external
to the individual.

The distinction between the two is obviously not always clear-
cut. However, it can be a useful distinction in some cases.

See also *psychosocial stressors*; *psychotic disorders*; *schizophrenia*.

prognosis: The predicted course of a mental disorder (or a disease).
Based on such data as symptoms, existing knowledge about the
disorder, psychiatric interviews, psychological tests, hospital observation, and case history material, the skilled clinician establishes
a probability of success or failure for treatment. The prognosis
is, of course, an inference. Therefore, in an individual case, the
eventual outcome may be at substantial variance from the prognosis.
However, when making predictions about groups, statistical statements, prognostic statements tend to be accurate.

When a prognosis is poor, a family should try to avoid an
attitude of utter despair. As indicated previously, in an individual
case, there is usually a realm of hope.

See also *diagnosis*.

projection: A kind of ego defense mechanism in which a repressed
idea or motive is unconsciously placed on an external source,

such as a person or thing. The name is aptly chosen. It is as if the mind acts like a slide projector and the outer world is the screen. What is perceived as external is put there by the individual's psychological and emotional needs.

The ego is defended in the sense that projection allows the individual to deny ideas or motives that are at variance with his or her superego, the agent of moral values. Thus the ego avoids the criticism of the superego. For example, Mabel has repressed hostile feelings toward her employer. However, she tells friends, "My boss doesn't like me." For a second example, Harris has repressed sexual desire for his sister-in-law. He thinks, "She has a crush on me. I better not encourage her." In both of these examples, the individual can easily maintain a feeling of psychological innocence.

See also *ego defense mechanisms*; *superego*.

projective test: A kind of personality test that takes advantage of a person's tendency to use the ego defense mechanism of projection. An *ambiguous stimulus*, a stimulus that can be perceived in two or more ways, is presented to the subject. These are usually cards with visual figures. Then the subject is asked to relate to the examiner perceptions of each stimulus. The assumption is that these perceptions are colored by unconscious ideas and motives and that they, in turn, reveal the latent aspects of the individual's personality.

Two of the principal projective tests are the Rorschach inkblot test and the Thematic Apperception Test (see below).

See also *personality test*; *projection*; *Rorschach test*; *Thematic Apperception Test (TAT)*.

psilocybin: A drug belonging to the class hallucinogens. Psilocybin is an alkaloid substance obtained from a fungus called *psilocybe mexicana*, or Mexican mushrooms. Street names for psilocybin include *mushrooms*, *businessman's acid*, and *magic*. About ½-hour after taking the drug, it produces alterations in perception and thought. There is a long tradition among the people of Mexico going back to the time of the Aztecs of using psilocybin to alter consciousness and open perceptual doors to religious experiences. (Mescaline has a similar tradition in Central and South America.)

Psilocybin is somewhat similar in its effects to lysergic acid diethylamide-25 (LSD). And the same reservations associated with the recreational use of LSD apply to the use of psilocybin.

See also *hallucinogens*; *lysergic acid diethylamide-25 (LSD)*; *mescaline*.

psyche: The original meaning of the word *psyche* in terms of its ancient Greek origins is "soul." Plato, for example, taught that the soul is a temporary sojourner on the earth, that it comes from a higher realm, an ideal world. In Greek mythology, the soul is personified in the form of the goddess Psyche. Her gossamer wings symbolize a butterfly with the potential to fly to a higher realm.

Contemporary usage of the word *psyche* is derived from the ancient usage. In psychoanalysis, *psyche* refers to the personality or the mind. General usage in behavioral science also suggests that *psyche* means the self.

The principal use of the word *psyche* today is as a root for such words as *psychiatry*, *psychology*, and *psychoanalysis*. In fact, this encyclopedia has entries for more than 30 words of this kind.

See also *ego*.

psychedelic drugs: See *hallucinogens*.

psychiatric nurse: A nurse who specializes in the care of mental patients. Such a nurse has had the regular medical nursing training plus additional training in the mental health field. On a psychiatric unit in a mental hospital, the charge psychiatric nurse is usually second in command after a psychiatrist and will normally direct the work of neuropsychiatric technicians. Psychiatrists are often absent from a given unit, and usually a great deal of responsibility is assigned to the head nurse.

A psychiatric nurse needs to have a substantial amount of knowledge about mental disorders, drug therapy, psychotherapy, and the care of patients in general. The American Nurses' Association (ANA) gives formal status to psychiatric nursing as a specialty.

See also *clinical psychologist*; *psychiatric social worker*; *psychiatric technician*; *psychiatrist*.

psychiatric social worker: A social worker who specializes in working with mental patients and their families. A psychiatric social worker usually holds a master's degree in social work (MSW) and has had special training in family problems and community resources. Also, many contemporary psychiatric social workers are trained psychotherapists.

Psychiatric social workers usually work in mental hospitals or community mental health centers. However, some of them are in private practice.

See also *clinical psychologist*; *psychiatric nurse*; *psychiatric technician*; *psychiatrist*.

psychiatric technician: An aid, or helper, usually to a charge psychiatric nurse on a mental hospital ward. The psychiatric technician's position is a paraprofessional one, meaning that it is thought of as secondary to the position of a more completely trained professional person (e.g., a psychiatrist, psychologist, social worker, or nurse). Some years ago, the psychiatric technician was hired with very little qualification and training. However, it is presently recognized that psychiatric technicians are on the "front lines" with mental patients. Psychiatric technicians provide a great deal of direct care, frequently talk to patients, and often make observations of great value to professionals. Therefore, formal training programs are becoming more and more the norm. At present, it is common to find that the position of psychiatric technician requires a 2-year college program leading to a state license.

See also *paraprofessionals*; *psychiatric nurse*.

psychiatrist: A medical doctor (M.D.) who specializes in treating mental disorders. The formal education required to become a psychiatrist involves 4 years of college, 4 years of medical school, an internship (1 or 2 years), and a residency in a mental hospital (1 or 2 years). At the completion of training, a psychiatrist may work in a private or state mental hospital, a community mental health center, or go into private practice.

The principal duties of a psychiatrist are diagnosis and treatment. Consequently, a psychiatrist is familiar with all of the mental disorders listed in the American Psychiatric Association's *Diagnostic and Statistical Manual of Mental Disorders*, their known or suspected causes, and their prognoses. In addition, he or she is familiar with drug therapy, somatic therapy, and psychotherapy.

A psychiatrist should not be confused with a clinical psychologist. This sometimes happens because they both, on occasion, do psychotherapy. However, because psychiatrists are medical doctors, they can prescribe drugs; clinical psychologists cannot. On the other hand, clinical psychologists are trained in the administration and evaluation of psychological tests, and this is usually not a part of a psychiatrist's educational background. In mental hospitals, psychiatrists and clinical psychologists are a part of a treatment team along with psychiatric nurses, psychiatric social workers, and psychiatric technicians.

See also *clinical psychologist*; *psychiatric nurse*; *psychiatric social worker*; *psychiatric technician*.

psychiatry: A field of medicine concerned with the diagnosis and treatment of mental disorders.

See also *psychiatrist*.

psychoactive drug: Any drug that has a significant effect on thinking, perception, or mood. (These drugs are also known as *psychotropic drugs*.) The concept of a psychoactive drug is a highly general one and includes a spectrum of agents such as antianxiety drugs (minor tranquilizers), antidepressant drugs, antipsychotic drugs (major tranquilizers), hallucinogens, narcotics, sedatives, and stimulants.

See also *antianxiety drugs*; *antidepressant drugs*; *hallucinogens*; *major tranquilizers (antipsychotic drugs)*; *narcotic drugs*; *psychoactive substance use disorders (substance use disorders)*; *stimulants*.

psychoactive substance use disorders (substance use disorders): A set of disorders characterized by the abuse of a drug that affects the central nervous system. Such drugs tend to modify arousal, thought processes, perception, and mood. Substance use in and of itself is not necessarily self-defeating or self-destructive. The American Psychiatric Association's *Diagnostic and Statistical Manual of Mental Disorders* identifies two basic criteria to distinguish *substance abuse* from substance use. These criteria are (1) a pattern of pathological use and (2) a duration of at least 1 month of the pattern.

In addition, the manual identifies a more serious condition called *substance dependence*. Several additional criteria are used to define substance dependence. Examples are (1) inability to quit or cut down, (2) investing excessive time in obtaining the substance, (3) withdrawal symptoms when an effort is made to quit or cut down, and (4) requiring increasingly large doses in order to obtain a drug effect (i.e., tolerance).

Specific substance abuse disorders are discussed elsewhere in this encyclopedia in connection with various drugs.

See also *alcoholism*; *amphetamines*; *barbiturates*; *cocaine*; *drug addiction*; *hallucinogens*; *marijuana*; *nicotine dependence (tobacco dependence)*; *phencyclidine (PCP)*.

psychoanalysis: Both a personality theory and a method of psychotherapy created by Sigmund Freud. A principal underlying theme running throughout psychoanalysis is that there is an unconscious mental life. A secondary theme of substantial importance is that the complexion of the unconscious mental life is shaped primarily by forbidden wishes of a sexual and aggressive nature.

The personality theory states that there are three major agents of the personality. The *id* consists of the basic inborn drives, and it is oriented toward pleasure. The *ego* is in contact with the external world, and it is oriented toward reality. The *superego* represents the values of one's parents and culture, and it is oriented toward morality. Conflicts between the id's wishes and the superego's prohibitions represent a neurotic process, and this neurotic process can be the basis for many psychological and emotional disturbances.

When the word *psychoanalysis* is used to refer to a kind of psychotherapy, it suggests an approach in which the unconscious aspects of mental life are explored and brought to a conscious level. The patient develops *insight*, meaning that he or she sees into the connections between repressed psychological information (e.g., painful childhood memories and forbidden wishes) and present moods and actions. It is anticipated that insight will relieve the patient of neurotic symptoms, particularly chronic anxiety.

The principal tool used to explore the unconscious aspects of a given patient's mental life is *free association*, a technique requiring that the individual talk at random, without censorship, about anything that comes to mind. Early in the development of psychoanalysis, Freud used hypnosis but eventually gave it up.

The words *psychoanalysis* and *psychotherapy* are not synonyms. Psychoanalysis is a *kind* of psychotherapy. Therefore the concept of psychotherapy is the broader one, and it includes psychoanalysis. However, it should be noted that psychoanalysis is accorded the high status of being historically the first of the modern kinds of psychotherapy.

See also *ego*; *free association*; *id*; *insight*; *psychoanalyst*; *psychotherapy*; *superego*; *unconscious mental life*.

psychoanalyst: A psychotherapist who uses psychoanalysis as a principal mode of treatment and who has received training at a psychoanalytic institute. In the United States, psychoanalysis is sometimes seen as a specialty within psychiatry. And it is correct that most psychoanalysts are physicians who hold a medical degree (M.D.). However, some psychoanalysts are also clinical psychologists, and these hold a doctorate (Ph.D.) with a concentration on psychology.

It has been something of an issue, particularly in the United States, whether or not nonmedical professionals can be qualified to practice psychoanalysis. This is often referred to as "the question of lay analysis." The implication is that the nonmedical professional is more or less equivalent to a layperson, one without particular qualification or skill. Freud himself took a distinct position on the issue and argued that nonmedical professionals could become qualified to practice psychoanalysis. Indeed, he directly encouraged such individuals if they seemed to have unusual talent. Among his protégés in this category were such famous psychoanalysts as Erik Erikson, Theodore Reik, and Otto Rank. Indeed, these individuals did not have their principal academic training in either medicine or psychology but in such diverse fields as art and history.

In sum, a psychoanalyst is usually a medical doctor but not necessarily.

See also *Erikson, Erik Homburger*; *psychoanalysis*; *psycho-therapy*; *Rank, Otto.*

psychobiology: The study of the relationship of biology to behavior. The two principal divisions of psychobiology are physiological psychology and comparative psychology. *Physiological psychology* studies the relationship of the nervous system (including the brain) and the endocrine system to behavior. *Comparative psychology* studies the behavior of organisms across species. Often the focus is on making comparisons between human behavior and the behavior of other living creatures.

Applying psychobiology to mental health, psychobiology makes certain key assumptions about the relationship of the mind to the body. The key assumption is that the living body is the physical basis of what we call *mind*. The activity of the brain and the nervous system give rise to the experiences that go by such names as *mental activity*, *consciousness*, *attention*, *memory*, and so forth.

It is important to understand that psychobiology is taking a position toward an ancient philosophical problem known as the mind–body problem. Essential aspects of the mind–body problem can be put forth in the form of a series of questions. Are the mind and the body separate and distinct entities in their own right? Does mind create body? Does body create mind? Do the mind and body interact, or do they simply travel along parallel lines? These questions have been answered quite differently by philosophers through the ages. It is not the present purpose to examine the various alternative ways of dealing with the mind–body problem but simply to point out that psychobiology "solves" the problem by assuming that the body comes first and that its processes produce the qualities we call mind. Thus mind is seen as secondary to the body. This position is formally known in philosophy as *materialistic monism*.

Taking the approach that mental states are caused by the action of the body, research from physiological psychology in particular makes a substantial contribution to the practice of psychiatry. Much of what has been learned about the brain and nervous system, and the endocrine system, is applied directly in drug therapy and somatic therapy. The biomedical viewpoint, a major viewpoint underlying the practice of psychiatry, has an allegiance with psychobiology.

See also *biomedical viewpoint*; *central nervous system*; *drug therapy*; *endocrine system*; *somatic therapy*.

psychodrama: A technique sometimes used as a part of the process of psychotherapy in which a patient is encouraged to directly express mental and emotional conflicts as if playing a role in a drama. The technique was pioneered by the psychiatrist J. L. Moreno and introduced by him in the United States in 1925. In its original form, psychodrama consisted of an actual stage, a small group of players, and an audience. In modified form, a psychodrama can be played out with as few as two people in an office setting.

Usually the troubled individual plays the part of himself or herself, and other people play significant figures such as a spouse, a parent, a close friend, or a child. The patient is in these cases the protagonist, and usually there is a principal antagonist. However, sometimes a technique known as *role reversal* is used, and the patient plays the part of the antagonist.

Psychodrama can be useful in more than one way. It allows for a catharsis, or release of emotion. It tends to foster increased insight into important human relations. On the whole, variations of psychodrama have been found to be a useful adjunct to psychotherapy. Gestalt therapy in particular has made much use of the specific technique of role playing.

See also *catharsis*; *Gestalt therapy*; *insight*; *psychotherapy*.

psychodynamic: A quality of mental life characterized by the interaction of psychological forces. Although the term can be used in a general way to describe the activity of any set of ideas, perceptions, or motives, in practice it is usually associated with psychoanalysis. The term *psychodynamic psychology* has become virtually synonymous with psychoanalysis.

In psychoanalysis, it is recognized that motives and ideas can either cooperate or be in conflict. The primary focus of attention has been on conflict. For example, a wish for forbidden sexual relations arising from the id can be in conflict with the superego's prohibitions. The conflict of the two opposing psychological forces, if severe, may in some cases produce neurotic symptoms. A key goal of psychoanalysis is to help a patient develop insight into psychodynamic processes in order to better place them under the control of the ego.

See also *ego*; *id*; *psychoanalysis*; *superego*.

psychogenic amnesia: Another name for *functional amnesia*, amnesia without a clear-cut biological basis.

See also *amnesia*.

psychogenic pain disorder: See *somatoform pain disorder (psychogenic pain disorder)*.

psychogenic viewpoint: The viewpoint in abnormal psychology and psychiatry that mental disorders are caused by psychological and emotional problems. It is difficult to specify an organic basis for many mental disorders. When this is the situation in a particular case, it is reasonable to entertain the hypothesis that the problem is psychological in nature. Disorders that appear to frequently have a psychogenic basis are anxiety disorders, somatoform disorders, dissociative disorders, personality disorders, and sexual disorders.

The psychogenic viewpoint does not rule out the possible importance of complicating organic conditions. However, when it is employed, it is based on the assumption that the primary cause of a disorder is psychological in nature, not organic.

The psychogenic viewpoint is often presented as being in conflict with the biomedical viewpoint, a viewpoint that assumes the cause of a mental disorder is primarily organic. However, the two viewpoints need not be thought of as necessarily in conflict. For some mental disorders, such as those previously identified, a psychogenic viewpoint is the more reasonable one. For other mental disorders, a biomedical viewpoint is the more reasonable one.

If the psychogenic viewpoint is accepted as the primary explanation of a given mental disorder, this provides a basis for the use of psychotherapy or behavior therapy. On the other hand, if a biomedical viewpoint is accepted as the primary explanation, this provides a basis for the use of somatic therapies such as drug therapy or electroconvulsive shock therapy. Thus the selection of one viewpoint over another is more than a pure theoretical problem.

See also *behavior therapy*; *biomedical viewpoint*; *functional disorders*; *psychotherapy*.

psychological addiction: The habit of using a drug on a regular basis even if there is little or no physiological need for the drug. A psychological addiction is experienced as a strong wish to continue using a particular drug, but cessation will not precipitate a physiological withdrawal crisis of significant proportions. In the case of certain drugs, the psychological addiction appears to be much more important than a physiological addiction. Among these drugs are amphetamines, cocaine, marijuana, lysergic acid diethylamide-25, and phencyclidine (PCP).

See also *addiction*; *drug addiction*.

psychological autopsy: A post-mortem investigation of a person's personality designed to determine if death was due to suicide. The procedure is used by some coroners in conjunction with the assistance of a clinical psychologist or psychiatrist.

See also *suicide*; *suicidology*.

psychological conflict: A clash between opposing agents or forces within the personality. One example of such a clash is the battle between the id and the superego described by psychoanalysis. The id represents primitive wishes based on the pleasure principle. The superego represents rules and restrictions based on the morality principle. If the struggle between the id and the superego is particularly intense, then neurotic symptoms can result.

Another type of psychological conflict is characterized by the need to make a choice between conflicting goals. An example of this kind of conflict is the *approach–avoidance conflict* in which a goal has simultaneously positive and negative aspects.

The kind of conflicts described here are called *intrapsychic conflicts* because they take place within the personality of a single individual. An *interpsychic conflict* takes place between at least two persons. An example is an argument between husband and wife. Both intrapsychic and interpsychic conflicts can be contributing factors to mental health problems.

See also *approach–avoidance conflict*; *id*; *superego*.

psychological test: An evaluation of an aspect of behavior conducted under controlled conditions. Examples of such aspects are intelligence, personality, creativity, aptitudes, and vocational interests. Various methods of testing exist. These include standardized interviews, observation of a subject through a one-way glass, and evaluating a subject's capacity to cope with a sham situation. However, in practice, most psychological tests are paper-and-pencil tests using a set of standardized materials.

These tests are usually published and copyrighted. They contain an instruction book for the examiner and tables of norms, averages of the performance of a reference group.

Two issues of critical importance for all psychological tests are those of validity and reliability. If a test has *validity*, it measures what it is supposed to measure. For example, an intelligence test should measure intelligence, not the ambition of the subject. If a test has *reliability*, it gives stable repeatable results. For example, if a subject is first evaluated with Form A of a given test and is subsequently evaluated with Form B of the same test, scores on the two tests should be very close together. Most standardized psychological tests have a fairly high level of both validity and reliability. This is established before publication through statistical procedures.

See also *intelligence tests*; *personality test*.

psychological traumata: Wounds to the personality caused by painful or highly unpleasant events. Examples of such events are being abused as a child, surviving a disaster, being assaulted, being raped, experiencing the death of a loved one, going through a divorce, losing status, and so forth.

Psychoanalysis in particular has stressed the importance of childhood traumata on the formation of the personality. It is hypothesized that traumata experienced early in life are poorly understood and are particularly damaging to the developing individual. It is likely that they are an underlying causal factor in mental health problems.

See also *life change units (LCUs)*; *posttraumatic stress disorder (traumatic neurosis)*; *psychosocial stressors*.

psychology: The science of the behavior of organisms. The word *science* is used in the definition instead of *study* in order to emphasize that contemporary psychology is based on research, not armchair speculation. The word *behavior* in the past used to refer only to observable actions. However, its present meaning has been broadened to include *covert behavior*, behavior that is contained within the subject. The most obvious example of covert behavior is the thinking process. The word *organisms* refers to any living creature ranging from birds to monkeys to human beings.

There are a number of fields of psychology. *Clinical psychology* concerns itself with psychological testing and psychotherapy. It is the single largest field of psychology. About 40% of of psychologists work in this field. *School psychology* concerns itself with the evaluation and placement of students, particularly in grammar school. *Counseling psychology* tends to focus primarily on the evaluation and placement of students, particularly in high school and college. However, counseling psychology also concerns itself with the personal and academic guidance of students. Also, counseling psychology overlaps with clinical psychology to some extent, and some professionals in the field engage in counseling with adults in the community. *Industrial psychology* concerns itself with both the welfare of employees and their productivity as workers. *Experimental psychology* concerns itself with basic research. In practice, most experimental psychologists are college professors who also have teaching duties.

See also *clinical psychologist*; *psychiatrist*.

psychomotor epilepsy: See *epilepsy*.

psychomotor retardation: An overall slowness of both reflexes and voluntary actions. For example, a puff of air to the eye will induce an eyeblink but less quickly than is generally expected. Or the subject may walk or speak more slowly than most people.

Psychomotor retardation is frequently a symptom associated with depression. However, it can also appear in other conditions and may be a sign of neurological problems.

See also *depression*; *neurology*.

psychopathic personality: Another term for antisocial personality disorder.

See also *antisocial personality disorder (psychopathic personality; sociopathic personality).*

psychopathology: The literal meaning of *psychopathology* is a "sickness of the mind or personality." The term is usually used to describe behavior that is destructive to oneself or to others. Thus, the symptoms of mental disorders are psychopathological in nature.

Although not all abnormal behavior represents psychopathology, the inverse statement is usually correct. If behavior is psychopathological, it is almost always abnormal. That is, it deviates significantly from a standard of reference for behavior used by a given group.

It is important to realize that, in the case of the word *psychopathological*, the concept of sickness is to some extent a metaphor. It is not so much that the person *is* sick as it is that the person acts *as if* he or she is sick. A number of critics of the concept of psychopathology as applied to mental disorders have pointed out that there is often no organic illness present. Thus it is critical to realize that the individual is not always "sick" in the medical sense but often "sick" only in the psychological sense.

See also *abnormal behavior; maladaptive behavior.*

psychopharmacological drugs: Drugs used to treat mental disorders. See also *drug therapy.*

psychophysiological disorders: See *psychosomatic disorders.*

psychosexual development: A maturational process involving both the sexual drive and the general personality. The basic idea is that one's thoughts, emotions, and actions from infancy to adulthood are to some extent influenced by sexual needs and interests.

The most famous single theory of psychosexual development was the one proposed by Freud, and it gave great impetus in this century to the study of the sexual life of both the child and the adult. Freud proposed a theory of infantile sexuality, and this was a somewhat unsettling notion, particularly around the early part of the twentieth century. However, Freud did not mean that infants have full-blown sexual interest as we understand it. Instead, certain signs and behaviors evident in both the infant and the child foreshadow mature sexuality.

Freud hypothesized that children go through five stages of psychosexual development. At first *libido*, or psychosexual energy, is concentrated in the oral zone. The *oral stage* lasts from birth to the end of infancy (i.e., about 18 months to 2 years). During the oral stage, the infant obtains a sort of erotic gratification from sucking, biting, chewing, and other oral activities. Then libido moves, because of maturation, to the anal zone. The *anal stage* lasts until the age of 3 or 4. During the anal stage, the child obtains a sort of erotic gratification from both the voluntary retention and eventual expulsion of fecal bulk.

Subsequently, the libido moves to the phallic zone. The *phallic stage* lasts from the third or fourth year to about the sixth year. During the phallic stage, the child obtains a degree of erotic gratification from self-manipulation of the phallus (i.e., the clitoris in a female and the penis in a male).

Now a crisis takes place. According to Freud, the child of either sex commonly develops an incest wish toward the parent of the opposite sex. There is almost immediate guilt arising from the punitive side of the child's recently formed superego. Also, there is fear of punishment from the parent of the same sex. The male in particular may develop the fantasy that the father will castrate him. The entire conflict herein described is called the *Oedipus complex*. (Sometimes, in females, the conflict is referred to as the Electra complex. However, it is correct to use the term *Oedipus complex* in reference to either sex.) As a consequence of the Oedipus complex, the child must repress sexual interest in order to be psychologically comfortable, and libido goes underground. This is the *latency stage* lasting from about 6 to 12 years of age. During the latency stage the child has no conscious interest in sexuality. On the contrary, at a conscious level, the normal child has many external interests manifested in play, avocations, friends, and school. These are sometimes referred to as "the golden years of childhood."

However, libido still exists, and it continues to work at an unconscious level. Thus when the child reaches puberty (around 12 or 13 years of age), libido will surface again at a conscious level. The adolescent will begin to develop in most cases a sexual interest in members of the opposite sex. This eventually expresses itself in marriage, sexual intercourse, the rearing of children, and so forth. This last stage, which starts at puberty, is called the *genital stage*.

Freud believed that if libido is fixated due to psychological traumata at one of the early stages of psychosexual development, the result can contribute to a neurotic process and have an adverse effect on the individual's adult personality.

Freud's theory of psychosexual development is open to criticism. Freud believed that the theory is universal and applicable to all children. This appears to be incorrect. The theory does seem to describe the development of some children in intact families with parents who play traditional roles. Also, not all children engage in autoerotic activity during the phallic stage. However, it does appear that the behavior is common and relatively normal. Although both sexes exhibit the behavior, it appears with somewhat more frequency in males.

To the therapist with a psychoanalytic orientation, behavioral traits such as excessive eating, sarcasm, and gullibility suggest oral fixations. Traits such as defiance or stinginess suggest anal fixations. Traits such as excessive dominance of others and self-absorption suggest phallic fixations. Thus the theory can be of some utility in therapy because it suggests to both the therapist and the patient possible explanations for maladaptive behavior. However, most contemporary psychiatrists and psychologists recognize that there are no universal explanations of specific behavioral traits. Thus, alternative explanations to Freud's psychosexual theory are, of course, possible.

See also *anal character traits*; *anal stage*; *genital stage*; *latency stage*; *libido*; *Oedipus complex*; *oral character traits*; *oral stage*; *superego*.

psychosexual disorders: See *sexual disorders (psychosexual disorders)*.

psychosocial stressors: Causes of stress arising primarily from interactions with other people. However, the concept also tends to include any general adverse impact from the environment, social or physical. Psychosocial stressors can range from mild to severe to catastrophic. An example of a mild psychosocial stressor is having a misunderstanding with a salesperson in a department store. An example of a severe psychosocial stressor is losing a majority of one's savings in a bad investment. An example of a catastrophic psychosocial stressor is barely escaping from flood waters and simultaneously losing one's home.

The concept of psychosocial stress plays a significant role in the American Psychiatric Association's *Diagnostic and Statistical Manual of Mental Disorders*. It explicitly recognizes that one of the important dimensions, or aspects, of a mental disorder is the severity of psychosocial stressors in a patient's life. Psychosocial stress can, in some cases, be a principal causal factor in a mental disorder. In other cases, it can aggravate the symptoms of a mental disorder.

Learning to cope with psychosocial stress is one of the great challenges of a person's life.

See also Diagnostic and Statistical Manual of Mental Disorders; *life change units (LCUs)*.

psychosomatic disorders: Physical illnesses either caused or aggravated by psychological and emotional factors. (These are also known as *psychophysiological disorders*.) The literal meaning of "psychosomatic" is *mind–body*, derived from the Greek words *psyche* and *soma*. Thus it could be said that a psychosomatic disorder is one in which a disturbance at a mental level causes a disturbance at a physical, or biological, level.

Almost any illness can, in a certain sense, be thought of as psychosomatic because virtually every illness can be aggravated by adverse psychological and emotional factors. Nevertheless, certain illnesses tend to be identified as the principal psychosomatic ones. These are tension headaches, migraine headaches, high blood pressure, peptic ulcers, spastic colitis, neurodermatitis, and obesity. It is also often noted that psychological factors may play a particularly important part in the prognosis for diseases such as rheumatoid arthritis and bronchial asthma.

Another way to look at psychosomatic disorders is to assert that they give evidence that any distinction between the mind and the body is arbitrary, primarily a matter of convenience. In fact there is only the organism, the living creature. The human organism has a nervous system with a brain, an endocrine system, and a group of biochemical processes. The action of the physical system gives rise to a certain set of experiences that we group together under the label *mind*. This orientation, known as the *holistic viewpoint*, argues that it is no wonder, and no mystery, that the "mind" can cause physical illness. It is, in a sense, an aspect of the physical system.

There is ample documentation establishing that emotional states such as fear, anxiety, anger, and depression can have an adverse effect on physical health, that they may even interfere with the effective action of the immune system. The same can be said of the impact of large life changes and psychosocial stressors in general.

An important source of stress can be one's own personality. Persons who display a great deal of Type A behavior, behavior characterized by self-imposed time pressure and aggressiveness, may generate much of their own stress.

The now-general recognition of the existence of psychosomatic disorders has led to more broadly based treatment approaches such as behavioral medicine in which psychological principles and methods are used in the treatment of organic disorders. Behavioral medicine incorporates such techniques as biofeedback training, relaxation methods, hypnosis, and behavior modification.

See also *asthma*; *behavioral medicine*; *behavior modification*; *biofeedback training*; *general adaptation syndrome*; *holistic viewpoint*; *hypnosis*; *life change units (LCUs)*; *psychosocial stressors*; *stress*; *Type A behavior*.

psychosurgery: Surgery performed on the brain to relieve the symptoms of a mental disorder. (It is also correct to use the term *psychosurgery* when the purpose of brain surgery is to relieve chronic pain.) The most well-known type of psychosurgery is the *lobotomy*, a procedure in which the frontal lobes of the brain are severed from the rest of the brain. Other psychosurgical procedures, less well-known, include (1) any severance of nerve fibers connecting two areas of the brain and (2) lesions produced in the *thalamus*, a relay center for the brain.

Psychosurgery has behind it a history of debate and controversy. Advocates of psychosurgery argue that, as a treatment of last resort, it can sometimes help to free a mental patient from chronic symptoms that have resisted other forms of treatment. Critics of psychosurgery argue that its effects are unpredictable and that it almost always leaves the patient with diminished cognitive capacities. They also argue that it is unethical to damage the very brain and nervous system on which recovery depends. On the whole, the critics of psychosurgery have been taken seriously, and these procedures, although legal, are seldom used today. Most psychiatrists avoid recommending psychosurgery and prefer to prescribe a major tranquilizing drug to relieve symptoms of psychotic disorders.

See also *lobotomy*; *major tranquilizers (antipsychotic drugs)*.

psychotherapy: Any kind of therapy that attempts to relieve the symptoms of mental disorders or general emotional distress through psychological means. An informal name for psychotherapy is "the talking cure." This name captures the essence of psychotherapy. It is possible to think of psychotherapy as a special kind of conversation between a therapist and a troubled person.

However, it needs to be noted that this "conversation" *is* indeed special because in practice it includes an array of techniques including free association, dream interpretation, role playing, deconditioning, hypnosis, and guided fantasies. Indeed, psychotherapy is one of the most creative and innovative areas of psychiatry and clinical psychology.

The first modern psychotherapy was psychoanalysis, its father was Sigmund Freud, and its birth coincides roughly with the early part of this century. However, it should be understood that today psychoanalysis has the status of one *kind* of psychotherapy among others.

A perennial question of importance is this one: Is psychotherapy effective? The question, unfortunately, cannot be answered with a simple *yes* or *no*. A tremendous amount of research has gone into various attempts to answer the question. However, the effectiveness of psychotherapy depends on too many factors to be able to respond categorically to any question concerning its effectiveness. The personality of the therapist, the nature of the disorder, the severity of the patient's symptoms, and the specific kind of psychotherapy used in a given case all have potent effects on outcomes. However, it can be said with assurance that psychotherapy is *often* effective. It offers real hope to persons with mental health problems. And, in many cases, it is an appealing alternative to drug therapy, electroshock therapy, and other somatic approaches.

This encyclopedia describes in some detail a number of different kinds of psychotherapies. These are listed in the following cross-references.

See also *aversion therapy*; *behavior modification*; *behavior therapy*; *client-centered therapy*; *cognitive-behavior therapy*; *cognitive therapy*; *controlled drinking therapy*; *desensitization therapy*; *directive therapy*; *existential therapy*; *Gestalt therapy*; *group therapy*; *humanistic therapy*; *hypnotherapy*; *implosive therapy*; *insight therapy*; *logotherapy*; *play therapy*; *psychoanalysis*; *psychodrama*; *rational-emotive therapy*; *reality therapy*; *sexual therapy*; *transactional analysis*; *will therapy*.

psychotic disorders: Disorders in which the individual is out of touch with reality as most of us understand it. It is rather clear-cut evidence of a psychotic disorder if a person is plagued with delusions (i.e., irrational beliefs) or hallucinations (i.e., false perceptions).

Psychotic disorders can be either functional or organic in nature, or a combination of both. If they are functional, there is no obvious biological process present. Causal factors appear to be basically psychological in nature. If they are organic, there is an apparent biological process at work. There may be an infection, a tumor, a stroke, or a biochemical imbalance. In practice, psychological and biological factors often interact in a complex way. For example, schizophrenia is usually thought of as functional. Nonetheless, there is considerable evidence to suggest that there is indeed a biological process at work in schizophrenia.

See also *autistic disorder (infantile autism)*; *delusional (paranoid) disorder*; *delusion*; *hallucination*; *mood disorders (affective disorders)*; *organic mental disorders*; *schizophrenia*.

psychotropic drug: See *psychoactive drug.*

pyromania: A disorder characterized by an impulse to set fires. Related symptoms include states of excitement and pleasure in association with the pyromanic act. A key feature of this disorder is that the individual does not set fires for financial profit. Instead, it appears that the act itself is intrinsically gratifying.

The personal history of the disorder in a given adult patient can usually be traced back to a desire to set fires as early as ages 7 or 8. Men appear to suffer from the disorder more than do women.

The explanation of pyromania depends on the life history of the particular patient. However, it is possible to speculate in a general way on psychological factors in the disorder. It is possible that some people use fire setting as a way to strike back at authority by doing something illegal. Others may use the behavior as a way of expressing pent-up hostility by doing something destructive. Psychoanalytic theory points out that fire and heat are used in a metaphorical way in connection with the sexual drive. For example, we say,"Your kisses set me on fire" or "He's a hot number." The person with confused or repressed sexual urges might find an erotic pleasure in the setting of fires.

One of the problems with pyromania is that the activities associated with it are illegal. A person with the disorder can often do a great deal of damage before being apprehended.

The treatment for pyromania usually consists of insight-oriented psychotherapy aimed at helping the individual understand the emotional roots of the disorder. A principal focus of therapy is on developing practical ways to gain self-control over irrational impulses.

See also *impulsive behavior*; *insight therapy*.

Q

Q-sort technique: A technique used in personality testing. The method was devised by the researcher William Stephenson in the 1950s. A Q-sort requires that the individual respond to a set of self-reference statements on cards. Examples of such statements are, "I have quite a bit of musical talent," "I think of myself as an introverted person," and "I'm a pretty aggressive individual when I want to be."

The cards are sorted by the person being tested into several piles ranging between two poles. One pole represents statements that fit the *self-concept*, the self as perceived by the subject. The other pole represents statements that do not fit the subject's self-concept. It is, of course, possible to also place cards in middle categories if the statement is only somewhat similar, or dissimilar, to a person's self-concept.

An analysis of the Q-sort will result in a rather coherent portrait of the subject's overall self-concept. It is possible to do a second sort based not on the subject's self-concept but on the subject's *ideal self*, the self the individual would like to become. Thus, at the completion of the analysis, the examiner has obtained not one, but two, portraits of the individual's self. The gap between the two portraits is referred to as *incongruence*. If there is a great deal of incongruence, there is also often present a substantial amount of anxiety, or distress, about one's existence, one's role in life, and one's relationships. On the other hand, if there is *congruence*, a high level of agreement between the self-concept and the ideal self, this suggests that the individual has a fairly relaxed attitude toward himself or herself and often toward life in general.

The Q-sort technique is a useful tool in personality research. It is also useful in assessing the progress of psychotherapy. At the beginning of therapy, the self-concept and the ideal self are often far apart. If they move toward each other after a number of therapy sessions, this gives a sort of face validity to the hypothesis that therapy is having a beneficial effect. This approach to assessment has been used in particular by Carl Rogers in connection with client-centered therapy.

See also *client-centered therapy*; *personality test*; *Rogers, Carl Ransom*; *self-concept*.

R

Rank, Otto (1884–1939): A psychoanalyst who contributed a treatment approach known as will therapy. At one time, a member of Freud's inner circle of associates, Rank was one of the first "lay analysts," meaning a psychoanalyst without a medical degree. Rank's academic training was in literature and history, and Freud approved of the rich and general background that Rank brought to psychoanalysis.

Rank and Freud parted as professional associates over the issue of the importance of the birth trauma. Rank believed that the emotional pain associated with the loss and separation from the mother at the moment that one came into the world was a prototype for anxiety in general; it was also the root of most neuroses seen in patients. Freud thought that the birth trauma might be of some importance, but he refused to assign to it the paramount role given by Rank.

Rank emigrated to the United States in the 1920s, after his break with Freud, and worked out the practical aspects of will therapy.

One of Rank's principal works is *The Trauma of Birth* (1923).

See also *Freud, Sigmund*; *psychoanalysis*; *will therapy*.

rape: An aggressive sexual act in which one person forces a second person to engage in sexual intercourse. The concept of force can include both physical and psychological force. Twisting a victim's arm is an example of physical force. Threatening to mutilate or kill a victim provides an example of psychological force. Some observers include the use of deception, such as a false promise of marriage, as a kind of psychological force. However, this may be carrying the concept of force substantially beyond its original meaning.

The essential theme in rape is not so much sex as aggression. Numerous studies have shown that an underlying motive of the rapist is to act in both a powerful and a hostile way toward another person. Thus rape is best understood as a form of assault. It is quite possible, in many cases, that forcing another person into the victim role makes the rapist sexually excited. However, it should be noted that numerous would-be rapists are unable to achieve an erection adequate for sexual intercourse.

Sexual relations between consenting adults are not, of course, rape. However, this raises the question of sexual relations between a minor and an adult. This is often referred to as *statutory rape* if the minor is younger than the age of consent. Statutory rape is a crime, and the adult can be prosecuted.

The victim in a rape is in the vast majority of cases a female. However, it can be argued that if a male is forced to engage in sexual relations that he has been assaulted and raped. Therefore, it is possible to speak of raping either sex.

A concept of increasing interest is *date rape*, a rape that takes place under conditions where the rapist has had at least some degree of invitation to be alone with the victim. If a rape takes place between strangers, then the victim's claims tend to be taken seriously by authorities. However, if a rape takes place between two people on a date, the victim's claims are clouded. Nonetheless, the existence of date rape should not be denied. And it should be looked upon as a psychosocial problem that merits exploration. It has been argued by some sociologists that date rape is more common than rape between strangers.

It is important to recognize that rape is a kind of criminal behavior and a social problem of substantial importance. Almost 80,000 rapes are committed each year. And this statistic is probably low because rape is an underreported crime. Many victims are ashamed to report the offense. And victims of date rape in most cases probably remain silent.

There is no standard personality profile that describes most rapists. However, a few general observations can be made. All of the statements that follow refer to male rapists. Most rapists are young adults; many are younger than 25 years of age. They tend as a group to have lower incomes, fewer vocational skills, and lower intelligence quotient (IQ) scores than most men. Around 50% of rapists are husbands in an intact marriage. The two principal psychological themes in rape appear to be power and aggression. Dominating a woman, forcing her to submit to his desires, feeds the rapist's need for power. Hitting or otherwise hurting a woman feeds the rapist's need for aggression. Once again, the element of assault in rape is as significant as the sexual element.

The rapist may receive treatment in prison or as a condition of probation. Rapists are usually seen as suffering from a personality disorder. Therefore the most common treatment used is psychotherapy aimed at helping the individual understand and control hostile impulses.

The victim of a rape frenquently suffers from a posttraumatic stress disorder and often benefits from psychotherapy aimed at helping her cope with nightmares, sleep disturbances, obsessional memories of the rape, and loss of joy in life.

See also *legal aspects of mental health*; *personality disorders*; *posttraumatic stress disorder (traumatic neurosis)*.

rapid eye movement (REM) sleep: The kind of sleep associated with dreaming. During rapid eye movement, or REM, sleep, the eyes actually move about erratically under the eyelids as if the individual is watching a motion picture. Electroencephalogram (EEG) recordings taken during REM episodes in sleep laboratories have shown that REMs tend to take place during light sleep. During light sleep, the brain's cortex is very alert and active. For these reasons, REM sleep is sometimes referred to as "paradoxical sleep." (During deep sleep, the brain's cortex displays slower and less complex EEG patterns.)

There seems to be a need for REM sleep. When subjects in sleep laboratories are deprived of REM sleep for several days, their waking personalities begin to show signs of disorganization.

They become irritable and anxious. This is why it may not be advisable to depend on drugs such as barbiturates for sleep. They may, in some cases, interfere with REM sleep and consequently have an adverse effect on one's mental and emotional state.

See also *barbiturates*; *dream analysis*; *insomnia*.

rapport: A harmonious relationship between two or more people. The word *rapport* is a French word, and its literal meaning is "in close accord." It is important that rapport exist between a husband and a wife, a psychologist and a person being tested, or a therapist and a patient. If rapport is present, then there is a feeling on the part of all parties concerned that understanding is present, that communication is taking place. If rapport is absent, then there is a feeling on the part of all parties that time is being wasted, that nothing is being accomplished.

Psychotherapists have paid a substantial amount of attention to the conditions required to create rapport. Listening to another person with interest, making good eye contact, responding with meaningful remarks, avoiding the making of moral judgments, are all ways a healing person can foster a state of rapport. Reality therapy and client-centered therapy in particular have stressed the essential role that rapport plays in therapy.

See also *client-centered therapy*; *psychotherapy*; *reality therapy*.

rational-emotive therapy: A kind of psychotherapy pioneered by the psychotherapist Albert Ellis. The essential assumption of rational-emotive therapy is that one can gain voluntary control over irrational thoughts and thereby acquire the capacity to regulate adverse emotional reactions. In other words, the *rational* power of the mind can be used to influence the *emotive* side of life.

Ellis was originally trained to conduct psychotherapy along psychoanalytic lines. However, he became dissatisfied with the highly indirect methods of psychoanalysis and its generally slow rate of progress. He developed rational-emotive therapy as a way of more directly addressing a patient's problems and bringing about a more rapid recovery. Ellis notes explicitly that the philosophy of stoicism was a forerunner of rational-emotive therapy. *Stoicism* teaches that the wise person rises above the passionate extremes of life such as excessive elation or profound depression. Epictetus (A.D. 60?–120?) and Marcus Aurelius (A.D. 121–180), respectively a slave and an emperor of ancient Rome, were two of the principal stoics.

Ellis has developed an ABC method of coping with adverse emotions. He notes that the initial element in an emotional chain is an activating event, or A. This activating event is something that takes place in the real world. Examples include an insult, a request to do something challenging, or a broken agreement. The activating event triggers a belief, or B. If the belief is rational, in accord with the facts of the event, then there is no problem. However, irrational beliefs are all too common. Thus a person might think in response to an insult, "He's a hateful, spiteful person. He's never liked me." Or a person might think in response to a request to do something challenging, "Why is Mrs. Smith asking me to give an oral book report? Doesn't she know I'll fall through the floor, that I'll die if I have to speak in front of the class?" Or a person might think in response to a broken agreement, "She has no consideration for me at all. She treats me like a thing, like a worthless object."

All of the thoughts in the preceding examples may be identified as irrational because they represent oversimplifications and over-generalizations of the facts. The individual is usually jumping to conclusions and not thinking clearly.

The belief now generates the emotional reaction, or C. (The emotional reaction is labeled *C* to suggest that it is a *consequence* of the thought.) If the thought is rational, then the emotional reaction is appropriate. On the other hand, if the thought is irrational, then the emotional reaction is too strong.

Ellis's work suggests that people who suffer from chronic anxiety, anger, or depression are also people who do not reflect on their own irrational thought processes. They assume that what they think is the truth, that their own irrational idea is the same thing as an activating event.

Therapy consists of helping a troubled person develop the new habit of reexamining irrational thoughts. Ellis calls this step *dispute*, or D. At first, the patient and the therapist together dispute, or argue with, the irrational thought. After therapy is complete, the former patient now has the acquired skill of disputing thoughts, of not taking them for granted.

Ellis first developed and published his concepts around 25 years ago. Of late there has been quite a bit of interest in innovations in psychotherapy such as cognitive-behavior modification and cognitive therapy. However, it should be noted that Ellis's rational-emotive therapy is a forerunner of these later developments and that he anticipated contemporary trends by a number of years.

See also *cognitive-behavior therapy*; *cognitive therapy*.

rationalization: A kind of ego defense mechanism in which either an irrational idea or irrational behavior is made to seem rational through the use of a chain of superficial logic. The basic theme of rationalization is the *making of excuses* in order to maintain self-esteem. For example, let us say that a person engages in sexual relations on a date and that this goes against his or her moral training. The next day the individual thinks, "It's not my fault. That so-and-so fed me too many drinks." The rationalization is a way of avoiding responsibility for one's own actions.

Two basic kinds of rationalization are sour grapes and sweet lemons. *Sour grapes* is characterized by thinking that something that one cannot have is undesirable anyway. Therefore, "I can't have it" is translated into "I don't want it." The fox in Aesop's fable could not reach a bunch of grapes high on the vine. As he skulked away, he muttered, "They were probably sour anyhow." A man proposes marriage to a woman and is rejected. Later he tells his friends, "I was lucky things didn't work out with Erica. I can see now she would have been a nag."

Sweet lemons is characterized by trying to convince oneself that an unfortunate event is in fact a fortunate one. There is a proverb that states, "When God hands you a lemon, make lemonade." For example, an investor loses a substantial sum of money on a stock. A few weeks later, he or she is rationalizing, "I learned a valuable lesson from this. It was worth the loss just to find out once and for all that it never pays to buy on margin."

Rationalization is a common ego defense mechanism used frequently by all of us and, employed in moderation, it probably helps to maintain mental health. However, the troubled person may use rationalization to excess and thus avoids a realistic confrontation with real problems that require practical solutions. Psychoanalytic theory suggests that a chronic dependence on rationalization indicates the presence of a neurotic process.

See also *ego defense mechanisms*; *neurosis*.

reaction formation: A kind of ego defense mechanism in which a repressed idea reappears at the conscious level in opposite form. For example, let us say that Eileen has a substantial amount of repressed hostility toward her husband. She also is a traditional wife who feels that it is essential she continue to love her husband. Her moral code demands this. The hostility expresses itself at the conscious level in masked form as sweetness and docility. She compulsively and rigidly carries out all wifely duties without fail as a way of proving to herself that she is *not* hostile, that she dearly loves her husband.

Here are a few more examples of reaction formation. A compulsive eater goes on a rigid diet. A person who abuses alcohol goes "on the wagon." A person who has previously spent money impulsively decides to follow a strict budget.

A reaction formation can often be useful, helping a person to control impulsive or irresponsible behavior. The danger resides in the fact that reaction formations often break down. The dieter goes on an eating binge. The drinker falls off of the wagon. The person following a strict budget suddenly goes on a spending spree. Unfortunately, when the reaction formation breaks down, the behavior may temporarily be more impulsive and erratic than before. That is why a reaction formation should be looked upon as a psychological crutch, sometimes useful, but not usually an adequate solution to the problems of living.

Psychoanalysis interprets some cases of overprotection on the part of a parent as an example of reaction formation.

See also *ego defense mechanisms*; *overprotection*.

reactive schizophrenia: See *process schizophrenia.*

reading disorder: See *developmental reading disorder (dyslexia).*

realistic anxiety: See *anxiety.*

reality contact: A quality of human experience characterized by an individual's perception of the world in the same way as most other people do in a given culture. Thus, in our culture, if a person believes that he or she can flap his or her arms and fly through the air like a bird, we would say that the individual has poor reality contact.

Poor, or inadequate, reality contact is one of the principal characteristics of psychotic disorders.

Some care should be given to the use of the word *reality.* From a philosophical viewpoint, reality is quite difficult to define. Therefore, as indicated in the first paragraph, the concept of reality used for practical purposes in psychiatry and clinical psychology is *consensual reality*, meaning the agreed-upon beliefs and perceptions of a given group of people.

See also *delusion*; *hallucination*; *psychotic disorders.*

reality principle: According to psychoanalytic theory, the operating principle of the ego. The ego, in contrast to the id that follows the pleasure principle, is in contact with reality in the healthy personality. Thus the ego is the agent of the personality that is functioning when we wait in a cafeteria line for food. The id, if it could have its way, would simply go to the head of the line. It is through the ego's employment of the reality principle that we can cope with frustration, plan for the future, estimate likelihoods of success and failure, and think in rational terms.

See also *ego*; *id*; *pleasure principle.*

reality testing: Behaving in such a way as to discover the acceptable boundaries of behavior. Examples are a school-age child disobeying a rule, a teenager violating a curfew, and a mental patient refusing to cooperate with a psychiatric technician. It is assumed, of course, in these examples that the subject's goal, conscious or unconscious, is to find out what limits an authority figure will set on behavior.

It is important for persons in positions of authority to realize that subordinate individuals may not be only "trying to get away with something" when they break rules. At a deeper psychological level, they are evaluating the constraints of their life situation.

See also *reality contact*; *reality principle*.

reality therapy: A kind of psychotherapy developed by the California psychiatrist William Glasser. Glasser equates mental health with the concept of responsibility. Conversely, mental illness is associated with irresponsibility. Persons are being responsible when they act in such a way as to further long-range interests. They are being irresponsible when they act in such a way as to obtain immediate gratification without regard for long-range interests. For example, Shane, an adolescent, wants to become an accountant. This will require at least 2 years of college. If he drops out of high school at 17 to make payments on a new car, he is behaving in an irresponsible manner in terms of his own stated ambition. Emotionally mature persons tend to focus not only on the present but on future goals. They can defer some of their gratification.

Glasser says that there are two basic psychological needs. First, there is the need to love and be loved. Second, there is the need to feel that we are worthwhile to ourselves and others. The concept of responsibility includes behaving in such a way as to meet these needs.

In order to help troubled persons, Glasser first focuses on establishing rapport with the patient. The patient must feel that real communication is going on and that the therapist has some genuine concern for his or her welfare. If rapport can be established, then the therapist is in the position to give guidance. *Guidance* consists of pointing out to a patient the explicit consequences of behavior. The patient is directly encouraged over and over again to do the responsible thing. Consequently, reality therapy is to some degree directive in contrast to the nondirective quality of client-centered therapy.

Reality therapy does not, like psychoanalysis, explore the past at length. The aim is not to analyze unconscious mental processes. On the contrary, any analysis that takes place is of the individual's life situation and its relationship to personal goals. The central question for reality therapy is not "Where have you been?" Instead, it is, "Where are you going?"

Although reality therapy can be of use with many kinds of patients and problems, it seems to be of particular value for persons with personality disorders. These individuals often act in an impulsive and irresponsible manner with very little guilt. Reality therapy helps them to see that they are not serving their own self-interests.

See also *client-centered therapy*; *personality disorders*; *psychoanalysis*; *psychotherapy*; *rapport*.

recidivism: The disposition of a person who has committed a crime to commit a similar crime again. The term *recidivism* is derived from the Latin word for *relapse*. Recidivism is often loosely used to describe relapses of mental patients and their return to a mental hospital, although some professional persons avoid this particular usage.

The *recidivism rate* is the repeat rate for a given offense or disorder. Thus, if 80% of individuals convicted of a given offense repeat that offense, then the recidivism rate is 80%.

reciprocal inhibition: In the context of desensitization therapy, the tendency of relaxation to have an extinguishing effect on an unwanted emotional reaction (e.g., anxiety). The aim is for relaxation to gradually inhibit or "hold back" anxiety. Because the interaction between the two factors is a sort of give-and-take, it is referred to as "reciprocal." However, the aim is for relaxation to eventually win out and suppress the adverse emotional reaction.

See also *desensitization therapy*.

regression: A person's return to behavior associated with an earlier level of development. Thus, if an adult cries, sucks a thumb, pouts, whines, urinates or defecates in clothing, and so forth, the behavior can be described as regressive. Regression is associated with some mental disorders. For example, patients who suffer from a schizophrenic disorder, disorganized type, often act in infantile ways. Also, regression is associated with senile dementias.

In psychoanalysis, regression is identified as a kind of ego defense mechanism. The basic idea is that when we are subjected to too much stress we sometimes go backwards in psychological time seeking old comforts. Thus, if eating brought great satisfaction as an infant, a person who feels somewhat overwhelmed by various responsibilities might find himself or herself looking for food.

See also *ego defense mechanisms*; *schizophrenia*; *senile dementia*.

reinforcer: See *operant conditioning*.

relaxation response: According to the physiological researcher Herbert Benson, a natural response that is antagonistic to excessive central nervous system arousal. Excessive arousal is associated with such emotional states as anxiety and anger and is believed to play a role in psychosomatic diseases. Instead of lowering arousal with antianxiety agents and narcotics, Benson has found that the relaxation response can be induced by meditation.

Benson has discovered that meditation can be detached from its associations with religious rituals and specific traditions such as Yoga or Zen. Taking a secular view, Benson says that the relaxation response can be induced if four conditions are present. First, the subject should have a quiet place to meditate. Second, the subject should have a mental device to assist concentration. This can be a word such as *one* or *relax*. The word, for example, can be repeated mentally with each respiration. Third, the subject needs a passive attitude, not aggressively pushing for relaxation. (One can get tense trying too hard to relax!) Fourth, the subject needs to be in a comfortable position. It is not necessary to adopt the kinds of special positions advocated in such traditions as Yoga and Zen. Sitting in a chair with both feet on the floor is fine. Sessions should be limited to 10 or 20 minutes in duration once or twice a day.

Again, the practical purpose of inducing the relaxation response is to combat the adverse effects associated with excessive physiological arousal.

See also *general adaptation syndrome*; *psychosocial stressors*; *psychosomatic disorders*.

reliability: See *psychological test*.

remission: A reduction in the intensity or severity of symptoms associated with a physical illness or mental disorder. Remissions can take place in one of two principal ways. First, they can take place as a result of a treatment such as the prescription of drugs or the use of psychotherapy. Second, they can take place spontaneously. Under these conditions, there is no obvious external agent. However, it is assumed that the self-restorative powers of the organism are at work.

In the context of mental disorders, it is important to understand that remissions are not cures. They are common in chronic disorders. However, relapses are also common. Nonetheless, remissions are worth working and hoping for because they buy a patient time and improve the quality of life. Sometimes remissions last for years.

See also *prognosis*.

repression: A kind of ego defense mechanism in which unpleasant memories and forbidden motives are directed toward the unconscious level of mental life. Unpleasant memories may include early childhood events that were emotionally traumatic. Forbidden motives often have an aggressive or sexual component. The basic idea of repression is that, in terms of the conscious self, certain ideas are threatening to its integrity and status. Therefore, protection of the ego is perceived in terms of attempting to rid oneself of these threatening agents. The entire repressive action is itself unconscious and involuntary.

Freud hypothesized that it is the mechanism of repression that actually creates the unconscious level of the personality. The unconscious dimension may be thought of as a psychological netherworld, a world populated by banished ideas.

However, banished ideas have a way of working their way back to consciousness. Freud spoke of the *return of the repressed*. Thus repressed psychological material often makes itself known in adverse ways such as slips of the tongue, disturbing dreams, compulsive behavior, chronic anxiety, and so forth.

The thrust of psychoanalysis as a form of therapy, as Freud originally conceived it, is to explore repressed material and make it accessible to conscious evaluation.

See also *ego defense mechanisms*; *Freud, Sigmund*; *psychoanalysis*; *unconscious mental life*.

reserpine: See *major tranquilizers (antipsychotic drugs)*.

resistance: A psychoanalytic concept with several related meanings. First, resistance refers to self-erected barriers to getting well. Freud noted that a patient often finds a certain amount of satisfaction in symptoms. For example, depression can be used to manipulate a spouse. A phobia may make it possible to avoid having to cope with certain demanding situations. Or a compulsion often reduces the intensity of chronic anxiety. Freud referred to this kind of resistance in terms of the *secondary gains* of an illness, meaning the peripheral benefits derived from symptoms.

Second, Freud used the concept of resistance to refer to obstacles to exploring the unconscious level of the personality. Because ideas at this level are repressed, there is a sort of psychological wall between the conscious and unconscious levels. The purpose of this wall is to keep repressed ideas in their proper place. When the conscious self attempts to explore in this realm, it is usually rebuffed as an unwanted intruder. Fortunately, this kind of resistance can be overcome with special techniques. Freud favored free association. Other techniques include hypnosis and narcotherapy. However, even with the use of the techniques mentioned, the uncovering of significant repressed information can be a slow and uncertain process.

It is possible to use the notion of resistance in other ways. The psychoanalyst Wilhelm Reich developed a concept called *character armor*, meaning the individual's character can also act as a resistant force in therapy. For example, let us say that a patient always arrives late for therapy sessions, frequently becomes peevish in response to the therapist's comments, and appears to be impatient with the process of therapy. Such an individual is using the personality trait of hostility as a device to resist therapy.

The psychotherapist needs to be aware of the existence of resistance in any form and must seek ways to help the patient overcome it. Often the resistance itself is analyzed, interpreted, and discussed with the patient.

See also *free association*; *Freud, Sigmund*; *hypnosis*; *narcotherapy*; *repression*; *unconscious mental life*.

retrograde amnesia: A kind of amnesia in which there is an impairment of memory for events *before* the beginning of the amnesia. For example, Heather was a victim of verbal child abuse. Her parents often told her that she was ugly and stupid, that no man would ever want to marry her. As an adult, she has a very difficult time clearly recalling actual incidents when she was insulted or criticized. It is all a vague blur. She is using the ego defense mechanism of repression to block the details because they are too emotionally painful.

See also *amnesia*; *anterograde amnesia*; *psychogenic amnesia*; *repression*.

risk-taking behavior: Behavior that carries with it a substantial likelihood of death, injury, or great personal loss. Such behavior is often informally described as suicidal, self-destructive, or flirting with death. Clear examples of such behavior include reckless driving, playing Russian roulette, and gambling all of one's life savings on a single play at a gaming table. Less clear examples include hang gliding, race car driving, and compulsive eating. Risk-taking behavior is sometimes a mental health problem because it is often maladaptive.

One general interpretation of risk-taking behavior comes from classical psychoanalysis. It is possible to hypothesize that the risk taken represents a counterphobia. The underlying phobia is the fear of death, injury, or loss. To prove to himself or herself that the fear is groundless, the individual takes the unnecessary risk. If all turns out well, the fear is temporarily put to rest.

A second interpretation of risk-taking behavior comes from general psychology. It is possible to hypothesize that some people find life understimulating. They perceive everyday activities as boring and tedious. Under the conditions of conventional living, they suffer from somewhat less than optimal central nervous system arousal. Thus they seek ways to increase arousal. And risk taking is certainly one of these ways. It is essential to realize that, in this interpretation, the individual's goal is not death, injury, or loss but merely excitement. An adverse consequence is, of course, the price that may have to be paid in the long run.

See also *counterphobic behavior*; *suicide*.

Ritalin: See *methylphenidate*.

Rogers, Carl Ransom (1902–1987): An American psychologist and father of client-centered therapy. Rogers was granted a Ph.D. degree in clinical psychology in 1931 by Columbia University Teachers College. He served for more than 10 years as the director of Rochester Guidance Center in New York. He taught psychology at several universities, including the University of Chicago. In 1946, he was elected president of the American Psychological Association. When he was 54 years of age, the association honored him with its Distinguished Scientific Contribution Award.

Rogers became disenchanted early in his career with traditional psychoanalysis. First, he believed that it focuses too much on the past and not enough on the present and the future. Second, it is too deterministic. The person's behavior is seen as reactive, a result of biological forces and painful experiences. Rogers wanted to introduce an element of voluntarism, suggesting that the individual has the capacity to make choices and effect changes. Third, it proceeds too slowly because it tends to minimize the individual's current problems in favor of exploring childhood and early developmental experiences. Fourth, the therapist is too much of an authority figure. He or she should be seen as a helper but not an all-wise judge.

Borrowing to some extent from ideas earlier expressed by Alfred Adler and Otto Rank, Rogers formulated client-centered therapy. One of the key ideas contained in client-centered therapy is the assertion that human beings have a basic self-actualizing tendency, an inborn inclination toward personal growth and mental health. This viewpoint Rogers held in common with Abraham Maslow. Therapy, according to Rogers, should provide a nurturing environment, making it possible for the individual's self-actualizing tendency to emerge.

Two of Rogers's books are *Psychotherapy and Personality Change* (1954) and *On Becoming a Person* (1961).

See also *Adler, Alfred*; *client-centered therapy*; *humanistic therapy*; *Maslow, Abraham Harold*; *Rank, Otto*; *self-actualization*.

Rorschach test: A projective test utilizing 10 standard inkblot patterns as stimuli. Five of the cards are black and white, and 5 of the cards have some color. Developed by the psychoanalyst Hermann Rorschach, the test was first published in 1921.

Subjects are asked to look at the 10 cards one at a time. The examiner asks the subject, "What do you see on this card? We both know it's just an inkblot, but you are free to use your imagination." A subject may say, "Oh, this looks just like two witches stirring a pot." Or another subject may say, "This looks like a bat flying." A huge spectrum of responses to the cards is possible. Answers are recorded in substantial detail.

The basic inspiration of the test arises from the ego defense mechanism of projection. An inkblot is an ambiguous stimulus, one that can be perceived in two or more ways. In view of the fact that such a stimulus is relatively structureless and meaningless in and of itself, it is assumed that any structure or meaningful perception of it by a subject arises as a projection from the unconscious level of mental life. In other words, one "sees" in the cards what one needs to see in terms of forbidden wishes, repressed hostility, or unconscious motives in general. Rorschach conceived of his test as a sort of X-ray of the mind.

Scoring of the test is based on one of several standard methods, including one proposed by Rorschach himself. It takes a certain amount of training to score the test with any kind of confidence or reliability. Because a certain amount of personal judgment is called for, two examiners, even if they are experienced clinical psychologists, do not always obtain identical results. They will, however, on the whole obtain similar results, just as two English teachers scoring a composition will obtain similar grades.

The Rorschach test is usually administered as a part of a battery of psychological tests including a standard intelligence test, the Thematic Apperception Test, and the Minnesota Multiphasic Personality Inventory.

See also *intelligence tests*; *Minnesota Multiphasic Personality Inventory (MMPI)*; *personality test*; *projection*; *projective test*; *Thematic Apperception Test (TAT)*.

Rotter Internal-External Scale: See *locus of control*.

rumination disorder of infancy: An eating disorder characterized by bringing back into the mouth previously swallowed food. The disorder obtains its name from a class of animals known as ruminants; these animals swallow food and then regurgitate it. The behavior of chewing this regurgitated food is known as "chewing the cud."

Although the behavior is normal for ruminants, it is certainly not normal for infants. Rumination in an infant can sometimes lead to significant malnutrition and death. The disorder is an uncommon one. It appears with equal frequency in males and females.

If regurgitation is due to illness or any organic disorder, it is not rumination disorder of infancy. The disorder is a functional condition and is best thought of as a maladaptive habit.

Sometimes a drug that inhibits vomiting is prescribed to treat the disorder. Another treatment consists of small and more frequent feedings. Overstuffing the infant distends the stomach, and this may become a cue for regurgitation in some children. A combination of medical care and behavior modification is likely to be effective in bringing the condition under control. Although spontaneous recovery from the condition is quite possible, it is unwise to count on this because of the very real danger to the child.

See also *behavior modification*; *eating disorders*.

Rush, Benjamin (1746–1813): An American physician, chemist, politician, and psychiatrist. Rush is traditionally called "the father of American psychiatry." He earned his M.D. degree at the University of Edinburgh in Scotland, was an innovator in the treatment of mental patients at Pennsylvania Hospital, signed the Declaration of Independence, and was in charge of hospitals during the Revolutionary War.

In one sense, Rush was ahead of his time because he looked upon mental illness as a treatable disease. On the other hand, his methods were harsh and of doubtful value. They included bloodletting, laxatives, and restraint with straps in a chair. In fairness to Rush, it must be said that, on the whole, he was looking for practical ways to help mental patients recover their health.

Rush wrote a book that was influential for many years, *Medical Inquiries and Observations upon the Diseases of the Mind* (1812).

See also *Beers, Clifford Whittingham*; *Dix, Dorothea Lynde*; *Pinel, Phillipe*; *psychiatrist*.

S

sadism: The tendency to obtain pleasure by inflicting pain or suffering on another person. In *sexual sadism*, the individual derives pleasure from the punishment or humiliation of a partner during sexual activity. When someone has *sadistic personality traits*, he or she tends to be insulting and abusive in a personal relationship. The word *sadism* is derived from the name of Donatien Alphonse François, the Marquis de Sade (1740–1814), a writer who whipped, chained, and otherwise abused his sexual partners.

Sexual sadism is classified as a sexual disorder. Individuals with this disorder find that their principal way of becoming sexually excited is to tie down, insult, hit, or otherwise abuse a sexual partner.

There is a tendency to think of sadism as taking place in a situation where the partner consents to it. This does, of course, occur. And, in this instance, the consenting partner may suffer from masochism. The term *sadomasochistic* is used to describe such relationships. However, a certain amount of sadism is forced on a nonconsenting partner. The partner may consent to sexual activity but not to the sadistic actions. Under these conditions, the sadistic actions may be thought of as sexual assault. Also, persons with the disorder may be tempted toward, or engage in, the crime of rape.

Men are quite a bit more likely to suffer from sadism than are women.

A number of causal factors have been associated with sadism. Psychoanalysis notes that infants often obtain pleasure from biting during the oral period. This is known as *oral-aggressive behavior*. Also, some toddlers obtain pleasure from the willful withholding of fecal bulk during the anal period. They can display their resentments toward their parents in this way. This is known as *anal-retentive behavior*. Fixations of libido (i.e., psychosexual energy) in the oral or anal zones due to emotional wounds in early childhood may result in sadistic behavior as an adult.

Other factors include being raised in a hostile and abusive home, harboring hostile feelings toward the opposite sex, believing that one is physically unattractive, and overcompensating for a sense of social inadequacy. Not all of these factors may be operative in an individual case.

As indicated, sadistic tendencies often start in childhood. Once established, they tend to be quite persistent. Psychotherapy may help an individual reduce the intensity of sadism.

See also *masochism*; *paraphilias*; *psychosexual development*; *rape*; *sexual disorders (psychosexual disorders)*.

scapegoating: A way of expressing aggression in which the aggression is diverted from an original source to a substitute one. The name is derived from an ancient practice of the Jewish people. On Atonement Day, a goat was chased out of the community. It symbolically carried the sins of the group.

Assume that Karl has been frustrated and criticized by his boss. He comes home from a bad day at work and begins to insult and verbally abuse his wife and children. He is scapegoating his aggression. It pays to be alert to scapegoating because it is a behavior that often has an adverse effect on a personal relationship.

schizoaffective disorder: A psychotic disorder presenting a mixed set of symptoms that resemble both schizophrenia and a mood disorder. Although the category exists in the American Psychiatric Association's *Diagnostic and Statistical Manual of Mental Disorders*, it exists primarily to provide a practical compromise when a clearer diagnosis cannot be made. A number of mental health professionals feel that the term *schizoaffective disorder* is either unnecessary or too vague.

See also Diagnostic and Statistical Manual of Mental Disorders; *mood disorders (affective disorders)*; *schizophrenia*.

schizoid personality disorder: A personality disorder characterized by an impairment in the ability to form emotional bonds with others. Words often used to describe the traits of an individual with this disorder are *cold*, *distant*, *detached*, *callous*, and *indifferent*. Related symptoms include a reluctance to express hostile feelings, a lack of direction in life, self-preoccupation, absent-mindedness, and prolonged fantasizing.

A schizoid personality disorder handicaps the individual in several ways. The individual may find it quite difficult to become sufficiently close to someone else to ever get married. If he or she does marry, the disorder can have an adverse effect on the marital relationship. One's career can be negatively affected, particularly if promotions require making a good impression on others. On the other hand, it must be admitted that if the career requires intense work in isolation, then a schizoid personality disorder may not be a significant impairment. If a person with this disorder ever becomes a parent, the symptoms of the disorder will interfere with bonding and the formation of emotional closeness between parent and child. A number of recluses, vagrants, and social derelicts suffer from the disorder.

The signs of a schizoid personality disorder are often evident in childhood. Males and females seem to be afflicted in equal numbers. No reliable statistics exist establishing the frequency of the disorder. However, both informal and clinical observation suggest that the disorder is fairly common.

Causal factors in the disorder are by no means clear. However, it seems quite possible that the individual may be disposed to some degree by temperament to have a preference for social isolation. In addition, it is reasonable to speculate that a parental style combining authoritarianism with emotional distance may foster a tendency on the part of the child toward withdrawal. There is some research evidence to support this general hypothesis.

Drug therapy is not recommended for the disorder. The principal treatment of choice is psychotherapy. The therapy should aim to help the individual find ways to obtain at least some gratification from interactions with others. A kind of psychotherapy that emphasizes guidance and gives some practical suggestions (e.g., reality therapy or rational-emotive therapy) may be of some help to the individual.

See also *personality disorders*.

schizophrenia: A mental disorder characterized by a gross impairment in the ability to think in logical and rational terms. Related symptoms frequently include delusions, hallucinations, odd use of language, and loss of touch with reality as most of us understand it. The behavior of persons suffering from this disorder is often, but not always, bizarre. Schizophrenia represents what has been informally called "madness" in the Western world.

A common error is to believe that persons with schizophrenia suffer from a "split personality." However, the term *multiple personality disorder* is reserved for this condition. It is true that "schiz" means split, and that "phrenia" means head. However, a proper reading of the term *schizophrenia* is to think of it as a "head" (i.e., mind) that has "split" from reality.

Five types of schizophrenia have been identified. However, it should be understood that, in reality, the clinical picture is often confusing and shifting. Therefore, a diagnosis according to a type is based on what appears to be the most prominent symptoms.

The *disorganized type* of schizophrenia is characterized by infantile and regressive behavior. Speech is often unintelligible. The individual is frequently silly and inappropriate. An older term for this type is *hebephrenic schizophrenia*. The word *hebephrenic* is derived from Hebe, the goddess of youth in Greek mythology. The implication is that the patient has returned to "youth."

The *catatonic type* of schizophrenia is characterized by such behaviors as mutism (i.e., not talking), odd posturing, and lack of cooperation. Sometimes the individual adopts an odd posture and remains immobile for a long interval. At other times, the individual may display *catatonic excitement* and engage in restless movement without an apparent goal. The impression that one obtains from observing the patient is one of great social withdrawal and hostile resistance.

The *paranoid type* of schizophrenia is characterized by suspicion and mistrust. The individual may have the delusion that he or she is being abused or victimized by others. Another common delusion is to believe that one is a great or famous person. A distinction is made between a *paranoid type* of schizophrenia and *delusional (paranoid) disorder*. In delusional disorder, the delusions are more systematic and well-organized than they are in the paranoid type of schizophrenia.

The *undifferentiated type* of schizophrenia is the diagnosis assigned to a patient when symptoms are confusing and overlap. The individual displays the principal signs of schizophrenia, but specific classification is difficult.

The *residual type* of schizophrenia is the diagnosis assigned to a patient who has a history of suffering from schizophrenia but who is at present showing only mild signs of the disorder.

Schizophrenia is relatively common. The rate of schizophrenia among adults is approximately 1%. A practical measure that is applied to prognosis and recovery is called the "rule of thirds." About ⅓ of patients will become chronic cases, about ⅓ will have off-and-on bouts with their disorder, and about ⅓ will make a full recovery. Males and females are affected in equal numbers. There is a strong tendency for schizophrenia to make its first appearance in young adulthood.

Schizophrenia is thought of as a functional disorder, not an organic one. It is usually said to be the most severe kind of functional mental disorder. It is classified as functional, however, *not* because biological and organic factors are absent, but because their presence and action are subtle. As research evidence has been gathering, the importance of biological and organic factors is becoming increasingly evident. Therefore, one cannot really say that this disorder is clearly and simply functional in nature.

A tremendous amount of thought and research has gone into attempting to explain schizophrenia. Next are listed some of the principal explanations. However, it should be realized that the explanations overlap. Also, multiple causal factors may be operating in a given case.

1. It is possible that schizophrenia has a genetic basis. Studies of families have clearly revealed that if one identical twin has schizophrenia, a second identical twin is more likely to have the disorder than a nontwin sibling. Because identical twins have identical hereditary structures, this suggests strongly that genetic factors make a contribution to this disorder.

2. It is possible that an inherited defect in the brain of persons with schizophrenia makes it difficult for them to process information in the same way as normal persons.

3. There is evidence to suggest that one of the causal factors in schizophrenia is excessive activity of the neurotransmitter dopamine. This is known as the *dopamine hypothesis*.

4. Psychoanalysis suggests that fixations of libido at the oral stage of development may contribute to the formation of schizophrenia. The oral stage is the most primitive level of psychosexual development, and much of the behavior of persons with schizophrenia is regressive and infantile. This is particularly true in the case of the disorganized type.

5. There is some research data to suggest that some parents are *schizophrenogenic*. That is, they inadvertently do things to bring out the disorder. They mix up and confuse the child during the developmental years. In particular, it is believed that they tend to use double-bind communication patterns that create insolvable psychological problems for their children.

6. Severe psychosocial stressors may be important precipitating factors in schizophrenia. If a person believes that he or she cannot cope with reality, then the individual may take flight into a fantasy world.

As indicated before, a substantial amount of effort has been expended in an attempt to explain schizophrenia. An equally great effort has gone into treatment. Although there is no "cure" for schizophrenia, treatments are often effective and can ameliorate the worst symptoms of a given patient's disorder. Below are listed some of the principal treatments for schizophrenia.

1. Electroconvulsive therapy (ECT) was frequently used in the past to treat this disorder. It is sometimes still used but infrequently.

2. Lobotomies, a kind of psychosurgery in which the frontal lobes of the brain are severed from the rest of the brain, were also used with some frequency in the past. Today the lobotomy is seldom a treatment of choice.

3. Drug therapy is the most prominent approach used at the present. Antipsychotic drugs (i.e., major tranquilizers) are frequently prescribed.

4. Psychotherapy has been used with varying degrees of success. Psychoanalytic therapy explores the unconscious roots of a patient's disorder. One aim is to free the libido from its oral fixations. A therapy that aims at making the patient think more clearly (e.g., cognitive therapy) may be quite helpful. Drug therapy and psychotherapy can work together. The drug may make the individual more lucid and able to take advantage of psychotherapy.

It is important to realize that there is real hope for persons with schizophrenia. According to the "rule" of thirds, a large percentage recover completely. In more stubborn cases, the disorder *is* treatable, if not curable. And through the use of psychotherapy, the individual can learn many practical and effective ways to cope with this disorder. In most cases, the patient will not be a resident of a mental hospital for life but will be helped to live in the larger world.

See also *biomedical viewpoint*; *Bleuler, Eugen*; *cognitive therapy*; *delusional (paranoid) disorder*; *dementia praecox*; *dopamine*; *double-bind communication*; *electroconvulsive therapy (ECT)*; *functional disorders*; *genetic predisposition*; *hebephrenic schizophrenia*; *lobotomy*; *major tranquilizers (antipsychotic drugs)*; *multiple personality disorder*; *oral stage*; *psychoanalysis*; *psychosocial stressors*.

schizophrenogenic parents: See *double-bind communication*.

schizotypal personality disorder: A personality disorder characterized by symptoms that are somewhat similar to, but milder than, the symptoms of schizophrenia. Although persons with this disorder are not psychotic, they are sometimes described as "bor-

derline" psychotic. They, unlike persons suffering from schizophrenia, maintain reality contact.

Specific signs of the disorder include thinking in magical terms,
holding strange ideas, lack of closeness with others, talking in
circles, lack of trust in others, and acting "touchy" when criticized.
There is also a tendency to experience illusions such as the feeling
that one is floating or that one is being looked at by an invisible
presence. However, these are *not* delusions because the individual
recognizes that they are almost certainly distortions of perception.

Causal factors in this disorder are almost certainly similar to
the causal factors in schizophrenia. It seems likely that genetic
and biochemical factors play a fundamental role. Research suggests
this disorder and schizophrenia are often associated in families.
It also seems likely that adverse developmental experiences and
psychosocial stressors aggravate the disorder. It is estimated that
the incidence of the disorder in the general population is about
3%. It is not known if one sex is more affected than the other.

The recommended treatment for the disorder is psychotherapy.
The therapy should aim primarily at helping the individual to
think more clearly and maintain reality contact. In most cases,
drug therapy is not indicated. However, if symptoms become
severe, a major tranquilizer is sometimes prescribed.

See also *schizoid personality disorder*; *schizophrenia*.

seasonal affective disorder (SAD): See *seasonal pattern*.

seasonal pattern: An aspect of either bipolar disorder or major
depression in which the appearance of symptoms can be linked
to a given season of the year. Commonly, this is identified as
winter. The general assumption is that deprivation of light triggers
a biological process that has an adverse effect on mood. It has
been speculated that living in Alaska or in northern regions can
aggravate mood disorders. The mood generally improves in the
spring and summer when more light is available.

Seasonal pattern has also been called seasonal affective disorder
(SAD). This clinical label does not have formal status in the

American Psychiatric Association's *Diagnostic and Statistical Manual of Mental Disorders*. Instead, as indicated before, seasonal pattern is treated as an *aspect* of already recognized mood disorders. See also *bipolar disorder*; *major depression (unipolar disorder)*.

secondary gain: See *resistance*.

sedatives: Drugs that depress the activity of the central nervous system. They have the general effect of lowering arousal and alertness. All sedatives are addictive at both a physiological and psychological level. The two principal kinds of sedatives are alcohol and barbiturates.

See also *alcoholism*; *barbiturates*.

self-actualization: As formulated by the personality theorist Abraham Maslow, an inborn tendency to maximize one's talents and potentialities. The concept of self-actualization was first proposed by the psychiatrist and neurologist Kurt Goldstein in connection with the striving tendencies of individuals with brain damage. However, it is in connection with Maslow's humanistic personality theory that the idea has really blossomed in psychology.

Maslow ranks human motivation on an ascending order in terms of needs as follows: basic physiological needs, stimulation needs, safety needs, love and belongingness needs, esteem needs, and self-actualization. All of the needs with the exception of self-actualization represent deficiency motivation; they are experienced as gaps in human existence. Self-actualization, on the other hand, represents a being need, or growth motivation. It is a great natural tendency in people to *become*, to do something with their lives that takes advantage of their abilities, aptitudes, and interests. For example, Martha feels that her true vocation in life is to become a music teacher. She works part-time while in college, earns good grades, defers marriage, and so forth, all in the interests of her goal. It can be said that much of her behavior is growth motivation, that she is a self-actualizing person.

Although Maslow believed that the need for self-actualization is inborn, he also believed that it is rather easily thwarted. Parents may unfeelingly criticize an adolescent or young adult's choices and decisions, friends may make arbitrary evaluations, opportunities may be difficult to obtain, or doubts may exist concerning one's talents. All of these obstacles, and more, may derail the impetus of self-actualization.

The concept of self-actualization is an important one in the context of mental health. If the need for self-actualization is frustrated, then the individual can fall into a state of depression. The individual may need to rediscover the path toward self-actualization. Reading inspiring books, taking small steps in the direction of personal growth, and humanistic therapy may all be helpful.

See also *depression*; *humanistic therapy*; *growth motivation*; *Maslow, Abraham Harold*.

self-concept: A set of related ideas that one holds about oneself in terms of intelligence, creativity, interests, aptitudes, behavioral traits, and personal appearance. The self-concept may be generally positive or generally negative. If it is generally positive, then the individual usually feels able and attractive. If it is generally negative, then the individual usually feels inadequate and unattractive.

It is important to realize that the self-concept often exists independent of the self as perceived by others. For example, in an extreme case, an individual may have a negative self-concept and be perceived as able and attractive by most other people.

The role of the self-concept plays an important part in Carl Rogers's client-centered therapy. A principal goal of this kind of therapy is to help an individual develop a more positive self-concept.

See also *client-centered therapy*; *Q-sort technique*; *Rogers, Carl Ransom*; *self-esteem*.

self-esteem: An evaluation of the self, a sort of self-ranking in terms of personal worth. Obviously the concept of self-esteem is related to the self-concept. Persons with a negative self-concept tend to have low self-esteem. Persons with a positive self-concept tend to have high self-esteem. Studies conducted by the research psychologist Stanley Coopersmith suggest that some of the important antecedents to self-esteem reside in childhood. On the whole, parents who tend to be democratic, authoritative (not authoritarian), and affectionate foster self-esteem in their children. As an adult, a series of failures in important life tasks can undermine self-esteem. Conversely, a series of successes can bolster self-esteem.

William James said that self-esteem can be thought of in terms of a formula:

$$\text{Success } \textit{divided by} \text{ Pretensions} = \text{Self-esteem}$$

Success refers to actual accomplishments. Pretensions refers to goals and dreams. Essentially, James's formula communicates the idea that self-esteem is subjective, not objective. If one has a low level of aspiration, then it does not take much real success to maintain self-esteem. However, if one has a high level of aspiration, then it takes much more real success to maintain self-esteem. As a consequence, odd as it may seem, many people who have substantial accomplishments often suffer from low self-esteem. In terms of James's formula, it is perhaps because they demand too much of themselves.

See also *James, William*; *self-concept*.

self-instructional training: A technique used in connection with cognitive-behavior therapy in which one gives oneself overt instructions. Pioneered by research psychologist Donald Meichenbaum, self-instructional training is derived from the observation that children often tell themselves out loud what to do. For example, a preschooler might announce to himself or herself, "I'm going to make my bed before I brush my teeth." The open statement apparently helps children follow a plan of action.

When modifying a maladaptive line of thinking or attempting to change an unwanted habit, it can be useful to return to the preschooler's approach. A person who keeps thinking depressing thoughts can use self-instructional training by saying aloud, "I'm going to stop this dead-end reasoning. I'm going to stop thinking in circles and start looking on the brighter side of things. I'm going to count a few of my blessings right now."

A person who is trying to lose weight can say aloud, "I'm going to skip dessert tonight."

Of course, it is a good idea to be alone when speaking aloud to oneself. Otherwise, the behavior is odd in the social sense. The self-instructions can also be written out on a piece of paper. The key is to take some sort of *action* in the right direction. Self-instructional training has been found to be an effective tool in therapy.

See also *cognitive-behavior therapy*.

Selye, Hans (1907–1982): A Canadian physician, endocrinologist, and early explorer of the effects of stress on health. Selye was born in Austria. He earned an M.D. degree in 1929 and a Ph.D. degree in 1931, both from the University of Prague. For most of his professional life, Selye was associated with the University of Montreal.

Early in his career, Selye conceived the idea that he did not want to study a particular sickness but sickness itself. In the same way that a given illness has a syndrome (i.e., set of symptoms) that is unique to it, the state of being sick also has a syndrome. Selye wanted to study this general pattern. At first, Selye's approach met with some skepticism. However, over the years, he succeeded in his general goal and was able to introduce into the scientific world the very powerful and useful concept of the general adaptation syndrome.

Two of Selye's principal works are *The Stress of Life* (1956) and *Stress in Health and Disease* (1976).

See also *general adaptation syndrome*; *psychosomatic disorders*; *stress*; *syndrome*.

senile dementia: A deterioration in functional intelligence and mental ability associated with old age. Old age in and of itself is not thought to be a cause of the dementia. Over time, neurons in the brain and nervous system tend to die. It is not completely clear why this process tends to take place. Several causal factors appear to exist. The body may attack itself through an autoimmune activity. Or a viral infection may have a gradual effect. Or there may be a lack of adequate blood supply to the brain due to arteriosclerosis. Or heavy smoking may deprive the brain of some blood by constricting arteries. Or the excessive consumption of alcohol may have a similar effect. Two or more of the causal factors may work in combination in a given case.

See also *Alzheimer's disease*; *presenile dementias*.

sensate focus learning: See *sexual therapy*.

sentence-completion test (sentence-completion method): A test requiring that the subject supply a conclusion to an incomplete sentence. The subject may be asked to respond orally or in writing. The method can be used as a projective personality test. The assumption is that the conclusion provided by the subject is a projection from the unconscious level of the personality. For example, let us assume that the following stem is provided: "I really believe . . . . " Jim writes, "I really believe that it's a wonderful life." Harry writes, "I really believe that most women can't be trusted." Both subjects may have revealed something significant. Jim's response suggests an optimistic attitude toward life. Harry's response suggests that he may have problems in male–female relationships. Of course, the conclusion to one sentence is merely suggestive. However, 20 or 30 sentences might be given. The group of responses often reveals one or two common themes. And the results of the sentence-completion test are usually compared with other test results.

See also *personality test*; *projective test*; *psychological test*.

sexual deviations: Sexual behaviors that are at odds with the norms and expectations of a given culture. In the past, sexual deviations have often been referred to as *perversions*, suggesting that the sexual drive has been turned in the direction of an improper or unnatural purpose. Of late, there has been a tendency among clinicians to avoid the negative emotional connotations of "deviations" and "perversions." Consequently, it is often recommended that the more neutral term *sexual variance* replace the older terms. This language indicates that not all deviations are pathological. For example, in the early part of this century, both cunnilingus and fellatio were thought to be perversions. Today's sexologists include them as normal sexual practices. And sexual surveys indicate that a large percentage of people in all walks of life engage in oral-genital contact.

On the other hand, it is agreed that much behavior varying from traditional standards is indeed pathological. Examples are incest, masochism, pederasty, pedophilia, and sadism.

See also *cunnilingus*; *fellatio*; *incest*; *masochism*; *paraphilias*; *pederasty*; *pedophilia*; *sadism*.

sexual disorders (psychosexual disorders): A large group of disorders characterized by eccentric sexual activity and/or sexual dysfunctions. These are discussed on an individual basis in this encyclopedia and are identified in the following cross-references.

See also *bestiality*; *dyspareunia*; *exhibitionism*; *frigidity*; *gender identity disorder of childhood*; *gender identity disorders*; *hypoactive sexual desire disorder (inhibited sexual excitement)*; *masochism*; *paraphilias*; *pedophilia*; *premature ejaculation*; *sadism*; *transsexualism*; *transvestic fetishism (transvestism)*; *vaginismus*; *voyeurism*.

sexual response cycle: According to the physiological research of William H. Masters and Virginia E. Johnson, a four-stage pattern consisting of (1) excitement, (2) plateau, (3) orgasm, and (4) resolution. During the *excitement* phase, erotic stimulation induces an increase in both heart rate and blood pressure. A *sex flush* in which the skin acquires a reddish color in the area of the neck and breasts is common in about 75% of women and 25% of men. Tumescence (i.e., swelling in size) of the clitoris takes place in females. Erection of the penis takes place in males.

During the *plateau* phase, both heart rate and blood pressure remain at increased levels. The sex flush may cover a larger surface of skin. In women, the clitoris withdraws. In men, the penis expands somewhat. The third stage, the *orgasm*, is brief in duration and is experienced as the peak of sexual pleasure in both females and males. Both heart rate and blood pressure briefly reach higher levels. The sex flush becomes more intense. In women, the clitoris remains retracted, and there are involuntary contractions of the *pubococcygeus (PC) muscle* surrounding the vaginal channel. In men, the penis undergoes involuntary contractions. (See *orgasm* for a more complete description.)

During the *resolution* phase, both heart rate and blood pressure return to normal levels. The sex flush fades rapidly. Both sexes are temporarily unresponsive to sexual stimulation.

However, it should be noted that some people have the ability to experience multiple orgasms. A *multiple orgasm* may be defined as two or more orgasms within a given period of sexual activity. Either the individual does not enter the resolution phase following the orgasm or comes out of it very quickly. It is estimated that almost 15% of women frequently have multiple orgasms. About 7% of men have multiple orgasms, and these are usually young men. Women state that their second orgasm is more pleasurable than their first one. Men, conversely, state that the first orgasm is more pleasurable than the second one.

See also *erectile disorder (erectile insufficiency)*; *frigidity*; *hypoactive sexual desire disorder (inhibited sexual excitement)*; *orgasm*; *sexual disorders (psychosexual disorders)*; *sexual therapy*.

sexual therapy: A broad general concept referring to any kind of therapy, or technique in therapy, that aims to relieve sexual dysfunction. William H. Masters and Virginia E. Johnson are considered pioneers in sex therapy and have introduced a number of innovative techniques. One of these is *sensate focus learning* in which both individuals are trained through touch and feeling to increase their level of sexual pleasure. This may be through self-stimulation or through mutual stimulation by partners. Another innovation is the *squeeze technique* used to control premature ejaculation. This involves the female masturbating the male almost to orgasm and then squeezing the penis in order to inhibit the ejaculatory reflex. Training with the squeeze technique is often effective in giving the male the capacity to extend the duration of the excitement phase of the sexual response cycle.

It should be clear that specific techniques in therapy, although of great value, usually must be combined with more general approaches involving self-understanding and more effective communication between a couple.

See also *erectile disorder (erectile insufficiency); frigidity; hypoactive sexual desire disorder (inhibited sexual excitement); orgasm; premature ejaculation; sexual disorders (psychosexual disorders); sexual response cycle*.

sheltered workshops: A vocational environment designed to provide training and encouragement to persons with either physical or mental disabilities. A sheltered workshop is more than occupational therapy because the individual is helped to learn a useful skill and is often paid. The basic idea is to help the individual to become more self-sufficient. Sheltered workshops can be of great value to mentally retarded persons, persons with mental disorders, persons with visual impairments, and so forth.

In order to be effective, a sheltered workshop requires trained personnel who specialize in working with disabled persons.

See also *halfway house; occupational therapy*.

Sherrington, Charles Scott (1861–1952): An English physiologist, Sherrington conducted the bulk of his research at Cambridge University. In 1932, he was recognized with a Nobel Prize for his contributions to our understanding of how neurons function.

Contemporary psychiatry explains some mental disorders in terms of difficulties in functioning at the neuronal level. For example, both schizophrenic disorders and depression appear to be linked to irregularities in neurotransmitter levels. Drug therapy is based on this general premise. The importance of Sherrington's work for psychiatry should be seen in this general framework. He was the principal pioneer who opened up the pathway leading to today's spectrum of understanding.

Two of Sherrington's works are *The Integrative Action of the Nervous System* (1906) and *Man and His Nature* (1940).

See also *biomedical viewpoint*; *dopamine*; *drug therapy*; *neuron*; *neurotransmitters*.

shyness: A common personality trait characterized by a tendency to be self-conscious and ill at ease in social situations. The shy person often feels embarrassed, tongue-tied, confused, and anxious when meeting people for the first time or when asked to speak in front of a group. Philip G. Zimbardo, a social psychologist, makes a distinction between situational shyness and chronic shyness. Persons who suffer from *situational shyness* have problems some of the time and only under certain circumstances. Persons who suffer from *chronic shyness* are distressed in almost all social situations. A study conducted by Zimbardo found about 80% of subjects admitted to situational shyness. About 25% admitted to chronic shyness.

Although shyness is by no means a mental disorder, it *is* a distressing trait. Shyness is so common that there is no single way to explain it. However, it is possible that a developmental history in which one was constantly criticized and found wanting may be a causal factor contributing to what Alfred Adler called an *inferiority complex*, and what today is usually referred to as low self-esteem.

Zimbardo found by working with groups of students that acquired social skills could diminish the intensity of shyness. Approaches such as assertiveness training can be helpful.

See also *Adler, Alfred*; *assertiveness training*; *self-esteem*.

sick role: A role we are allowed to play when we are suffering from a physical illness or a mental disorder. The sick role allows us to withdraw for a time from conventional responsibilities, to become more demanding of others, to become more self-absorbed, and so forth. The sick role has its obvious value, and it plays a functional part in the process of getting well.

Unfortunately, a sick role also provides *secondary gains*, peripheral benefits derived from symptoms. A person may find that he or she enjoys the control and power associated with being ill. Another person may find that he or she finds it very pleasant to avoid work and other responsibilities. It is possible for the sick role to be reinforced by friends and family who are too sympathetic or otherwise attentive to a patient's needs. In the case of mental disorders, Freud observed that the existence of secondary gains may lead to resistance to improvement.

See also *conversion disorder*; *factitious disorders*; *malingering*; *resistance*.

significant others: As formulated by the psychiatrist Harry S. Sullivan, other people who play important roles in either our development as children or ongoing adult life. In the case of children, the most significant others are usually the parents. Older brothers and sisters who exert authority and influence may also be significant others. When we are adults, the most important significant others are usually our partners. To a lesser extent, friends and our own children may also be significant others.

It is clear that interpersonal relationships often play an important role in mental health. It is now a commonplace observation that a disturbed relationship with parents in childhood is a contributing factor to mental disorders. A troubled relationship with a husband or wife may aggravate a problem such as depression.

See also *Berne, Eric*; *child abuse*; *family therapy*; *Sullivan, Harry Stack*; *transactional analysis*.

situational stress reaction: A transient reaction characterized by the inability to cope effectively with the demands of a new or unusual situation. Ineffective and/or maladaptive responses such as crying, screaming, pouting, refusing to cooperate, mental confusion, anxiety, anger, and depression may appear. A situational stress reaction is usually thought of as an acute problem and tends to spontaneously disappear without treatment.

It is also possible to make a distinction between a mild reaction and a gross one. For example, the kinds of demands involved in moving to a different home might precipitate a *mild reaction* involving crying and irrational bickering with one's spouse. On the other hand, living through a severe earthquake in which one observed injury and death might precipitate a *gross reaction* involving mental disorientation and emotional numbness.

See also *posttraumatic stress disorder (traumatic neurosis)*; *regression*; *stress*.

Skinner, Burrhus Frederic (1904–): An American psychologist who conducted pioneer work in operant conditioning. Skinner received a Ph.D. degree in psychology from Harvard University in 1931. He subsequently taught psychology, and did research, first at the University of Minnesota and then at Indiana University.

Sixteen years after he earned his Ph.D., Skinner returned to Harvard to occupy the prestigious William James Chair in psychology. It is somewhat ironic that Skinner was granted this position in view of the fact that William James was a cognitive psychologist who placed great value on conscious processes such as thinking and perception. Skinner, on the other hand, is a radical behaviorist who denies the importance of consciousness as an explanatory concept.

As indicated before, Skinner's main domain of research has been operant conditioning. In his early research, his principal experimental subjects were rats and pigeons. Later he was able to demonstrate how principles of operant conditioning could be extended to human beings. For example, he is the inventor of the teaching machine, a programmed approach to learning that is incorporated into much of today's computer-assisted instruction.

Skinner takes the general position that most behavior, including maladaptive behavior, is learned. What is learned can be unlearned or modified. Thus there is hope for troubled persons. Their behavior is not fixed and unalterable. Although Skinner is not a therapist himself, his formulations and findings are the foundation upon which behavior modification are built.

Skinner is considered a giant of psychology. His status is similar to that of Freud's. His impact upon the course of contemporary psychology has been profound.

Three of Skinner's books are *The Behavior of Organisms* (1938), *Beyond Freedom and Dignity* (1971), and *About Behaviorism* (1974).

See also *behavior modification*; *James, William*; *operant conditioning*.

sleepwalking disorder (somnambulism): A disorder characterized by walking about in one's sleep with open eyes and an expressionless face. Sometimes the individual engages in goal-oriented actions such as putting on shoes or obtaining food. The disorder is more common in children than in adults. When it is present in adults, it was also usually present in their childhood.

Episodes take place during deep sleep, and the subject is resistant to being awakened. Contrary to folklore, it is possible for a person who is sleepwalking to injure himself or herself. The sleepwalker needs protection.

Biological factors that may play a role in sleepwalking disorder include epilepsy and infections of the brain. A psychological factor that may be operative is chronic anxiety. When this is the case, some psychotherapists identify sleepwalking disorder as a dissociative disorder.

In most cases, children who have the disorder do not have it when they are adults. Spontaneous recovery from the disorder is common. If treatment is required, anticonvulsive medication or an antianxiety agent is sometimes prescribed. Often psychotherapy with the goal of reducing anxiety is recommended.

See also *brain pathology*; *dissociative disorders*; *epilepsy*; *insomnia*.

social introversion: A maladaptive behavioral trait characterized by an extreme tendency to avoid contact with other persons. The trait is measurable on the Minnesota Multiphasic Personality Inventory (MMPI). Social introversion and the familiar concept of shyness are overlapping categories. Essentially, they are on the same psychological continuum. Social introversion suggests a somewhat stronger withdrawal and avoidance response than does shyness.

See also *Minnesota Multiphasic Personality Inventory (MMPI)*; *shyness*.

social learning (observational learning): Learning by observation and contact with others. Social learning requires a high level of consciousness and the ability to copy the behavior of a model. A number of studies have demonstrated that it is a very important learning modality for human beings. Children, for example, often use their parents as models and mimic their behavior. If one's parents model behavioral pathology, then their actions can have an adverse effect on the mental health of the child.

Experiments conducted by Albert Bandura, a former president of the American Psychological Association, and his colleagues clearly demonstrate that aggressive patterns of behavior can be learned from models. Such experiments suggest that the role of social learning in the acquisition of an antisocial personality disorder may be quite important.

See also *antisocial personality disorder*; *classical conditioning*; *operant conditioning*.

sociopathic personality: See *antisocial personality disorder (psychopathic personality; sociopathic personality)*.

sociotherapy: A general term for any approach to therapy that focuses on *interpersonal factors*, psychological processes between two or more persons. In contrast, individual psychotherapy tends to focus on *intrapsychic factors*, psychological processes within one person.

It is possible to look on many mental health problems as reactive ones in which the troubled person is to a large extent disturbed because of the way in which he or she is treated by a significant other person. For example, let us say that Julia is suffering from chronic depression. She is a traditional woman, a full-time homemaker, and the mother of three children. She is married to an overcontrolling husband who takes her for granted and often discounts her opinions. It is clear that much of her depression is a response to her husband's high-handed treatment.

It is becoming increasingly common to recognize that it "takes two to tango." As a general approach, sociotherapy has inspired psychotherapists to take human relationships seriously.

See also *Berne, Eric*; *couple counseling*; *family therapy*; *psychodrama*; *significant others*; *Sullivan, Harry Stack*; *transactional analysis*.

sodium Pentothal (thiopental sodium): A drug belonging to the class barbiturates. (Sodium Pentothal is the well-known trade name for a drug with the generic name thiopental sodium.) When injected intravenously, sodium Pentothal can be used as an anesthetic. It also can produce effects similar to a medium or deep trance in hypnosis. This altered state of consciousness can be useful as a psychotherapeutic strategy in the treatment of amnesia, the recovery of repressed memories, or in the exploration of a patient's unconscious mental life. When sodium Pentothal is used in this way the procedure is referred to as *narcoanalysis*.

See also *barbiturates*; *hypnotherapy*; *narcotherapy*.

sodomy: In general, any "unnatural" sexual act. The name is derived from the ancient city of Sodom. The Bible relates in Genesis that Sodom and its companion city Gomorrah were destroyed because their people were evil.

In most cases, when the term *sodomy* is used, the implication is that it refers to anal intercourse. To a lesser extent, the term is sometimes used to refer to sexual relations with animals.

See also *bestiality*; *homosexuality*; *paraphilias*; *pederasty*.

somatic therapy: Any treatment approach in which a procedure is administered to the body in an effort to alleviate the symptoms of a mental disorder. The term *somatic* is derived from the Greek word "soma," meaning body. Somatic therapy should be contrasted with psychotherapy in which the treatment is administered to the personality directly, not the body.

Both somatic therapy and psychotherapy are used in contemporary treatment approaches. Although the two are different, they are by no means opposed. For example, a person suffering from a schizophrenic disorder who is helped to become more lucid with an antipsychotic agent may be further assisted with psychotherapy.

Although there are several kinds of somatic therapies, the one most used today is drug therapy. With the advent of effective drugs for many mental disorders, the use of electroconvulsive therapy and lobotomy has greatly diminished.

See also *drug therapy*; *electroconvulsive therapy (ECT)*; *hydrotherapy*; *lobotomy*; *psychotherapy*.

somatization disorder: A kind of somatoform disorder characterized by symptoms of physical illness without organic basis. (An earlier term for this disorder was *Briquet's syndrome*.) In order to receive a diagnosis of somatization disorder, a person must present a history of multiple complaints starting prior to 30 years of age and spanning a number of years. In most cases, the disorder starts in adolescence. Symptoms include the conviction that one suffers from poor health, false neurological signs such as blurred vision or difficulty in walking, digestive distress, complaints of pain, symptoms of heart trouble, and sexual problems. In women, there are frequently complaints related to the menstrual cycle.

Somatization disorder needs to be distinguished from hypochondriasis and conversion disorder, both related and somewhat similar somatoform disorders. In hypochondriasis, the person's focus is on *fear* of contracting an illness. In conversion disorder, the person's symptoms produce *impairment* such as blindness or deafness. In truth, the three disorders have much in common, and an actual patient may present a confusing symptomatic picture making classification difficult.

Somatization disorder is a diagnosis seldom applied to males. In the case of women, estimates concerning its incidence vary from 2 or 3 per thousand to 20 per thousand (i.e., about 2%).

Another problem is that physical symptoms must be taken seriously. Before a diagnosis of somatization disorder is made, actual organic illness must be ruled out.

Causal factors in somatization disorder have not been clearly identified. This is a relatively new diagnostic category, and its understanding requires more study. However, it can be said, in general terms, that the disorder appears to be primarily functional in nature, not organic. It is possible to speculate that its underlying cause is a neurotic process by which the individual extracts some sort of psychological benefit from physical symptoms. It allows him or her to control others, to exert power, to avoid having to cope with unpleasant challenges, and so forth. The psychoanalytic theory of the secondary gains of an illness can be helpful here (see *resistance*).

The most common treatment for somatization disorder is psychotherapy. The therapy is usually insight-oriented, helping the patient to understand the roots of the neurotic process and the ways it is kept alive. Although persons with the disorder usually display quite a bit of resistance to improvement, there is hope. If the therapist and the patient have good rapport, then substantial improvement can result.

See also *Briquet's syndrome*; *conversion disorder*; *hypochondriasis*; *hysteria*; *insight therapy*; *resistance*.

somatoform disorders: A group of five related disorders. The term *somatoform* is used to suggest that psychological and emotional difficulties have expressed themselves in a bodily form. (The Greek word for body is "soma.") The five disorders are body dysmorphic disorder (dysmorphophobia), conversion disorder, hypochondriasis, somatization disorder, and somatoform pain disorder.

See also *body dysmorphic disorder (dysmorphophobia)*; *conversion disorder*; *hypochondriasis*; *somatization disorder*; *somatoform pain disorder (psychogenic pain disorder)*.

somatoform pain disorder (psychogenic pain disorder): A disorder characterized by the presence of pain without any apparent organic cause. Somatoform pain disorder is hypothesized to have its origins in psychological and emotional conflicts. The pain is a symptom of an underlying neurotic process. It is common for persons with the disorder to resist this interpretation. The pain is quite vivid and real, and it seems impossible that its origin could be psychological.

Often in the case of somatoform pain disorder, the presence of pain allows the patient to evade some task or responsibility. Even though this is so, it does not mean that the patient is malingering in any conscious or voluntary way. It is not, of course, easy to distinguish an actual disorder from malingering.

The disorder is more common in young adults than in other age groups, and it is identified more often in females than in males. Although it is assumed that the underlying cause is a neurotic process, stress may trigger, or aggravate, the symptoms of the disorder.

Treatments for the disorder include tricyclic antidepressants, hypnosis, biofeedback training, and pain-reduction training programs. Of course, psychotherapy aimed at helping the individual better understand the psychological roots of the disorder is also useful.

See also *neurosis*; *somatoform disorders*.

somnambulism: A term with two related meanings. First, somnambulism is often used as a synonym for sleepwalking disorder. Second, the term is sometimes used to describe the state of consciousness associated with a deep trance in hypnosis.

See also *hypnosis*; *sleepwalking disorder (somnambulism)*.

spontaneous remission: See *remission*.

stage of exhaustion: See *general adaptation syndrome*.

stage of resistance: See *general adaptation syndrome.*

Stanford–Binet Intelligence Scale: A standardized test of intelligence developed at Stanford University by the psychologist Lewis M. Terman in the 1910s. Terman based the Stanford–Binet scales on the original work of Alfred Binet and Theodore Simon in France. The Stanford–Binet scale was the first intelligence test widely used in the United States.

Originally designed to measure the intelligence of children, the Stanford–Binet Scale, because of two revisions, is now capable of measuring the intelligence of both adolescents and adults.

Test items are arranged in order of difficulty from easy to difficult, an approach innovated by Binet and Simon to reveal a subject's mental age. The items themselves consist of questions and short tasks designed to assess vocabulary, memory, reasoning, attention, mathematical ability, social awareness, and perceptual-motor ability. The Stanford–Binet Scale provides an intelligence quotient (IQ), which gives an overall measure of an individual's cognitive functioning.

See also *intelligence*; *intelligence quotient (IQ)*; *intelligence tests*; *Wechsler intelligence scales.*

statutory rape: See *rape.*

stigma: A red mark on the skin due to internal bleeding. Some persons with mental disorders display stigmata. (*Stigmata* is the plural form of the term.) These blemishes are believed to be due to localized congestions of blood in capillaries related to extreme emotional tension.

There is also a religious tradition that when stigmata appear on particularly devout or reverent persons that they correspond to the wounds Christ received when he was crucified.

See also *neurodermatitis*; *somatoform disorders.*

stimulants: Drugs that have the effect of increasing alertness or arousal. People who have recently taken a stimulant often talk more, become more active, feel more confident, and sometimes experience a loss of appetite. Of course, these effects are temporary. When the effects of the drug wear off, there is often a boomerang effect, and the individual feels lethargic and somewhat depressed. The quickest way to obtain relief is to take a stimulant again. And a vicious circle commences. Because of their capacity to bring quick relief from feelings of boredom or depression, stimulants have a high potential for abuse.

See also *amphetamines*; *caffeine*; *cocaine*.

stress: The rate of wear and tear on the organism. Also, as defined by the stress researcher Hans Selye, the sum of all nonspecific changes caused by function or damage.

It is important to distinguish stress from a stressor. A *stressor* is the cause of stress. Stress is the effect. Thus if one feels mentally and physically exhausted after working in a factory that is filled with loud clanging sounds, the loud clanging sounds are stressors. The toll taken on the person is stress.

It is now generally recognized that stress is an important factor in both mental and physical illnesses. Persons who want to maintain health at both levels need to pay attention to practical ways to reduce stress.

See also *general adaptation syndrome*; *life change units (LCUs)*; *psychosocial stressors*; *psychosomatic disorders*; *Selye, Hans*.

stress-inoculation training: A technique associated with cognitive-behavior modification in which a person learns to cope with stress through the use of a three-step procedure. Step 1 is the *educational phase* in which the person is encouraged by the therapist to develop new ways of looking at situations that generate stressful responses. This may involve changing beliefs and expectations. One's ideas and attitudes are examined closely during this phase. (This phase is very similar to rational-emotive therapy.) Step 2 is the *rehearsal* *phase* in which the person prepares to cope with challenging situations. The individual actively thinks through what will have to be done and convinces himself or herself that it is possible to cope. It is recommended that the individual avoid the common tendency to focus on negative emotions but simply give attention to what has to be done. Step 3 is *application training* in which the person actually uses new coping skills in real situations.

The range of applications of stress-inoculation training is wide. Donald Meichenbaum, a leading researcher in cognitive-behavior modification, points out that the technique has been used to help people deal with problems varying from phobic disorders to control of anger to toleration of pain.

See also *cognitive-behavior therapy*; *rational-emotive therapy*; *self-instructional training*.

stressor: See *stress*.

stroke: See *cerebrovascular accident (CVA)*.

stupor: A condition characterized by a general lack of responsiveness. Alertness, perception, comprehension, and orientation are often significantly impaired. Words frequently used to describe a state of stupor are *in a daze*, *lethargic*, and *sluggish*.

A stupor can have an organic basis (e.g., a neurological problem), or it can be due to a mental disorder. Persons suffering from the catatonic type of a schizophrenic disorder are often mute and unresponsive, and this is referred to as a *catatonic stupor*.

See also *delirium*; *dementia*; *schizophrenia*.

stuttering (stammering): Stuttering is a general term for a group of specific speech problems distinguished by involuntary interruptions in verbal fluency. The three most common problems are as follows. *Repetition* is characterized by the uttering of word fragments several times. This is also informally referred to as "bouncing." An example is Porky Pig's sign-off in the Merry Melodies cartoons when he says, "Th-th-th-th-that's all folks!" There may be a *blocking* of the ability to speak. The person is often stopped cold and has a hard time saying the next word. *Prolongation* is characterized by the drawing out of words. For example, "gravy" becomes "graaaavy."

Persons who stutter usually feel embarrassed when speaking. Their faces often redden and take on a strained expression. Naturally, most persons with the difficulty feel anxiety when approaching situations in which they will have to meet persons for the first time. It would seem reasonable to observe that shyness can aggravate stuttering and that stuttering can in turn aggravate shyness.

Stuttering is a very common problem, often making its first appearance in early childhood. About 1% of children are affected. It cannot be taken for granted that they will outgrow the problem. In a very large number of instances, the condition continues into adolescence and adulthood with very little relief. It is estimated that the combined number of persons who stutter in the United States, including both adults and children, is over 2 million. Males are more likely to stutter than are females. The ratio is about 4 to 1.

There is no single clear-cut explanation of stuttering. It is possible that neurological problems and constitutional factors play causal roles in stuttering. However, the bulk of evidence suggests that a psychogenic explanation is the more important one. Stuttering appears to result primarily as a combination of emotional conflicts and maladaptive speech habits. Broadly speaking, the spontaneous appearance of lack of fluency during early childhood (quite normal) is often "selected" by the reinforcement principle. Some parents pay too much attention to these early involuntary speech errors; they may be overly solicitous or overly critical. They make the child self-conscious and anxious. The child begins to feel caught in a psychological trap. Joseph G. Sheehan, a leading speech therapist, theorized that the child is experiencing an approach–avoidance conflict. The child wants to speak to attain the rewards associated with communicating with others (approach), and he or she, at the same time, does not want to speak because of the emotional pain associated with being criticized and too closely observed (avoidance). The result is a state of anxiety that expresses itself in the form of stuttering.

It is also possible to look upon stuttering in psychoanalytic terms as a form of passive-aggressive behavior. The child who stutters is often a "good" child, a socialized child. The child observes that the parents are distressed by stuttering. When the child feels hostile, stuttering may be a "safe" way of expressing aggression. Note that the psychoanalytic explanation does not contradict the behavioral explanation previously offered. In fact, they are quite complementary.

Persons who stutter are often temporarily fluent, particularly when they sing or play a role in a play. These observations also lend credence to the view that the problem is primarily psychogenic in origin, not organic.

Therapy for stuttering usually consists of a combination of insight-oriented psychotherapy (mainly for adolescents and adults) and behavior modification in the form of speech-training procedures. When these approaches are combined, a high rate of success is often obtained. An example of a speech-training procedure is *syllable-timed speech* in which the person speaks to the beat of a metronome. Another example is *voluntary stuttering* in which the person consciously practices the speech error. Both of these methods help to bring stuttering, which is involuntary, under better voluntary control.

See also *aphasia*; *approach–avoidance conflict*; *behavior modification*; *psychogenic viewpoint*; *shyness*.

sublimation: A kind of ego defense mechanism in which an unacceptable primitive impulse is converted into a socially acceptable one. Thus raw aggressive impulses find expression in business competition, sports, games, debating contests, and so forth. And raw sexual impulses find expression in romance, fine arts, dance, and marriage.

The basic theory is that the id is pleasure oriented. It wants its way now, without regard to reality. However, the superego is morality oriented and says "no" to instant gratification. The reality-oriented ego mediates between the two and finds a middle road, making it possible to express the energy of the id's impulse in a way that is acceptable to one's family and culture.

Sublimation is one of the classical defense mechanisms identified by Freud. He described it as the psychological process that makes civilization possible. If we were unable to renounce infantile impulses, we could not build an organized social world.

The individual who is unable to adequately sublimate impulses has mental health problems. He or she will have unpleasant confrontations with parents, sexual partners, friends, and the law. One way to look at personality disorders, particularly the antisocial type, is to think of them as failures of sublimation.

See also *antisocial personality disorder (psychopathic personality; sociopathic personality); ego; ego defense mechanisms; Freud, Sigmund; id; personality disorders; superego.*

substance use disorders: See *psychoactive substance use disorders (substance use disorders).*

suicide: The act of killing oneself. Suicide can be thought of as self-murder. (The Latin root *sui* means "of oneself.") Suicide is usually thought of as a voluntary act bringing sudden death. However, the psychiatrist Karl Menninger makes a distinction between *acute suicide*, characterized by an abrupt end to life, and *chronic suicide*, characterized by a slow self-destructive process. The second type is not clearly voluntary. The psychologist and suicidologist Norman L. Farberow uses the term *indirect self-destructive behavior*, and, by this, he means approximately the same thing that Karl Menninger means when he speaks of chronic suicide. Indirect self-destructive behavior covers a large range of behaviors including diabetics not following dietary restrictions, drug abuse, alcoholism, overeating, cigarette smoking against a physician's orders, self-mutilation, accident proneness, and participating in high-risk sports.

Obviously, indirect self-destructive behavior is a very important aspect of the concept of suicide. Unfortunately, it is difficult to assess its statistical incidence. However, it can be safely said that it is much more frequent than acute suicide. For the balance of this entry, unless otherwise stated, the term *suicide* standing alone will refer to what Menninger calls "acute suicide," or the common conception of suicide in terms of sudden death.

Many statistical surveys of suicide have been attempted, and they have yielded a large amount of information. Some highlights are listed next. The data are for the United States.

1. It is estimated that between 25,000 to 60,000 suicides take place each year. The range is wide because of unknown factors. For example, it is believed that many victims of auto accidents are actually suicide victims.

2. Approximately 1 in 100 persons has made a suicide attempt.

3. As a cause of death among adolescents and young adults, suicide ranks number 3. Accidents and acts of violence (including murder) are numbers 1 and 2.

4. Elderly persons (over 75 years of age) are more likely to take their own lives than are adolescents and young adults. However, suicide does not have a high rank as a cause of death for the elderly because they are more prone to serious illnesses than are younger persons.

5. White males are the principal victims of suicide. They outnumber white females by 4 to 1.

6. Black males are about one-half as likely to commit suicide as are white males. Only a very small percentage of black females take their own lives.

7. There are about 10 suicide attempts for every successful suicide. Some of these attempts are believed to be *sham attempts*, attempts in which the actual intentions of the victim are in question. For example, an attempt might be a way of manipulating a partner into marriage. However, suicidologists recommend that all suicide attempts be taken seriously. Often people with a history of seemingly sham attempts eventually do commit suicide.

8. Overall, suicide ranks number 10 as a cause of death.

Why do some people take their own lives? There is no single answer to this question. However, a number of theories have been advanced, and a number of causal factors have been identified. Taken together, a general understanding of suicide emerges.

Classical psychoanalysis sees suicide as the failure of a struggle between *Eros*, the life instincts, and *Thanatos*, the death instinct. The life instincts are a cluster of forces that express themselves in the form of hunger, thirst, pain avoidance, elimination, and sexual desire. The death instinct is a single force that expresses itself either in the form of destruction (outwardly directed) or self-destruction. Under certain conditions, such as great frustration, loneliness, chronic depression, and prolonged illness, Thanatos can get the upper hand over Eros. At that point, the individual may commit suicide or engage in indirect self-destructive behavior.

Psychoanalysis sees suicide not only in self-destructive terms but also as destruction directed toward others. Suicide is not only a self-aggressive act; it frequently is also a socially aggressive act. A suicide victim punishes others. Sometimes the act of suicide is a way of saying, "Look what you've done to me. Now cry and suffer the way you've made me cry and suffer."

Humanistic psychology views suicide in commonsense terms. When people find themselves unable to become the persons they were meant to be, to have the marriages they believe that they were meant to have, to bring their hopes and dreams to fruition, they become depressed and sometimes self-destructive. When one is convinced that existence has lost its meaning, that life is closing in, that there are no roads to happiness, then suicide may begin to look like an answer to the problems of life.

The theory of learned helplessness advanced by behavioral psychology contributes to the understanding of suicide. If a person learns that he or she is helpless in situation A, then he or she may feel helpless in situation B. The person is not necessarily actually helpless in situation B but *believes* that he or she is helpless. In consequence, the individual will not act in a constructive manner. Learned helplessness has been shown to play a role in chronic depression. Chronic depression in turn has been shown to play a role in suicide.

The theories advanced here are based on individual psychology. However, it is possible to look at suicide in sociocultural terms. The great sociologist Emile Durkheim said that there were three basic types of suicides. *Egoistic suicide* takes place when the individual is alienated from another person or a group (e.g., a spouse or a family). *Altruistic suicide* takes place when an individual sacrifices himself or herself for a group. Examples are *kamikaze* pilots in World War II, martyrs, and the heroic acts of some warriors. *Anomic suicide* takes place under conditions of great change in the society. The term *anomie* means without norms or standards. Thus, when people feel that their stable anchors are gone, when traditions fail, when they are tossed into a turbulence they cannot control, they may opt for suicide as a way out of the social storm.

The various theories and causal factors identified are not mutually exclusive. They overlap and give a general view of the kinds of processes involved in suicide.

In recent years, a great deal of effort has been directed toward suicide prevention. Suicide prevention can be divided into two general categories. These are (1) general preventive measures and (2) crisis intervention. General preventive measures involve helping parents to raise children with high self-esteem, helping adults overcome depression, discovering ways to cope with aggressive and self-aggressive impulses, developing ways to deal with learned helplessness, and so forth. Crisis intervention has led to the establishment of suicide and crisis intervention centers. Many cities and large communities have hot lines to these centers. Trained volunteers answer telephones 24 hours a day. A professional staff of psychiatrists and clinical psychologists backs up the volunteer crew. If one is particularly despondent or thinking of suicide, the use of a crisis service is recommended. Help is available. In 1966, the Center for Studies of Suicide Prevention was established by an agency of the federal government, and a broad network of support is in place.

The survivor of a failed suicide attempt is in need of counseling and psychotherapy. It is not recommended that the person be allowed to return to the same situation as if nothing much is wrong. A suicide attempt is always a serious affair. Sometimes it is a "cry for help," and this cry should not be ignored. Sometimes family members are convinced that the attempt was an effort to manipulate or seek attention. However, even if this is so, the attempt itself is a maladaptive way of attaining these ends, and the individual is in need of help in order to find more mature ways of coping with life.

See also *alcoholism*; *behaviorism*; *crisis intervention*; *drug addiction*; *humanistic therapy*; *learned helplessness*; *nicotine dependence (tobacco dependence)*; *psychoanalysis*; *risk-taking behavior*; *suicidology*; *Thanatos*.

suicidology: The study of suicide and self-destructive behavior. An expert who makes a study of suicide is called a *suicidologist*. The principal aims of suicidology as a field of study are to describe important aspects of suicide, to gather statistical data, to explain suicide, to seek ways to prevent suicide, and to develop effective treatments for persons who are contemplating, or who have attempted, suicide.

See also *suicide*.

Sullivan, Harry Stack (1892–1949): An American psychiatrist and psychoanalyst who stressed the importance of interpersonal factors in development and adjustment. In 1917, Sullivan earned an M.D. degree from the Chicago College of Medicine and Surgery. For 10 years he was the president of the William Alanson White Foundation, an important psychoanalytic training institute. He edited the journal *Psychiatry* for a number of years.

Sullivan asserted that personality could not be studied or understood in a social vacuum. The individual is a result of interactions with important other people, or *significant others*. Examples of these significant others are parents (or parent surrogates), a spouse, siblings, relatives, friends, and peers. In some cases, even imaginary figures can be important (e.g., "my dream girl" or "my prince charming"). Even a person living in isolation such as a recluse may relate to imaginary figures or the memories of persons known in the past.

The approach to understanding the personality recommended by Sullivan does not discredit the importance that Freud placed on biological and sexual factors. However, it does attempt to place them in proper perspective, emphasizing that they exert their influence in the context of a family and other people.

Sullivan's general line of thinking is identified as the principal antecedent to transactional analysis, the method of therapy developed by the psychiatrist Eric Berne.

Conceptions of Modern Psychiatry (1947) was published when Sullivan was alive. Other books by him, based on his lectures and notes, were published after his death. Two of these books are *The Interpersonal Theory of Psychiatry* (1953) and *The Psychiatric Interview* (1954).

See also *Berne, Eric*; *significant others*; *transactional analysis*; *White, William Alanson*.

superego: According to Freud, the morality-oriented agent of the personality. The superego has two aspects: (1) the ego ideal and (2) the conscience. The *ego ideal* sets goals and a level of aspiration in life. It points the way toward the future. The ego ideal was acquired during childhood by identification with one's parents and is a reflection of their dreams for the child. It is important to understand that the ego ideal may be at a variance with one's own self-actualizing tendencies. For example, assume that a child has artistic talent. Also assume that the parents want the child to have a profession as an accountant. The superego would reflect the wish to be an accountant, and it might actively suppress the individual's artistic nature. Thus a clash between one's ego ideal and one's own inborn talents and potentialities can be a source of personal conflict.

The *conscience* sets standards of right and wrong. It says, "Yes, this is the right thing to do" or "no, you must not do that." The feeling that one is about to violate one's own superego's prohibitions produces anxiety. Thus, an important aspect of a neurotic process contributing to anxiety disorders is the nagging feeling that one is on the verge of acting-out impulses forbidden by the superego. If one does actually do the forbidden thing, the resulting feeling is guilt. The superego says in essence, "That was a terrible thing to do. You have failed yourself and your family."

In psychoanalytic theory, anxiety disorders are seen as cases in which the superego development is too strict. The superego acts like a straitjacket on the personality. Personality disorders, on the other hand, are seen as cases in which the superego development is inadequate. The individual may lack a well-defined sense of right and wrong.

See also *anxiety disorders*; *ego*; *Freud, Sigmund*; *id*; *neurosis*; *personality disorders*; *psychoanalysis*.

symptom: The visible sign of an underlying illness, disorder, or disease process. For an example of a physical illness, tenderness in the right lower abdomen is one of the symptoms of appendicitis. For an example of a mental disorder, delusional thinking is one of the symptoms of a schizophrenic disorder. Symptoms are useful in making a diagnosis. However, a diagnosis is seldom made on the basis of a single unrelated symptom.

See also *biomedical viewpoint*; *syndrome*.

syndrome: A set of related symptoms suggesting the presence of an underlying illness, disorder, or disease process. For example, the syndrome suggesting the presence of a schizophrenic disorder consists of delusional thinking, hallucinations, inappropriate emotional responses, confusion concerning one's sense of identity, inability to make and carry out long-term plans, withdrawal from others, and odd or bizarre behaviors. The more of the elements of a syndrome are present, the more likely that a given diagnosis is reliable.

See also *biomedical viewpoint*; *symptom*.

syphilis: See *general paresis*.

systematic desensitization: See *desensitization therapy*.

T

tarantism: A disorder associated with the Middle Ages characterized by an uncontrollable desire to dance wildly to the point of exhaustion. Tarantism originated in southern Italy, and the condition was believed to be caused by the bite of the tarantula, a species of European wolf spider. Oddly, the cure for tarantism was thought to be voluntary dancing to the *tarantella*, a melody played in either ⅜ or ⁶⁄₈ time. The tarantella steadily gains speed as it is played and danced. The memory of tarantism survives today in the fact that the tarantella is still performed at wedding ceremonies associated with the Italian culture.

Tarantism is of historical interest because it demonstrates how odd behaviors are often falsely explained. It is very doubtful that the bite of the tarantula has the capacity to induce a dancing mania. In the absence of adequate explanations at a biological or psychological level, there is a strong tendency to explain deviant behavior in somewhat fantastic terms such as a spider's bite, the kiss of a wolf, the seduction of a satyr, the influence of demons, or the practice of witchcraft.

See also *demonology*; *lycanthropy*; Malleus Maleficarum.

tardive dyskinesia: A neurological disorder characterized by involuntary movements. At first, these are facial twitches and tongue thrusts. If the disease progresses, unwanted motions and actions are displayed in the upper body; eventually the whole body is affected.

Tardive dyskinesia is one of the adverse side effects of antipsychotic drugs. It appears after the individual has been taking a drug for a fairly long period of time—usually a number of months or years. This is why the term *tardive* is used. It is related to the familiar word *tardy* and means late appearance. Sometimes tardive dyskinesia does not appear while the patient is taking a drug but after withdrawing from the drug.

The probable cause of tardive dyskinesia is irregular activity of the neurotransmitter dopamine. The problem is somewhat more likely to show up in patients who are over 40 years of age than in younger patients. The incidence of tardive dyskinesia is unknown. Some estimates place it as high as 10% to 20% (or more) among mental patients who have been taking antipsychotic drugs for prolonged periods of time.

Once tardive dyskinesia appears, it is very difficult to reverse or treat successfully. It is possible that the problem represents, in some cases, irreversible damage to the nervous system. For this reason, it is important that certain precautions be observed. First, antipsychotic drugs should be prescribed only if necessary. Second, the smallest dose required for effective treatment should be prescribed. Third, patients taking these drugs should be observed very closely for any hint of adverse side effects.

See also *dopamine*; *major tranquilizers (antipsychotic drugs)*; *neurology*.

tension headache: See *migraine headache*.

Terman, Lewis Madison (1877–1956): An American psychologist who introduced practical intelligence testing into the United States. Terman earned a Ph.D. from Clark University in 1905 under the sponsorship of Granville Stanley Hall. From 1910 until his death, Terman was associated with Stanford University.

Terman adapted the Binet–Simon Intelligence Scale, developed in France, for English use. This led to the publication of the Stanford–Binet Scale, the first standardized individual intelligence test used in the United States. Terman conducted longitudinal studies of development and intelligence. One of his principal conclusions was that gifted children are, contrary to the folklore of the time, emotionally healthy and socially competent.

During World War I, Terman was a leading figure in the development of intelligence tests used in the assessment and placement of recruits. The two well-known intelligence tests that resulted from his work, and that of his colleagues, were the Army Alpha and the Army Beta tests. The Army Alpha was used to test persons with conventional reading and language abilities. The Army Beta was used to evaluate persons with reading or language difficulties.

Terman was the author of *The Measurement of Intelligence* (1916). He coauthored, with M. A. Merrill, *Measuring Intelligence* (1937).

See also *Binet, Alfred*; *intelligence tests*; *Stanford–Binet Intelligence Scale*.

testosterone: See *androgens*.

Thanatos: The ancient Greek god of death. According to Freud, we have an inborn death instinct just as we have an inborn group of life instincts. Freud called the death instinct *Thanatos* and the life instincts *Eros* (after the ancient Greek god of love). The conflict between Thanatos and Eros starts at birth. In one's youth, Eros is stronger than Thanatos, and the death instinct is driven away from the self. Not destroyed, only redirected, it expresses itself outwardly in the form of aggressive behavior toward others. In old age, Thanatos gains ascendance over Eros, turns inward, and brings about the eventual decay and organic death of the person.

Freud and other psychoanalysts (e.g., Karl Menninger) used the death instinct to explain suicide and self-destructive behavior. They reasoned that pathological personality development and adverse life situations can turn Thanatos inward prematurely.

Freud's use of Thanatos to explain natural organic death, suicide, and self-destructive behavior has met with only limited acceptance among mental health professionals. The concept of a death instinct seems to be vague and overly general.

See also *Freud, Sigmund*; *psychoanalysis*; *suicide*.

Thematic Apperception Test (TAT): A personality test consisting of a set of cards with drawings of human beings. The test was devised by the Harvard psychologist Henry A. Murray and first published in 1938. The Thematic Apperception Test (TAT) has proven to be one of the workhorses of psychological testing. It is used extensively in both research and diagnosis.

In most instances, the drawings on the cards suggest people interacting with each other. The TAT is a projective test because the drawings are *ambiguous*, meaning they can be seen in two or more ways. For example, in some cases, a person can be thought of as either male or female. Or an object on an end table might be an ashtray or a gun. Thus what a subject says is happening, or seems to see, is thought to be a projection from the unconscious level of the personality.

An examiner giving the test asks the subject to relate a brief story about each card presented. The story is to have a beginning, a middle, and an end. And the subject is also asked to tell what the people are thinking and feeling.

The principal aim of the test is to uncover the intensity levels of a set of social motives. These include needs for achievement, abasement, affiliation, aggression, autonomy, dominance, exhibition, nurturance, order, and power. When the test is analyzed, it provides a profile of high and low measures in these areas, giving a substantial amount of insight into the individual's reasons for acting in certain ways. If the test is given to a person with a mental disorder, as it often is, the results provide a partial explanation of pathological behavior.

The results of the TAT are seldom interpreted alone. They are combined with the outcomes of a battery of tests and psychological interviews.

See also *Minnesota Multiphasic Personality Inventory (MMPI)*; *personality test*; *projective test*; *Rorschach test*.

therapy: A general process characterized by either an effort to cure an illness or relieve its symptoms. (The word *therapy* is derived from a Greek word meaning "to take care of.") In the case of mental disorders, there are two basic kinds of therapy. *Biological therapy* is based on the assumption that mental and emotional problems are often caused by difficulties at an organic level. (This is known as the *biomedical viewpoint.*) Examples of difficulties at an organic level are neurotransmitter imbalances, endocrine imbalances, hypoglycemia, brain tumors, and infections of the central nervous system. The principal kinds of biological therapies are drug therapy, electroshock therapy, and psychosurgery.

Psychotherapy is based on the assumption that mental and emotional problems are often caused by difficulties at a psychological level. (This is known as the *psychogenic viewpoint.*) Examples of difficulties at a psychological level are a troubled developmental history, unconscious motivational conflicts, maladaptive habits, and distressed interpersonal relationships. The principal kinds of psychotherapies are insight-oriented therapies and behavior therapy.

See also *behavior therapy*; *biomedical viewpoint*; *drug therapy*; *electroconvulsive therapy (ECT)*; *insight therapy*; *psychogenic viewpoint*; *psychosurgery*.

tic disorder: The word *tic* refers to repeated actions and movements of an involuntary nature. Examples are jerking or twisting of the head, blinking of the eyes, smacking of the lips, and facial grimaces. There are also *vocal tics* involving grunts, clicks, and other sounds. Although tics can affect both children and adults, the term *tic disorder* is reserved for tic problems first evident in childhood or adolescence.

There are three principal kinds of tic disorders. *Transient tic disorder* waxes and wanes in intensity and usually disappears within a year. *Chronic motor* or *vocal tic disorder* is more enduring. The tics are a problem for more than 1 year. *Tourette's disorder* is characterized by multiple tics. The tics may appear together, or they may alternate in appearance. In many cases, foul language is used. This is referred to as *coprolalia*. In many cases, Tourette's disorder persists into adulthood. It cannot be taken for granted that the child or adolescent will automatically grow out of the condition. Treatment is recommended.

All three tic disorders appear more frequently in males than in females at a ratio of about 3 to 1.

A transient tic disorder appears to be an expression of nervous tension. Often the child is in a state of emotional conflict, and the family environment may be an unhappy or oppressive one. The involuntary performance of the tic appears to bring momentary relief from tension, and this, unfortunately reinforces the tic. The recommended treatment for a transient tic disorder is child psychotherapy combined with parental counseling. The aim of the treatment is to relieve the child of unnecessary stress.

In the case of chronic motor or vocal tic disorder and Tourette's disorder, neurological problems often play a complicating role. For example, the child may suffer from epilepsy or minimal brain dysfunction. The recommended treatment for the two disorders identified in this paragraph is also a combination of child psychotherapy and parental counseling. However, this may be combined with drug therapy designed to treat neurological problems.

A tic disorder is not to be confused with tardive dyskinesia (see reference).

See also *developmental disorders*; *epilepsy*; *minimal brain dysfunction (MBD)*; *tardive dyskinesia*.

tobacco dependence: See *nicotine dependence (tobacco dependence)*.

token economy: A system used in some mental hospitals, prisons, juvenile homes, and schools to shape the behavior of patients, prisoners, and children in desired directions. The approach is based on principles of operant conditioning and is essentially a form of behavior modification. Approved behaviors are reinforced with tokens. (In some cases, the actual tokens may be replaced by points earned on paper.) The tokens function somewhat like money. They can be saved to earn privileges such as the right to go see a movie, to have a special dessert, to have white linen on the dining table, to make a long-distance telephone call, and so forth. As in a country's economy, the inmate of an institution can better his or her standard of living by willingly participating in the token economy.

Token economies in mental hospitals have been criticized on the basis that they are not a cure for mental disorders. Improvement is superficial and merely a matter of conformity. Critics say that the patients are being treated like conditioned robots. However, it can be argued that token economies have a generally therapeutic effect because they help patients to become more responsible. Steps taken in the direction of more responsible behavior tend to foster self-esteem, and self-esteem is certainly a component of mental health. Like any system, a token economy is useful only if it is applied with humanity and respect for others.

See also *behavior modification*; *behavior therapy*; *operant conditioning*.

toxic delirium: A clouding of consciousness caused by a poisonous substance. The poisonous substance may have entered the body directly by mouth or injection. Or it may have been absorbed indirectly by inadvertent exposure.

See also *delirium*.

tranquilizer: A drug that has a beneficial effect on the symptoms of mental disorders. A tranquilizer is not a cure but a treatment for a mental disorder. There are two basic classes of tranquilizers. The *major tranquilizers* (i.e., antipsychotic drugs) are used to treat severe mental problems such as schizophrenic disorders. The minor tranquilizers (i.e., antianxiety drugs) are used to treat behavioral and emotional problems in which the control of anxiety is an important goal.

See also *antianxiety drugs*; *drug therapy*; *major tranquilizers (antipsychotic drugs)*.

transactional analysis: A kind of psychotherapy characterized by a detailed analysis of communication patterns in troubled relationships. The father of transactional analysis was the psychiatrist Eric Berne (1910–1970). Berne based much of transactional analysis's personality theory on Freud's thought. The importance of interpersonal behavior in transactional analysis was inspired by the work of the psychiatrist Harry S. Sullivan.

The basic personality theory proposed by Berne states that the whole personality consists of three ego states: the Parent, the Adult, and the Child. (The ego states are capitalized to distinguish them from actual parents, adults, and children.) The term *ego state* is chosen to suggest that the Parent, the Adult, and the Child are more than theoretical abstractions. They are actual "states" entered by the ego. Thus one may act as a controlling parent by being dogmatic and giving orders. Or one may act as a rational adult by planning ahead and thinking clearly. Or one may act as a spoiled child by pouting or whining.

The Parent represents the *taught* aspect of life. It stands for what actual parents tried to teach, society's rules, religious values, and so forth. The Adult represents the *thinking* aspect of life. It stands for reason and logic. The Child represents the *feeling* aspect of life. It expresses pain and pleasure, joy, anger, and depression. It is evident that the Parent, the Adult, and the Child are quite similar to Freud's concept of the superego, the ego, and the id. A principal difference, according to Berne, is that, in psychoanalysis, these are theoretical propositions. In transactional analysis, they are actual behavior patterns experienced by the individual.

Transactional analysis steps outside of the boundaries of classical psychoanalysis by noting that the three ego states in Person 1 communicate with the three ego states in Person 2. Thus the Parent of Person 1 might criticize the Child of Person 2. This leads to the concepts of *transactions*, exchanges of information and recognition between at least two people.

Three kinds of basic transactions are identified. *Parallel transactions* take place when people agree (or seem to agree). *Crossed transactions* take place when people disagree by arguing or bickering. *Ulterior transactions* take place when communication patterns have two levels, one of them evident and the other hidden. Ulterior transactions have a "sneaky" quality, allowing one person to snipe at a second person.

Although parallel transactions are free of obvious conflict, they are not necessarily desirable. For example, in a marriage, a first partner might be very dominating and critical, constantly sending negative messages from the Parent to the other person's Child. The second person, wanting to be agreeable, may not fight, regularly sending apologetic messages back from the Child to the other person's Parent. The second person may eventually pay a heavy price in the form of depression. The first person pays a less obvious price in the form of becoming an emotionally alienated hostile tyrant.

Berne believed that the greatest danger in relationships resides in ulterior transactions. Complex recurrent patterns involving ulterior transactions he labeled *games*, and this became the basis of his best-selling book *Games People Play*. Games are self-defeating in nature. Played over and over, they undermine a relationship, making people become increasingly distant and remote from each other. In marriages plagued by game playing, the partners tend to lose the sense that they are real persons, not things to be manipulated.

When transactional analysis is used to help a troubled couple improve a relationship, two principal goals exist. The first goal is to assist each partner to develop greater *autonomy*, the conviction that one is really in charge of one's own life. The second goal is to assist the partners to develop greater *intimacy*, a sense of emotional closeness and authentic communication.

Transactional analysis is an important approach to mental and emotional problems because it recognizes that many of our troubles do not arise in a social vacuum. Other people are involved, and many times the "sick" person is reacting adversely to the behavior patterns of another person who is exerting psychological power. This insight is not, of course, exclusive to transactional analysis. It is also contained in family therapy, psychodrama, and sociotherapy.

See also *Berne, Eric*; *family therapy*; *Freud, Sigmund*; *psychoanalysis*; *psychodrama*; *sociotherapy*; *Sullivan, Harry Stack*.

transference: In psychoanalysis, a projection from the unconscious level of the patient's personality onto the person of the therapist. The patient, for example, may perceive the therapist as an all-wise and all-knowing person. This is certainly not because the therapist is actually omniscient but because of the patient's unconscious wish that the therapist holds the magical keys to making the patient well.

Three important kinds of transferences are positive transference, negative transference, and countertransference. *Positive transference* involves "good" feelings toward the therapist. One example is given in the first paragraph. For a second example, sometimes the patient develops a crush on the therapist, thinking of the therapist as a potential lover. From the point of view of psychoanalysis, this "love" is only an illusion arising from the positive transference. In most cases, if not too strong, a positive transference can be taken advantage of to assist the process of therapy.

Negative transference involves hostile feelings toward the therapist. For example, the patient may perceive the therapist as an overcontrolling authority figure who is trying to take the fun out of life. A negative transference can be a serious problem and may play a role in galvanizing a patient's resistance to the process of therapy.

Countertransference involves projections from the unconscious level of the therapist's own personality onto the person of the patient. For example, the therapist may develop a crush on the patient and indulge in sexual fantasies. For a second example, the therapist may have hostile feelings toward the patient because he or she reminds the therapist of someone who is disliked or who treated the therapist badly as a child. In both of the examples given, the countertransference may interfere with the therapist's effectiveness.

Although the term *transference* tends to be associated primarily with psychoanalysis, it can be seen that the kinds of feelings involved can present a potential problem in any relationship between a therapist and a patient.

See also *Breuer, Josef*; *Freud, Sigmund*; *psychoanalysis*; *psychotherapy*.

transsexualism: A kind of gender identity disorder characterized by unhappiness with one's biological gender. The person suffering from transsexualism wishes that he or she could have the genitals and social role of the opposite sex.

Although this disorder has received a great deal of publicity, it is relatively uncommon. It is estimated that about 1 in 30,000 men and 1 in 100,000 women suffer from the disorder. The individual with the disorder is often depressed and suicidal.

Adult transsexuals often have a history of gender identity confusion in their early years. Boys and girls who consistently display behavioral traits and interests that are the opposite of their own sex fit in this general category.

Although it is possible that genetic factors play a role in this disorder, it seems relatively unlikely that they are its principal cause. As far as is known, the person suffering from transsexualism is, in most cases, genetically normal. On the other hand, there is almost always a history of significant problems between parents and the child.

It seems reasonable to assume that conventional gender identity forms to a large extent out of identification with the parent of the same sex. If, for example, a boy finds it difficult to emotionally bond with his father, or if no father is present in the household, he may identify more strongly with his mother. If the identification is strong enough, his wish will be to be a woman, not a man. The same statements can, of course, be made about females. However, it is clear from a large body of child development research that the favorite parent of either sex, male or female, is usually the mother. In view of this fact and in view of the fact that many contemporary households consist of a single female parent, this may explain in part why transsexualism is more common in males than in females.

There are two basic general approaches to the treatment of transsexualism. The first is sex-change surgery. The second is psychotherapy. Although the successes of sex-change surgery have been popularized, it must be remembered that transsexualism is a disorder and that sex-change surgery is seldom a satisfactory treatment. Many persons who have had the surgery complain of dissatisfactions with the outcome of the surgery and continuing problems in adjustment. Most researchers who have studied the pros and cons of sex-change surgery consider it a last resort when no other treatment has been effective.

Psychotherapy is usually insight oriented with two principal aims. First, the individual is helped to understand the psychological and emotional roots of his or her transsexualism. Second, ways are sought to help the individual foster identifications and emotional bonds with persons of the same sex. Some research suggests that group therapy consisting of persons with similar problems may be particularly helpful in the case of transsexualism. Although therapy does not necessarily cure transsexualism, it may help the individual live with the problem with less emotional discomfort.

See also *gender identity disorder of childhood*; *gender identity disorders*.

transvestic fetishism (transvestism): A sexual disorder characterized by cross-dressing on the part of a male. In most cases, the purpose of the cross-dressing is to obtain sexual excitement. Some males find it an erotic experience to put on the clothes of a female.

If transvestic fetishism becomes entrenched, it often becomes generalized, and the male may begin to go to public places dressed as a woman. Also, he may use cross-dressing as a way to relax, as a way of reducing anxiety or nervous tension.

One way to understand transvestic fetishism is to place it within the framework of sexual fetishism in general. Fetishism is the obtaining of sexual arousal by an object of stimulation (i.e., a fetish) not commonly thought to be particularly erotic such as a pair of shoes or other article of clothing. A common practice is for the individual to masturbate while looking at, or contacting, the object. Transvestic fetishism can be thought of as a more direct form of contact with the object or objects.

It is important not to confuse transvestic fetishism with transsexualism. The male suffering from transvestic fetishism is distinctly heterosexual in orientation. He is clearly aroused by females and, in spite of the wish to cross-dress, does not wish to become a woman. Only infrequently does transvestic fetishism eventually become transsexualism.

Varying attitudes have been taken toward transvestic fetishism. If the disorder causes the individual no particular difficulty in daily living, then it is sometimes looked upon as a relatively harmless eccentricity. However, transvestic fetishism may be a source of distress. For example, a man's wife may strenuously object to the behavior. Or the man dressed as a woman may enter public rest rooms reserved for women. If transvestic fetishism is causing problems in adjustment, then the recommended treatment is psychotherapy. Drug therapy and the use of hormones is usually avoided in treatment.

See also *fetishism*; *paraphilias*; *sexual disorders (psychosexual disorders)*; *transsexualism*.

transvestism: See *transvestic fetishism (transvestism)*.

traumata: See *psychological traumata*.

traumatic neurosis: See *posttraumatic stress disorder (traumatic neurosis*.

treatment contract: See *behavioral contracting*.

tricyclic antidepressants: See *antidepressant drugs*.

Turner's syndrome: A set of symptoms caused by a chromosomal anomaly in which there is a missing X chromosome on the twenty-third pair in the female (i.e., monosomy 23). (The syndrome derives its name in honor of original research conducted by the physician H. H. Turner.) Persons with the syndrome usually display lack of development of the ovaries; in some cases, the ovaries are absent. Other symptoms include infantile sexual development in general (e.g., small breasts and little or no pubic hair), stunted growth, webbing of the neck, a flattened nose, lack of menstruation, and impaired hearing. Diabetes is more common in people with Turner's syndrome than among people in general.

Mental retardation is associated with about 20% of the cases of Turner's syndrome. In many cases, the individual with Turner's syndrome has normal, or nearly normal, intelligence.

An important treatment for Turner's syndrome is the administration of estrogens prior to adolescence. Under these circumstances, although the female will remain sterile, other aspects of development will be close to normal.

See also *chromosomal anomalies*; *estrogens*; *mental retardation*.

Type A behavior: A behavior pattern characterized by aggressive behavior, impatience, and general hostility. Specific examples of Type A behavior are (1) trying to do two or more things at one time, (2) executing all actions at a rapid pace, and (3) feeling guilty when trying to relax. The behavior pattern was first identified by the cardiologists Meyer Friedman and Ray H. Rosenman in the 1970s. They contrasted it with Type B behavior characterized by a more relaxed, philosophical, and easygoing attitude toward life.

Friedman and Rosenman asserted that their research showed that Type A behavior was a risk factor in coronary heart disease. The logic was that the Type A behavior is a cause of self-induced stress. Although, on the surface, the idea that Type A behavior is a risk factor in heart disease is appealing, the results of various studies are controversial, and the importance of Type A behavior as a risk factor is at present somewhat uncertain. Nonetheless, it is probably prudent to avoid Type A behavior and to seek ways to keep the overall stress in one's life to a reasonable level.

See also *psychosomatic disorders*; *stress*.

U

unconscious mental life: According to Freud, ideas, motives, and memories existing in the personality at a level not accessible to normal conscious processes of memory, reflection, and will. Freud did not originate this idea. Antecedents to Freud's concept of an unconscious mental life can be found in the writings of philosophers such as Plato, Wilhelm Leibnitz, Johann Friedrich Herbart, and Friedrich Nietzsche. Freud was quite familiar with philosophical works and gave credit to his intellectual forebears. However, Freud is credited with elevating the concept of an unconscious mental life to a high status as an explanatory agent in abnormal psychology and investigating its applications for psychotherapy.

The concept of an unconscious mental life is a key one in classical psychoanalysis. It is assumed that a struggle between unconscious motives, often forbidden and half-understood and the prohibitions of the superego (i.e., the agent of society) represent a neurotic process. The fear that one may violate one's moral code and impulsively act out antisocial aggressive or sexual desires is experienced as anxiety. One way to explain the presence of emotional distress in anxiety disorders is to refer to this process.

Freud recommended that the word *unconscious* be used as an adjective, not a noun. Therefore, it is not good usage to refer to *the* unconscious as if it were a territory or a place. It is best to speak of unconscious wishes, unconscious motives, an unconscious level of the personality, or an unconscious mental life. (Freud did not make this distinction in his early writings but stressed it in his later works.)

Psychoanalysis as a form of therapy basically involves the exploration of the unconscious level of the personality. The idea is to escape being the victim of unknown forces. A basic assumption of psychoanalysis is that if an idea, a memory, or a motive is consciously understood, then the individual has a good chance of gaining greater voluntary control over both emotions and actions.

See also *free association*; *Freud, Sigmund*; *psychoanalysis*; *repression*.

undifferentiated schizophrenia (schizophrenia, undifferentiated type): See *schizophrenia*.

undoing: A kind of ego defense mechanism in which the individual engages in a thought or action designed to alleviate anxiety or guilt feelings relating to a prior thought or action. Essentially undoing is an atonement, an effort to make amends. The effort can be magical or realistic. For an example of a magical effort, let us say that Sebastian has recently punished his daughter both severely and unfairly. Now he is feeling guilty. He looks at his favorite photograph of his daughter and repeats to himself mentally three times, "I love you, dear. Forgive me." This ritual makes him feel that somehow he has reversed the ill effects of his rash behavior. This kind of undoing is very similar to the compulsions associated with obsessive-compulsive disorder.

For an example of a realistic effort, let us say that Inez feels she neglected her aging parents shortly before their death. Now, a few years later, she spends 15 hours a week working as a volunteer in a board and care facility for elderly persons.

See also *ego defense mechanisms*; *obsessive-compulsive disorder*.

unipolar disorder: See *major depression (unipolar disorder)*.

V

vaginismus: A sexual disorder characterized by an involuntary contraction of the muscles around the vagina. The contraction is painful, and it makes sexual intercourse either difficult or impossible. Vaginismus is induced either by the immediate expectation of intercourse or the act of intercourse. The condition being described here is not caused by an organic abnormality or a disease but is classified as a functional disorder.

Vaginismus has psychological and emotional roots. Causes that have been identified or hypothesized to exist include frustration because of an impotent partner, latent homosexual desires, having been raped or sexually abused, lack of emotional closeness with one's partner, the belief that sex is dirty, and inability to trust one's partner. In a given case, one or several of these causes may be operative.

The principal treatment for vaginismus is sexual therapy aimed at adapting the patient to the insertion of the penis in the vagina. An approach emphasizing desensitization can be helpful in this regard. This can be accomplished through guided fantasies and/ or through the graded insertion of dilators. The dilator can be inserted at home by the female under conditions of privacy and relaxation.

In addition, the patient should be helped to understand the emotional roots of her problem and encouraged to seek ways to cope with them. It is usually a good idea for the male partner to participate in some of the therapy sessions. Some males are excessively egocentric and aggressive during sexual relations. These males need to learn more effective ways to behave. Vaginismus should not be seen as the woman's problem but as the couple's problem.

See also *desensitization therapy*; *dyspareunia*; *sexual disorders (psychosexual disorders)*; *sexual therapy*.

validity: See *psychological test*.

Valium: See *diazepam*.

virilism: A relatively rare pathological condition characterized by the presence of male secondary sexual characteristics in a female. Examples of such characteristics are a beard and a deep voice. Other symptoms may included lack of breast development and absence of menstruation. Virilism has psychological and emotional ramifications. Females with the disorder may suffer from gender confusion, depression, shyness, and lack of sexual interest.

The cause of virilism is an imbalance in hormones. There appears to be an excessive production of androgens, probably because of malfunctioning of the pituitary gland. In the majority of cases, the recommended medical treatment is hormone therapy administered by an endocrinologist. In some cases, a tumor on the pituitary gland is discovered, and surgery is sometimes employed. In almost all cases, adjunct psychotherapy is recommended to assist the female in coping with the difficulties presented by the virilism.

See also *androgens*; *endocrine system*.

visual hallucination: See *hallucination*.

voyeurism: A kind of paraphilia (i.e., sexual variance) characterized by the act of looking at others in order to obtain either sexual excitement or gratification. (The term is from a French word meaning "to see.") A *voyeur* is a person who practices voyeurism. If sexual gratification is obtained, it is usually through masturbation.

Terms that are more or less interchangeable with voyeurism are *scopophilia* (sometimes written *scotophilia* and *scoptophilia*) and *inspectionalism*. Some authorities make a distinction between scopophilia and voyeurism. Scopophilia is sexual excitement obtained by looking at the sexual actions of others or at their genital organs. Voyeurism suggests looking at a person in the nude or undressing. Frequently, this is done compulsively and in secret. However, any distinctions that are made between scopophilia and voyeurism are fuzzy at best, and conventional usage usually employs voyeurism as a term that covers the general range of sexual eccentricities involving the act of looking.

Male voyeurs who look secretively at females in states of undress are sometimes referred to as "peeping Toms," and their behavior is referred to as "peepism." This usage derives from the legend of Peeping Tom of Coventry. In the eleventh century, Lady Godiva, wife of the Earl of Mercia in England, rode naked through town in exchange for his agreement to reduce the tax burden of the people. No one was supposed to look at her. Tom violated the agreement and developed blindness as a result.

A distinction can be made between pseudovoyeurism and voyeurism. *Pseudovoyeurism* is the kind of sexual pleasure obtained by looking at a cooperative partner. Also, probably most of the pleasure obtained looking at pornography falls into the class of pseudovoyeurism. *Voyeurism* can be thought of as a sexual disorder only under these conditions: (1) The voyeurism is causing the person practical problems in living, (2) the victims of the voyeurism are looked at in secret, and (3) the individual prefers the voyeuristic acts to actual sexual relations.

Most voyeurs are males. They outnumber women by about 9 to 1.

Voyeurism has psychological and emotional roots. Causes that have been identified or hypothesized to exist include shyness, low self-esteem, a desire to guard against sexual failure, infantile fixations, a fear of women, the wish to express hostility in fantasy, and a need to feel superior.

The recommended treatment for voyeurism is psychotherapy aimed at helping the individual to (1) understand his own behavior and (2) seek more realistic sexual outlets.

See also *paraphilias*; *sexual deviations*.

W

Watson, John Broadus (1878–1958): An American psychologist and father of the school of psychology known as behaviorism. In 1903, Watson received his Ph.D. degree in psychology from the University of Chicago. At the age of 30, he began teaching and doing research at Johns Hopkins University. In 1915, he was elected president of the American Psychological Association. In 1922, he resigned from his position at Hopkins and followed a career in the advertising industry. He was a principal founder of advertising psychology.

Watson had a strong grounding in academic philosophy and early in his career became convinced that psychology as then practiced was based on a false set of assumptions. One of these false assumptions was the importance of a subjective frame of reference, an individual's own distinctive way of perceiving the world. Another false assumption was the great value placed on consciousness, or self-awareness. Watson asserted that these, and similar, assumptions were leading psychology down a pathway toward sloppy science.

Watson argued that it is impossible to rigorously study inner experience and consciousness, key factors in what most of us call the mind. Thus the study of the mind is impractical because it relies too heavily on personal and private observation. Instead of studying the mind, Watson recommended that psychologists study observable behavior. Behavior itself is a legitimate object of study and has none of the drawbacks of consciousness or mental life. The actions of an organism are open to public observation. Two or more observers can agree, for example, that a rat, monkey, or person actually did, or did not, execute a given action.

This general line of thinking underlies behaviorism as a school of psychology, and it was a breath of fresh air for psychology in the 1910s. It inspired many young scientists to follow psychology as a career because they became convinced that it could eventually be a discipline as rigorous as physics or chemistry.

Watsonian behaviorism was inspired to a large extent by the earlier work of researchers such as Ivan Pavlov in Russia. Indeed, Watson took the conditioned reflex as the basic building block of acquired behavior. Obtaining his lead from Pavlov, Watson tended to focus his own research projects on the learning process. And this trend continued among behaviorists. For example, B. F. Skinner, a leading behaviorist, has conducted most of his research in the area of learning.

Watson exerted a tremendous influence on psychology. The two leading forces in academic psychology in the United States for many years were psychoanalysis and behaviorism. The behavioristic point of view is the one that resides behind behavior therapy.

Three of Watson's books are *Psychology as the Behaviorist Sees It* (1913), *Psychology from the Standpoint of a Behaviorist* (1919), and *Behaviorism* (1925).

See also *behaviorism*; *behavior therapy*; *classical conditioning*; *Pavlov, Ivan Petrovich*; *Skinner, Burrhus Frederic*.

Wechsler intelligence scales: A group of standardized tests of intelligence developed by the clinical psychologist David Wechsler (1896–1981). These tests are the Wechsler Adult Intelligence Scale (WAIS), the Wechsler Intelligence Scale for Children (WISC), and the Wechsler Preschool and Primary Scale of Intelligence (WPPSI). The WPPSI is intended for children between the ages of 4 to 6.

The Wechsler scales have been developed and revised over a number of years. Their forerunner was the Wechsler-Bellevue

Intelligence Scale, first published in 1939. The tests are administered individually and are widely regarded as instruments with a high degree of validity and reliability.

One of the principal advantages of the Wechsler tests is that they are divided into two mental areas: verbal and performance. The Verbal Scale for each test is divided into a set of subtests with titles such as *Information, Comprehension, Arithmetic, Similarities, Digit Span*, and *Vocabulary*. The Performance Scale for each test is divided into a set of subtests with titles such as *Digit Symbol, Picture Completion, Block Design, Picture Arrangement*, and *Object Assembly*. It is possible to obtain a Verbal IQ, a Performance IQ, and a Full Scale IQ.

What is the distinction between verbal and performance intelligence? The distinction is, of course, not precise, but general. Nonetheless, it is a distinction of some value. A high level of verbal intelligence suggests the individual has ability to think in abstract terms using both words and mathematical symbols. Attorneys and teachers are examples of persons who require a high level of verbal intelligence in their work. A high level of performance intelligence suggests the individual has ability to perceive relationships and to fit things together into organized wholes. Carpenters and cosmetologists are examples of persons who require a high level of performance intelligence in their work. Of course, the two kinds of intelligence are not mutually exclusive, and a person may have a high level of both kinds. A surgeon is an example of a person who needs high levels of both verbal and performance intelligence.

Because the Wechsler scales make a distinction between verbal intelligence and performance intelligence and because of the subtests, these scales are of particular value in making clinical assessments and diagnoses. The scales are helpful in evaluating relative degrees of impairment in patients due to functional deterioration associated with a nonorganic mental disorder, loss of faculties due to brain damage, or a combination of both.

For an example of neurological assessment, assume that Glen, age 52, is the victim of a cerebrovascular accident (i.e., a stroke). His physician recommends that he be given the WAIS before he is released from the hospital in order to assess the amount of loss of specific mental faculties and to make recommendations for outpatient therapy. He is given the WAIS 6 months later in order to evaluate his degree of recovery.

See also *cerebrovascular accident (CVA)*; *intelligence*; *intelligence quotient (IQ)*; *psychological test*; *Stanford–Binet Intelligence Scale*.

White, William Alanson (1870–1937): An American psychiatrist who was an early advocate of the use of psychoanalysis in the treatment of mental patients. White earned his M.D. degree from Long Island College, served as director of the Washington Government Hospital for the Insane, was a founder of the *Psychoanalytic Review*, and was a president, at different times, of both the American Psychiatric Association and the American Psychoanalytic Association.

Harry Stack Sullivan, Erich Fromm, and others founded a psychoanalytic training institute in 1943. They honored White's contributions by naming it the William Alanson White Institute.

Among White's books are *Outlines of Psychiatry* (1907) and *Principles of Mental Hygiene* (1919).

See also *Fromm, Erich*; *psychoanalysis*; *Sullivan, Harry Stack*.

will therapy: A kind of psychotherapy developed in the 1920s and 1930s by Otto Rank, an early associate of Freud. Rank asserted that the *birth trauma*, the emotional wound inflicted on the infant when separated from the mother's womb, was the basic pattern for all anxiety. Rank's assertion was based on original suggestions made by Freud, but Rank expanded greatly on them.

According to Rank, the symbolic expression of the birth trauma in adult experience becomes "fear of life." People with this underlying fear tend to be shy, conforming, withdrawn, and lack an individual identity. Unconsciously, Rank thought that such persons wish to return to the protection of the womb.

In therapy, Rank focused on the present and the future rather than on the past. He emphasized the faculty of the ego known as *will*, the power to make choices and to move ahead in life. He encouraged his patients to act, to do, and to overcome their inhibitions.

Although will therapy is seldom practiced as such at present, it was influential. It can be thought of as a forerunner of both assertiveness training and reality therapy. Also, Carl Rogers was impressed with Rank's ideas and incorporated some of them into client-centered therapy.

See also *assertiveness training*; *client-centered therapy*; *ego*; *Freud, Sigmund*; *psychotherapy*; *reality therapy*; *Rogers, Carl Ransom*.

withdrawal: A general process referring to any defensive strategy used by the person to retreat from a threat, a stressful situation, a challenge, other people, or reality itself. In mild instances, withdrawal is expressed as shyness, self-consciousness, remoteness from others, and so forth. In highly pathological instances, withdrawal is expressed as muteness, catatonic stupor, and regression to infantile behavior. Under these circumstances, it is associated with conditions such as autistic disorder, schizoid personality disorder, and schizophrenic disorders.

See also *ego defense mechanisms*; *schizoid personality disorder*; *schizophrenia*; *social introversion*.

withdrawal symptoms: Physiological and psychological symptoms experienced when a person dependent on a drug stops its use. Examples of physiological symptoms are headaches, upset stomach, significant changes in vital signs such as blood pressure and pulse, convulsions, shakiness, and lack of energy. Examples of psychological symptoms are irritability, depression, confusion, and delusions.

See also *delirium tremens*; *drug addiction*.

Wolpe, Joseph (1915–): A psychiatrist who originated systematic desensitization, a kind of behavior therapy. Wolpe was born in South Africa, earned his medical degree there, and served in World War II with the South African Medical Corp. In 1965, he was appointed a professor of psychiatry at Temple University in

Philadelphia. The American Psychological Association's Distinguished Scientific Award was granted to Wolpe in 1979.

It was during his tour of military service that Wolpe became disenchanted with traditional psychoanalysis as a method of treating neurotic disorders. He was working at the time with patients who were suffering from various kinds of emotional reactions to the stress induced by combat. The term *war neurosis* was used to describe their general condition. Wolpe discovered that lengthy explorations of childhood through free association had a very slow and uncertain therapeutic effect on this particular class of patients.

Wolpe decided that the emotional difficulties of his military patients could be more readily explained in terms of classical conditioning, a kind of learning studied extensively by Pavlov. In brief, Wolpe saw that the anxiety of his patients was *learned* through association with traumatic situations. He realized that his patients needed to be deconditioned and searched for a way to do it. Systematic desensitization was the result of his labors.

As he continued his research, Wolpe discovered that systematic desensitization has a broad range of application to a number of mental and emotional disorders.

Two of Wolpe's books are *Psychotherapy by Reciprocal Inhibition* (1958) and *The Practice of Behavior Therapy* (1974).

See also *behavior therapy*; *classical conditioning*; *desensitization therapy*; *Pavlov, Ivan Petrovich*.

word salad: A chaotic jumble of words and sentences that make little sense to the listener. Some of the words may be neologisms. The tendency to produce word salads is associated primarily with the schizophrenic disorders. It may also be displayed by patients suffering from neurological disorders.

Here is an example of a word salad produced by a patient suffering from a schizophrenic disorder: "I you perfect lakaloo insisting past tense science for now trust deeds no no no."

See also *clang associations*; *confabulation*; *flight of ideas*; *neologism*.

X Y Z

zoophilia: See *bestiality*.

zoophobia: See *phobia*.

INDEX OF AUTHORITIES

Boldface numbers indicate a full-length biography.